TOPICS IN PALLIATIVE CARE

Volume 4

Edited by

Russell K. Portenoy
Beth Israel Medical Center
New York, New York

Eduardo Bruera
University of Texas
M.D. Anderson Cancer Center
Houston, Texas

OXFORD
UNIVERSITY PRESS
2000

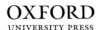

OXFORD
UNIVERSITY PRESS

Oxford   New York
Athens Auckland Bangkok Bogotá Buenos Aires Calcutta
Cape Town Chennai Dar es Salaam Delhi Florence Hong Kong Istanbul
Karachi Kuala Lumpur Madrid Melbourne Mexico City Mumbai
Nairobi Paris São Paulo Singapore Taipei Tokyo Toronto Warsaw

and associated companies in
Berlin Ibadan

Copyright © 2000 by Oxford University Press, Inc.

Published by Oxford University Press, Inc.
198 Madison Avenue, New York, New York 10016

Oxford is a registered trademark of Oxford University Press

Library of Congress Cataloging-in-Publication Data
Topics in palliative care / edited by Russell K. Portenoy, Eduardo Bruera.
p.   cm.—(Topics in palliative care : v. 4)
Includes bibliographical references and index.
ISBN 0-19-513219-X
1. Cancer—Palliative treatment.
I. Portenoy, Russell K.
II. Bruera, Eduardo.
III. Series.
[DNLM: 1. Palliative Care.   2. Neoplasms—drug therapy.
Pain—drug therapy.
WB 310 T674 1997] RC271.P33T664 1997
616.99′406—dc20 DNLM/DLC for Library of Congress 96-22250

9 8 7 6 5 4 3 2 1
Printed in the United States of America
on acid-free paper

To our wives,
Susan and Maria,
whose love and support
make our work possible.

Preface to the Series

Topics in Palliative Care, a series devoted to research and practice in palliative care, was created to address the growing need to disseminate new information about this rapidly evolving field.

Palliative care is an interdisciplinary therapeutic model for the management of patients with incurable, progressive illness. In this model, the family is considered the unit of care. The clinical purview includes those factors—physical, psychological, social, and spritual—that contribute to suffering, undermine quality of life, and prevent a death with comfort and dignity. The definition promulgated by the World Health Organization exemplifies this perspective.°

> Palliative care is the active total care of patients whose disease is not responsive to curative treatment. Control of pain, of other symptoms, and of psychological, social and spiritual problems is paramount. The goal of palliative care is the achievement of the best possible quality of life for patients and their families.

Palliative care is a fundamental part of clinical practice, the "parallel universe" to therapies directed at cure or prolongation of life. All clinicians who treat patients with chronic life-threatening diseases are engaged in palliative care, continually attempting to manage complex symptomatology and functional disturbances.

The need for specialized palliative care services may arise at any point during the illness. Symptom control and psychological adaptation are the usual concerns during the period of active disease-oriented therapies. Toward the end of life, however, needs intensify and broaden. Psychosocial distress or family distress, spiritual or existential concerns, advance care planning, and ethical concerns, among many other issues, may be considered by the various disciplines that coalesce in the delivery of optimal care. Clinicians who specialize in palliative care perceive their role as similar to those of specialists in other disciplines of medicine: referring patients to other primary caregivers when appropriate, acting as primary caregivers (as members of the team) when the challenges of the case warrant this involvement, and teaching and conducting research in the field of palliative care.

°World Health Organization. Technical Report Series 804, Cancer Pain and Palliative Care. Geneva: World Health Organization, 1990:11.

With recognition of palliative care as an essential element in medical care and as an area of specialization, there is a need for information about the approaches used by specialists from many disciplines in managing the varied problems that fall under the purview of this model. The scientific foundation of palliative care is also advancing, and similarly, methods are needed to highlight for practitioners at the bedside the findings of empirical research. *Topics in Palliative Care* has been designed to meet the need for enhanced communication in this changing field.

To highlight the diversity of concerns in palliative care, each volume of *Topics in Palliative Care* is divided into sections that address a range of issues. Various sections address aspects of symptom control, psychosocial functioning, spiritual or existential concerns, ethics, and other topics. The chapters in each section review the area and focus on a small number of salient issues for analysis. The authors present and evaluate existing data, provide a context drawn from both the clinic and research, and integrate knowledge in a manner that is both practical and readable.

We are grateful to the many contributors for their excellent work and their timeliness. We also thank our publisher, who has expressed great faith in the project. Such strong support has buttressed our desire to create an educational forum that may enhance palliative care in the clinical setting and drive its growth as a discipline.

New York, NY   R.K.P.
Houston, TX   E.B.

Contents

Contributors

JANET L. ABRAHM, M.D., F.A.C.P.
Department of Medicine
University of Pennsylvania School of
  Medicine
Philadelphia, Pennsylvania, USA

DINO AMADORI, M.D.
Department of Oncology
Pierantoni Hospital
Forli, Italy

ROBERT M. ARNOLD, M.D.
Section of Palliative Care and Medical
  Ethics and Center for Bioethics and
  Health Law
University of Pittsburgh School of
  Medicine
Montefiore University Hospital
Pittsburgh, Pennsylvania, USA

EDUARDO BRUERA, M.D.
Department of Symptom Control and
  Palliative Care
University of Texas, M.D. Anderson
  Cancer Center
Houston, Texas, USA

VICTOR T. CHANG, M.D.
Department of Medicine
New Jersey Medical School
Director of Palliative Care
Section Hematology/Oncology
VA New Jersey Health Care System
East Orange, New Jersey, USA

DEBORAH DUDGEON, R.N., M.D.,
  F.R.C.P.C.
Palliative Care Medicine Program
Department of Internal Medicine
Queen's University
Kingston, Ontario, Canada

ANNA R. DU PEN, A.R.N.P.
Pacific Northwest Pain Management
  Associates
Seattle, Washington, USA

STUART L. DU PEN, M.D.
Swedish Pain Services
Swedish Hospital- Seattle
Seattle, Washington, USA

ROBIN L. FAINSINGER, M.D.
Division of Palliative Care Medicine
Royal Alexandra Hospital
Edmonton, Alberta, Canada

GARY S. FISCHER, M.D.
Section of Palliative Care and Medical
  Ethics and Center for Bioethics and
  Health Law
University of Pittsburgh School of
  Medicine
Pittsburgh, Pennsylvania, USA

JULIE HEARN, M.Sc.
Department of Palliative Care and
  Policy
King's College School of Medicine &
  Dentistry, and St. Christopher's
  Hospice
London, United Kingdom

IRENE J. HIGGINSON, B.M., B.S.,
  Ph.D.
Department of Palliative Care and Policy
King's College School of Medicine &
  Dentistry, and St. Christopher's
  Hospice
London, United Kingdom

RUSSELL D. HULL, M.B., B.S.
Thrombosis Research Unit
University of Calgary
Calgary, Alberta, Canada

CHIRAG R. JANI, M.D.
Division of Geriatric Medicine
Department of Internal Medicine
University of South Florida College of
    Medicine
Tampa, Florida, USA

MARK N. LEVINE, M.D., M.Sc.
Department of Medicine
McMaster University
Hamilton, Ontario, Canada

MARCO MALTONI, M.D.
Palliative Care Unit
Department of Oncology
Pierantoni General Hospital
Forli, Italy

ISABELLE MANCINI, M.D.
Institut Jules Bordet
Brussells, Belgium

J. CAMERON MUIR, M.D.
Division of Hematology/Oncology
Northwestern University Medical School
Chicago, Illinois, USA

ORIANA NANNI, M.Sc.
Biostatistics Unit
Department of Oncology
Pierantoni General Hospital
Forli, Italy

JOSE PEREIRA, M.B., Ch.B.,
    C.C.F.P.
Edmonton Palliative Care Program
Grey Nuns Community Hospital &
    Health Centre
Edmonton, Alberta, Canada

GRAHAM F. PINEO, M.D.
Thrombosis Research Unit
University of Calgary
Calgary, Alberta, Canada

MARCO PIROVANO, M.D.
Department of Medical Oncology
S. Carlo Borromeo Hospital
Milan, Italy

SUSAN ROSENTHAL, M.D.
Department of Medicine
University of Rochester
Rochester, New York, USA

EMANUELA SCARPI, M.Sc.
Department of Oncology
Pierantoni General Hospital
Forli, Italy

RONALD S. SCHONWETTER, M.D.
    F.A.C.P.
Division of Geriatric Medicine
Department of Internal Medicine
University of South Florida College of
    Medicine
Tampa, Florida, USA

JAMES A. TULSKY, M.D.
Center for Health Services Research in
    Primary Care
Durham Veteran's Affairs Medical
    Center, and Center for Clinical Health
    Policy Research and the Center for
    the Study of Aging and Human
    Development
Duke University Medical Center
Durham, North Carolina, USA

CHARLES F. VON GUNTEN, M.D.
    Ph.D.
San Diego Hospice
San Diego, California, USA

SHARON WATANABE, M.D.
Edmonton Palliative Care Program
Grey Nuns Community Hospital &
    Health Centre
Edmonton, Alberta, Canada

DAVID E. WEISSMAN, M.D.
Palliative Medicine Program
Division of Hematology/Oncology
Medical College of Wisconsin
Milwaukee, Wisconsin, USA

I

SURVIVAL ESTIMATION IN PALLIATIVE CARE

1

Model for Estimation of Survival in Patients with Far-Advanced Cancer

MARCO MALTONI, ORIANA NANNI, EMANUELA SCARPI,
MARCO PIROVANO, AND DINO AMADORI

Research aimed at identifying prognostic factors of survival in a population of far-advanced and terminal cancer patients is a very delicate and risky matter. It involves a variety of implications and consequences that we deem necessary to examine and discuss, though briefly, at the very start.

First of all, we must emphasize the probabilistic value of the information acquired; the use of test results requires great caution in every case.[1,2] In fact, "the prognosis of any individual shall always be either better or worse than the median of a group of patients at the same stage of the same disease."[3] Therefore, the reply to the question "How long have I got, doctor?"[4] can be given only in terms of a probability percentage.

Another comment concerns the use of research findings. The objective is to obtain as much data as possible capable of suggesting an adequate treatment, avoiding the risks of over- or under-treatment. An Italian investigating group has identified a short life expectancy as a fundamental parameter when deciding to switch from cure to care.[5] Expected survival is only one of the factors that should assist physicians in decision making, since it contributes to the global staging and case-mix classification of these patients.[6] Other factors that have been suggested as criteria for moving from specific therapies to palliative care include current and expected quality of life, features of the primary tumor, patient characteristics (age, performance status, level of awareness, psychological and spiritual attitude), expected toxicity of conventional chemotherapies and availability of experimental drugs, and economic considerations.

Concerning the last factor, in the modern era of cost-driven therapies, the temptation to save money at all costs may induce physicians to consider palliative care, though less expensive than conventional therapies,[7,8] still too costly, and to think that the cheapest patient is a dead patient.[9] This risk of considering palliative treatment futile must be avoided.

The right to die with dignity may be transformed into a duty to die if patients come to the conclusion that they are a useless, unbearable burden on their families and society. Such a belief will easily induce them to ask for euthanasia. By contrast, if patients perceive sympathy, love, and benevolence in those closest to them, they will be induced to wish for optimal physical palliation in order to preserve that positive evaluation of themselves. Therefore, the promotion of communication among physicians, patients, and patients' families suggested by Lynn[10] becomes meaningful and may lead to a shared patient–doctor decision about the existential and economical choices to be adopted.

The patient's treatment preferences should not be ignored when making therapeutic decision. In Weeks' study,[11] patients wished for survival-prolonging treatments when life expectancy was more than 6 months; when life expectancy was shorter, they preferred therapies that would improve their quality of life. In regard to therapeutic and logistical choices, the literature shows that the median survival periods of hospice patients, all[12,13] or most[14] with advanced cancer, in Western Europe and North America, are practically identical. Christakis' study[14] of patients enrolled in hospice programs in the United States in 1990 showed a median survival of 36 days, whereas our two successive studies showed a median survival of 32 and 33 days, respectively.[12,13]

Within the studied cohorts, however, were subsets of patients with extremely different actual survival rates. In the Christakis study, 15.6% of patients survived for ≤7 days and 14.9% for ≥6 months; in our studies, 14.8–13.7% patients survived for ≤7 days and 4.4–2.4% for ≥6 months. This data shows that patients defined as terminal present different defined prognoses.

The *terminal stage* can be defined as a pathological condition leading the doctor, the patient, and the patient's family to expect death in the near future as a direct consequence of the illness, since no specific antitumor treatment appears to have any effect.[15] This definition is not precise since "near future" may refer to hours, days, weeks, or even months. However, it identifies two useful criteria: the ineffectiveness of specific therapies and the short life expectancy of the patient.

The primary purpose of prognostic studies of far-advanced cancer patients should be to identify prognostic factors that facilitate the decision to shift from cure to care and the consequent enrollment of the patient, duly financed, in a hospice program. It is also advisable to classify the patients within a large population into prognostically homogeneous subgroups. Last, but not least, counseling involving doctors, patients, and their families is to be fostered.

Guidelines have been suggested for evaluation of the methods used and of the findings from the studies on prognostic factors.[16] These guidelines, which appear in Table 1.1, are divided into three sections: (1) epidemiological validity, (2) biostatistical consistency, and (3) clinical applicability.[17] An analysis of the studies on

Table 1.1. Users guide for an article about prognosis

Are the results of the study valid?
Primary guides
Was there a representative and well-defined sample of patients at a similar point in the course of the disease?
Was follow-up sufficiently long and complete?
Secondary guides
Were objective and unbiased outcome criteria used?
Was there adjustment for important prognostic factors?
What are the results?
How great is the likelihood of the outcome event(s) in a specified period of time?
How precise are the estimates of likelihood?
Will the results help me care for my patients?
Were the study patients similar to my own?
Will the results lead directly to selecting or avoiding therapy?
Are the results useful for reassuring or counseling patients?

Reprinted with permission from: "User's guides to the medical literature. V. How to use an article about prognosis," *JAMA* 1994, 272:234–237, Copyright 1994, American Medical Association.

survival prognostic factors in terminally ill cancer patients demonstrates their strengths and weaknesses. The definition and staging of terminal cancer patients are still in the preliminary stage and the concept of *inception cohort* is often unclear, since patients who might be recruited are at different points in the course of their disease.

Only a few studies give information on referral patterns or sampling procedures, that is, on the mode of recruiting or selecting subjects. On the other hand, the length of the follow-up period is generally quite adequate in these studies and enables patients to be assisted up to the time of death, a matter of months. Therefore, the number of events occurring during this period helps to ensure the adequacy of the studies. Even the outcome, death in this case, is objective and measurable.

In regard to confusing factors, multivariate analysis and stratification of patients according to well-defined characteristics (treatments undergone and quality of the care setting) should ensure the adequacy of study results. Validation of the results of a preliminary study (training set), including an adequate number of patients for each prognostic factor, has been performed only in a few studies in an independent control group (testing set).

In the appendix to this chapter, the statistical methods most frequently used in the studies of prognostic factors are described. Then we discuss the factors we consider to be most useful in providing statistically correct and clinically useful information.

Based on the results of our two studies on prognostic factors in far-advanced

and terminal cancer patients, we have developed a predictive model, the Palliative Prognostic Score (PaP Score), which we shall now describe.

Patients and Methods

The training and testing procedure has been adopted in the development and
validation of a prognostic score for terminally ill cancer patients; therefore, two
consecutive, independent case series were recruited. The first series (training set)
of 519 eligible patients was recruited from October 1992 to November 1993 from
22 Italian centers, coordinated by our group and by the Oncological Department
of S. Carlo Borromeo Hospital in Milan. The cases were used to construct the
regression model and for the subsequent calculation of the prognostic index.

The second series (testing set) of 451 patients was recruited from January to
August 1996 from 14 Italian centers, some of which had provided the training set.
In this series the PaP Score was validated.

The same eligibility and exclusion criteria were adopted for both series. All
patients with an advanced solid tumor for whom antiblastic therapy was no longer
considered viable were accepted. Patients receiving palliative radiotherapy and
anabolic hormonal treatment were allowed; patients with myelomas, renal tumors, and hematological neoplasms were excluded because of possible interference of the neoplasia with some blood values. Table 1.2 shows the list of variables
collected for each training set patient. The variables are divided into clinical
(symptoms, weight loss, primary and metastatic cancer sites, Karnofsky Performance Status [KPS], Clinical Prediction of Survival [CPS]) and biological (hemoglobin, white blood cell count, proteins, albumin, tranferrin, ferritin, and pseudocholinesterase levels) categories.

Statistical Analysis

The statistical method used in our model has been described analytically in some
of our previous papers[12,13,18–20]; the fundamental points will be summarized here.
Since the chief purpose of prognosis is to gauge expected survival, the survival
periods were measured from the date of enrollment, and death due to all causes
was taken as the outcome. Survival curves were traced by the Kaplan-Meier
method, and the comparison among the curves relating to each prognostic factor
in the univariate analysis was based on the log-rank test. The simultaneous
analysis of several prognostic factors that proved to be significant by univariate
exploratory analysis of the training set made the choice of a multiple regression
model necessary. Since from a graphic viewpoint it became clear that the death
rate remains constant over time, a parametric multiple regression model appeared to be suitable for our case series. According to this model, the effect on
survival of the variables examined has been investigated by the linear predictor

Table 1.2. Clinical and biological parameters evaluated

Clinical parameters

Sex

Age

Primary site of neoplasia

Metastatic sites

Palliative hormonal treatment

Karnofsky Performance Status (KPS)

Clinical Prediction of Survival (CPS)

Hospitalization

Hemotransfusion in the last 15 days

Weight loss

Symptomatology

Pain killer treatment

Biological parameters

Serum albumin level

Serum prealbumin level

Proteinuria, 24 hr

Hemoglobin

Transport iron

Pseudocholinesterase

Transferrin

Total white blood cell count

Leukocyte count

$g(x_j) = (\beta_0 + \beta_1 x_{1j} + \ldots + \beta_p x_{pj})$, where, for the jth patient $_{(j\,=\,1,\,2,\,\cdots\,,\,n)}$, x_{ij} $_{(i\,=\,1,\,2,\,\cdots,\,p)}$ is the value assumed by each of the p variables and β_i is the pertinent regression coefficient, estimated by the maximum likelihood method.

For each clinical variable, the best survival was chosen as the reference, whereas for biological variables, the reference category is represented by the normal value class. From an initial model containing all clinical and biological factors that resulted independently in two previous separate analyses, a final parsimonious model was obtained by means of a backward selection procedure.

The quantity $g(x_j)$ was used to compute a score suitable for classifying each patient into groups with different prognoses at a given time. In this context, clinical considerations suggested that the study group should be divided into three cohorts based on 30-day survival of >70% (group A), 30–70% (group B), and <30% (group C). In order to obtain an easy-to-handle score, for the prognostic factors retained in the final model the value of each regression coefficient was divided by the smallest regression coefficient, and the results were rounded to the nearest integer or to the nearest integer +0.5. For each patient, a total score was calculated by summing up all the coefficients calculated above (partial scores). All analyses were performed using SAS software.

Results

The design of our study enables us to report synoptically the results of the training and testing trials described elsewhere.[12,13] The median survival in the 519-patient training set was 32 days; in the 451-patient testing set, it was 33 days. The final regression model, containing only those variables whose likelihood ratio test had $p < .05$, retains dyspnea, anorexia, KPS, CPS, total white blood cell count, and lymphocyte percentage. Table 1.3 reports the maximum likelihood estimate of the regression coefficient (β), its standard error [SE (β)], and the value of the partial score. Each patient was assigned a total score, the PaP Score, corresponding to the sum of all his or her appropriate partial scores.

Table 1.3 shows the PaP Score cutoff, which made it possible to classify each patient into an appropriate prognostic group. The same PaP Score was then applied to the second patient series (the testing set). In the training set, 178 (34.3%) patients were classified in risk group A, with a median survival of 64 days; 205 (39.5%) patients in risk group B, with a median survival of 32 days; and 136 (26.2%) patients in risk group C, with a median survival of 11 days.

In the testing set, as described in Table 1.4, the percentage of patients, the median survival, and the 30-day survival probability are similar to those in the training set. In addition, the total percentages of short (<7 days) and long (>180 days) survivors overlap (Table 1.5).

Figure 1.1a shows the different survival experience of the patients belonging to the three risk groups of the training set. This figure shows good agreement between survival curves estimated by the exponential model and those estimated by the Kaplan-Meier technique. Figure 1.1b shows the analogous curves for the three risk groups in the testing set.

Discussion

The studies that led to the development of the PaP Score and, later, to its validation on an independent cohort of patients were designed to identify, by multivariate analyses, clinical and laboratory parameters capable of integrating the CPS by increasing its predictive capacity. The efforts made to complement, not to substitute for, clinical experience have been reported by other researchers for various categories of patients.[1,21]

Our study deals only with very advanced cancer patients. Some authors[22,23]

Table 1.3. Training set: Multivariate survival analysis of the variables retained in the final model and partial score for each category of prognostic factors

		β	$SE\ (\beta)$	p	Partial score
Intercept		5.42	0.21		
Dyspnea	No	0.00	—		0
	Yes	−0.19	0.10	0.05	1
Anorexia	No	0.00	—		0
	Yes	−0.25	0.10	0.01	1.5
KPS	≥50	0.00	—		0
	30–40	0.03	0.11	0.79	0
	10–20	−0.44	0.20	0.03	2.5
CPS (weeks)	>12	0.00	—		0
	11–12	−0.33	0.18	0.06	2.0
	9–10	−0.56	0.19	0.004	2.5
	7–8	−0.49	0.16	0.003	2.5
	5–6	−0.83	0.17	<0.001	4.5
	3–4	−1.10	0.17	<0.001	6.0
	1–2	−1.61	0.20	<0.001	8.5
Total white blood cell count	Normal	0.00	—		0
	High	−0.14	0.12	0.24	0.5
	Very high	−0.28	0.12	0.02	1.5
Lymphocyte percentage	Normal	0.00	—		0
	Low	−0.19	0.11	0.10	1.0
	Very low	−0.49	0.13	<0.001	2.5

PaP Score: Classification of patients into three risk groups

Risk group		Total score
A	30-day survival probability >70%	0–5.5
B	30-day survival probability 30–70%	5.6–11.0
C	30-day survival probability <30%	11.1–17.5

have stressed the importance of soft factors in the early stages of the disease, but their hypothesis has not been widely accepted. By contrast, the prognostic importance of soft factors, which avoid incorrect assessment, is clearly demonstrated and generally accepted for patients with very advanced and terminal disease.

The purpose of the following review of several research models published over the years is to explain the choices made for our study. The bibliographical citations are as complete as possible; comments, however, are limited, especially when we deal with matters treated in other chapters of this volume.

Some authors judge the CPS alone to be biased by a high percentage of

Table 1.4. Successful validation of the PaP Score in terminally ill cancer patients: distribution and survival

	Training set			Testing set		
Score	Distribution N (%)	30-day survival (%)	Median survival (days)	Distribution N (%)	30-day survival (%)	Median survival (days)
0–5.5 (Group A)	178 (34.3)	82.0	64	127 (28.2)	86.6	76
5.6–11.0 (Group B)	205 (39.5)	52.7	32	206 (45.7)	51.6	32
11.1–17.5 (Group C)	136 (26.2)	9.6	11	118 (26.1)	16.9	14

incorrect predictions that often overestimate expected survival.[24–26] More recent studies emphasize the evaluator's experience with palliation, since it shows an optimal predictive capability,[27–31] sometimes higher than that of the KPS.[32]

Clinical survival prediction thus seems to have prognostic value, but since it is greatly influenced by the physician's experience and is a subjective estimate, it is poorly reproducible and unsuitable for use by nonpalliative physician and medical program managers, who must decide whether to admit a patient to a palliative care program.

In our study, carried out by trained, full-time palliative care people, the clinical predictivity of survival was shown to be reliable in both the training and test sets, even though the sets differed from each other. In fact, some centers participated in the first part of the study and not in the second, and vice versa.[12,13]

Integration of the CPS with objectivable parameters is therefore absolutely necessary. The most widely used performance status scores (the KPS[33] and the Eastern Cooperative Oncology Group Performance Status [ECOG PS][34]) proved to be reliable prognostic parameters, mainly for low score values predictive of short survival. By contrast, higher performance values are not always predictive of long survival.[29,30,35–41] Again, some indices of daily life activity have been found

Table 1.5. Successful validation of the PaP Score in terminally ill cancer patients: percentage of short- and long-survivors in the training and testing sets

	Training set (N = 519)		Testing set (N = 451)	
	≤7 days (%)	>180 days (%)	≤7 days (%)	>180 days (%)
Risk group A	3 (1.7)	21 (11.7)	4 (3.1)	9 (7.0)
Risk group B	28 (13.6)	2 (0.9)	23 (11.1)	2 (0.9)
Risk group C	46 (33.8)	0 (0)	35 (29.6)	0 (0)
Total	77 (14.8)	23 (4.4)	62 (13.7)	11(2.4)

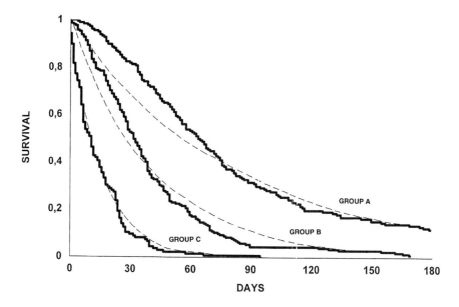

Figure 1.1a. Training set: survival experience of the three groups of patients identified by the PaP Score. Surviving probabilities are estimated by the exponential model (dotted lines) and by the Kaplan-Meier method (continuous lines). Log-rank = 294.8 (2 df), $p <$ 0.0001.

Risk groups	Total score
A (N = 178) 30-day survival probability >70%	0–5.5
B (N = 205) 30-day survival probability 30–70%	5.6–11.0
C (N = 136) 30-day survival probability <30%	11.1–17.5

Reprinted with permission from Elsevier Science from: "A new Palliative Prognostic Score (PaP Score): a first step for the staging of terminally ill cancer patients," by Pirovano M. et al., *Journal of Pain and Symptom Management* 17:231–239, Copyright 1999 by the US Cancer Pain Relief Committee.

to be predictive.[42] An ad hoc modification of the KPS [the Palliative Performance Scale (PPS)] for palliative use has shown reliable prognostic predictivity.[43] The predictive capacity of the KPS increases when it is integrated with certain clinical symptoms.[18,28,29,37,40,44–50]

   The presence of a series of physical symptoms constitutes a "terminal cancer syndrome" or "terminal common pathway" that is also prognostically meaning-ful.[40,51–53]

   Many symptoms in the terminal syndrome are related to the gastroenteric system and are somehow linked with the cachexia-anorexia cancer syndrome.[11,12,18,19,40,54,55] In our multivariate analysis, gastroenteric subjective symptoms proved to be significant, since they include the prognostic value of other

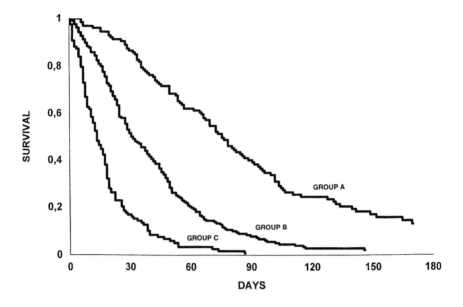

Figure 1.1b. Testing set: survival experience of the three groups of patients identified by the PaP Score (Kaplan-Meier estimates). Log-rank = 203.8 (2 df), $p < 0.0001$.
Reprinted with permission from Elsevier Science from: "Successful validation of the Palliative Prognostic Score (PaP Score) in terminally ill cancer patients," by Maltoni M. et al., *Journal of Pain and Symptom Management* 17:240–247, Copyright 1999 by the US Cancer Pain Relief Committee.

objective nutritional, biological, and/or integrated biological-clinical parameters, which are considered prognostically valuable in large case series, especially in geriatric populations.[19,30,56-62]

Among the clinical symptoms, delirium has been given increasing prognostical value.[37,50,61,63] We did not include it as a parameter in our original study, but we added it to the validation study in order to evaluate its impact. It proved to be significant, especially in the subgroup of longer-surviving patients (data not showed).[64]

In the literature, a quality-of-life assessment of terminally ill patients by validated instruments is considered to have dubious prognostic value. The general opinion is that these instruments are less important than organic and physical factors.[27,65] However, some authors believe that the quality of life has a statistically significant prognostic value.[39,66,67] Recently, it has been found that the prognostic relevance of quality-of-life multidimensional tests is due largely to the physical symptomatic component of these tests and its impact on the total score.[68,69]

Some biological factors have been found to have prognostic value, though in different degrees. These include certain characteristics of the leukocytic level (leukocytosis) and the neutrophil:lymphocyte ratio (lymphocytopenia), the hemoglobin level, and the levels of some plasma enzymes and electro-lytes.[11,12,19,30,59,61,62,70–76]

Exhaustive literature reviews have been published on prognostic factors in terminally ill cancer patients.[17,20,77–80] However, as far as we know, none of them shows either planned, designed methodological modes of systematic analysis or the comparison and analysis of results in a way that allows meta-analysis. Multivariate analyses of a factor series reveals the independent prognostic capacity of each parameter. Each factor can be integrated into a score after it is weighted and assigned a numerical value corresponding to its weight.

Scores have been produced for the purpose of defining the stage in disease progression, the probable outcome of a given clinical condition in an intensive care setting, and the probable outcome of chronic disease at a certain point in the future (6 months).[1,58,81–89] The PaP score is the first survival score in terminally ill cancer patients. The phases of our research[12,13] can be summarized as follows:

1. Identification of clinical and biological factors with independent prognostic capacity by multivariate analysis.
2. Development and validation of a prognostic score in an independent population.
3. Clinical utilization of the information obtained from the score to support therapeutic decisions.

With reference to the last item, the indications appearing in some studies[1,86,90] are not very encouraging. No significant changes have been noted in clinicians' willingness to adjust their therapies in light of the prognostic information obtained from specialized investigations. The authors conclude that doctors may decide, more or less consciously, to use their own diagnostic and therapeutic methods.[90] Our score, like others for other disease categories,[1,21] does not substitute for the doctor's judgment, but instead complements it by adopting easily gathered data on objective parameters. The attending physician maintains pre-eminence in both the prognostic evaluation and the doctor–patient therapeutic alliance and communication.[91] However, the integration of CPS with objective factors can correct an erroneous CPS; moreover, it facilitates clinicians' self-training and self-evaluation, which can be extended to nonspecialist palliative care operators.

Our PaP Score model contributes to the research on prognostic factors in the difficult process of staging very advanced cancer patients. This process must take into account organic, sociopsychological, qualitative, and quantitative life expectancy factors.

Appendix

When studying prognostic factors, it is necessary to both evaluate the effects of many variables and adjust the weight of each variable to the others. To do this, multiple regression models have been used in clinical research. The task, however, is not an easy one, since unique and correct assumptions, mathematical competence, and a large patient series are required. The estimations of prognostic values are valid only if the assumptions of the model are at least approximately true.

Before applying any multiple regression model, it is useful to perform a univariate analysis for each parameter in order to get some ideas of its relation to the outcome. In univariate analysis, survival curves are traced according to the Kaplan-Meier method, and a statistical test of the various categories of each variable (log-rank test or Wilcoxon test) is performed.[92,93] Univariate analysis can be used as a screening procedure, but its automatic use can cause problems because it does not account for possible correlation, possible interaction, or eventual joint effect of different variables. When many variables may be prognostic, in the model-constructing process the choice is based on the universally accepted principle of parsimony: the investigators should try to reduce the model's complexity and to summarize the major systemic effects in a few parameters. A parsimonious model excludes spurious or unnecessary parameters. In addition, it is clinically relevant, since the identification of a limited set of significant predictors avoids the collection of unnecessary data and allows the optimal use of costly medical tests.

Various regression models have been reported in the literature. The choice of the statistical model is seldom based on previous distributional examinations, but it is frequently based on maximizing how available information is used. When the outcome consists of a binary or discrete variable (e.g., alive/dead at a given time t), binary or ordinal logistic models are frequently used. The Cox proportional hazard model and parametric survival models[94] are often used for censored time-to event-data.[95]

The main characteristic of the Cox semiparametric model is that it does not assume anything about the survival function except the proportionality of hazard functions. Among parametric models, the exponential function is the one most commonly used in regression analysis due to its straightforwardness. In order to obtain a parsimonious model, it is convenient to use a systematic selection procedure that chooses a relatively small subset of all variables by excluding those with limited predictive value. The stepwise selection procedure, which can be based on either "forward" or "backward" selection, is one of the most widely used methods.[96] However, the uncritical application of these procedures for the selection of prognostic factors can lead to highly problematic results.

In developing a model of prognostic factors, generally too many variables are used in relation to the size of the patient set. In these cases, spurious prognostic associations can be found because of the "noise" in the data or because of multiple comparisons. Harrel et al.[97] suggest that in order to have predictive value for validation on a new patient sample, no more than $m/10$ predictors should be examined to fit a multiple regression model, where m is the number of uncensored event times (deaths) in the sample used to fit the model.

Another important aspect of prognostic factor analysis is the choice of the best cutoff for continuous characteristics. The median value or the quantiles of variable distribution are commonly used to divide patients into two or more groups if clear clinical-biological criteria are not available. However, it is not certain that this approach can identify the cutoff with the best discriminating capacity. Different approaches have been adopted in order to optimise the choice of the best discriminant value. Lausen[98] suggests a method for computing the correct p value related to the obtained classification rule.

When the model to be adopted and the variables with independent prognostic weight have been determined, it is necessary to know their predictivity.[99] To determine this, an indicator from 0 to 1, called the *multiple correlation coefficient* (R^2), is usually used in cases of linear regression. However, this procedure cannot easily be used in survival regressive models. In the recent literature, various methods have been proposed to measure the predictive strength of a given model in terms of the amount of explained variability.[100–102] Since likelihood is a measure of the explained variation, the difference between the log-likelihood of the selected model and the log-likelihood of the model with no covariates can be transformed into a measure of the proportion of explained variation.

A model's predictive value can be estimated during its development, with a study design consisting of training plus testing: one data set (training set) is used to develop the model according to standard methods, and a different data set (testing set) is used to validate the model. If the size of the training set is adequate, it is possible to validate the model's accuracy internally, using various approaches: (1) data splitting, which consists of subdividing the series at random into two unequal parts, one for model construction and the other for model validation; (2) cross-validation; or (3) bootstrapping. Cross-validation and bootstrapping are more sophisticated techniques: the data set is randomly and repeatedly subdivided using the data-splitting procedure.[103,104]

To quantify the prevision error, Harrel et al.[105] evaluated the model's discriminatory ability from the testing set, quantifying it with a concordance index in the area underlying the curve's *receiving operating characteristic (ROC)*, in which the outcome is dichotomized (alive/dead at a given time t). This index evaluates the probability that the predicted and observed outcomes are in agreement.

Another simple method used to determine a model's predictive capacity in the testing set consists of tracing the observed and predicted survival curves as a function of the covariates. Theoretically, it is expected that the influence of prognostic factors inserted in the final model is overestimated in the training set; this influence is reduced in the testing set, and the observed survival curves are closer to each other (the shrinkage effect[103]). If the observed and predicted curves are very similar, the model has predictive accuracy.

When the number of prognostic factors retained in the final model is relatively high, it is convenient to summarize the prognostic information by defining only a few risk groups. These groups should be formed in such a way as to produce prognostic homogeneity for patients within each group and heterogeneity among the various groups. Risk groups can be identified by developing a prognostic index based on the regression coefficient of each prognostic factor. For each subject, based on the function of his or her prognostic characteristics, it is possible to obtain a prognostic index by adding the values of the regression coefficients. According to the centiles of the prognostic index distribution, various risk groups can be defined.[96]

Acknowledgments

The authors thank Professor Felice Cenesi for the English translation of the paper and acknowledge the careful assistance of Alessandra Pizzigati.

References

1. Knaus WA, Harrell FE, Lynn J, et al. The SUPPORT prognostic model. Objective estimates of survival for seriously ill hospitalized adults. *Ann Intern Med* 1995; 122 (3):191–203.
2. Wagner DP, Knaus WA, Harrell FE, et al. Daily prognostic estimates for critically ill adults in intensive care units: Results from a prospective, multicenter, inception cohort analysis. *Crit Care Med* 1994; 22:1359–1372.
3. Selawry OS. The individual and the median. In: Stoll BA, ed. *Mind and Cancer Prognosis.* Chichester: Wiley, 1979:39–43.
4. Maher EJ. How long have I got doctor? *Eur J Cancer* 1994; 30A(3):283–284.
5. Working Expert Group on Guidelines of Specifical Medical Treatment in Advanced Cancer Patients. Amadori D, De Conno F, Maltoni M. (Eds). UTET, Milano, 1999, pp. 1–272.
6. Toscani F on behalf of the Italian Co-operative Research Group on Palliative Medicine. Classification and staging of terminal cancer patients: rationale and objectives of a multicenter cohort prospective study and methods used. *Support Care Cancer* 1996; 4:56–60.
7. Emanuel EJ. Cost saving at the end of life: what do the data show? *JAMA* 1996; 275:1907–1914.
8. Maltoni M, Nanni O, Naldoni M, et al.: Evaluation of cost of home therapy for patients with terminal diseases. *Curr Opin Oncol* 1998; 10:302–309.
9. Bilchik GS. Dollars and death. *Hosp Health Netw* December 20, 1996:18–22.
10. Lynn J, Knaus WA. Background for SUPPORT. *J Clin Epidemiol* 1990; 43(suppl): 1S–4S.
11. Weeks JC, Cook EF, O'Day SJ, et al. Relationship between cancer patient predictions of prognosis and their treatment preferences. *JAMA* 1998; 279:1709–1714.
12. Pirovano M, Maltoni M, Nanni O, et al. A new Palliative Prognostic Score (PaP Score): a first step for the staging of terminally ill cancer patients. *J Pain Symptom Manage* 1999; 17:231–239.
13. Maltoni M, Nanni O, Pirovano M, et al. Successful validation of the Palliative Prog-

nostic Score (PaP Score) in terminally ill cancer patients. *J Pain Symptom Manage* 1999; 17:240–247.

14. Christakis NA, Escarce JJ. Survival of Medicare patients after enrollment in hospice programs. *N Engl J Med* 1996; 335:172–178.

15. Di Mola G (ed). Il malato inguaribile: problemi di definizione. In: *Cure Palliative.* Milano: Masson, 1994:33–34.

16. Laupacis A, Wells G, Scott Richardson W, et al.: Users' guides to the medical literature. V. How to use an article about prognosis. *JAMA* 1994; 272:234–237.

17. Viganò A. Aspetti epidemiologici, statistici e clinici della ricerca sui fattori prognostici nei malati di cancro in fase terminale. *Quad Cure Palliat* 1997; 5:113–121.

18. Maltoni M, Pirovano M, Scarpi E, et al. Prediction of survival of patients terminally ill with cancer. *Cancer* 1995; 75:2614–2622.

19. Maltoni M, Pirovano M, Nanni O, et al. Biological indices predictive of survival in 519 terminally ill cancer patients. *J Pain Symptom Manage* 1997; 13:1–9.

20. Maltoni M, Pirovano M, Nanni O, et al.: Prognostic factors in terminal cancer patients. *Eur J Palliat Care* 1994; 1(3):122–125.

21. Fine MJ, Singer DE, Hanusa BH, et al. Validation of a Pneumonia Prognostic Index using the Medisgroups Comparative Hospital Database. *Am J Med* 1993; 94:153–159.

22. Piccirillo JF, Feinstein AR. Clinical symptoms and comorbidity: significance for the prognostic classification of cancer. *Cancer* 1996; 77:834–842.

23. Degner LF, Sloan JA. Symptom distress in newly diagnosed ambulatory cancer patients as a predictor of survival in lung cancer. *J Pain Symptom Manage* 1995; 10(6):423–431.

24. Parkes CM. Accuracy of predictions of survival in later stages of cancer. *Br Med J* 1972; 2:29–31.

25. Heyse-Moore LH, Johnson-Bell VE. Can doctors accurately predict the life expectancy of patients with terminal cancer? *Palliat Med* 1987; 1:165–166.

26. Forster LE, Lynn J. Predicting life span for applicants to inpatients hospice. *Arch Intern Med.* 1988; 148:2540–2543.

27. Addington-Hall JM, MacDonald LD, Anderson HR. Can the Spitzer Quality of Life Index help to reduce prognostic uncertainty in terminal care? *Br J Cancer* 1990; 62:695–699.

28. Hardy JR, Turner R, Saunders M, et al. Prediction of survival in a hospital-based continuing care unit. *Eur J Cancer* 1994; 30A(3):284–288.

29. Loprinzi CL, Laurie JA, Wieand HS, et al. Prospective evaluation of prognostic variables from patient-completed questionnaires. *J Clin Oncol* 1994; 12:601–607.

30. Rosenthal MA, Gebsky VJ, Keffor RF, et al. Prediction of life expectancy in hospice patients: identification of novel prognostic factors. *Palliat Med* 1993; 7:199–204.

31. Viganò A, Bruera E, Suarez-Almazor ME. Prognosis in terminal cancer patients: clinical estimation of survival (CES) compared with actual survival (AS) and a predictive model. *J Palliat Care* 1998; 14(3):127. Abstract 58.

32. Maltoni M, Nanni O, Derni S, et al. Clinical prediction of survival is more accurate than the Karnofsky Performance Status in estimating life span of terminally-ill cancer patients. *Eur J Cancer* 1994; 30A(6):764–766.

33. Karnofsky DA, Burchenal JH. The clinical evaluation of chemotherapeutic agents in cancer. In: Macleod CM, ed. *Evaluation of Chemotherapeutic Agents.* New York: Columbia University Press, 1949: 191–205.

34. Oken MM, Greech RM, Tormey DC, et al. Toxicity and response criteria of the Eastern Cooperative Oncology Group. *Am J Clin Oncol* 1982; 5:649–655.
35. Yates JW, Chalmer B, McKegney FP. Evaluation of patients with advanced cancer using the Karnofsky Performance Status. *Cancer* 1980; 45:2220–2224.
36. Miller RJ. Predicting survival in the advanced cancer patients. *Henry Ford Hosp Med* 1991; 39(2):81–84.
37. Bruera E, Miller MJ, Kuehn N, et al. Estimate survival of patients admitted to a palliative care unit: a prospective study. *J Pain Symptom Manage* 1992; 7:82–86.
38. Schonwetter RS, Teasdale TA, Storey P, et al. Estimation of survival time in terminal cancer patients: an impedance to hospice admissions? *Hospice J* 1990; 6(4):65–79.
39. Tamburini M, Brunelli C, Rosso S, et al. Prognostic value of quality of life scores in terminal cancer patients. *J Pain Symptom Manage* 1996; 1:32–41.
40. Reuben DB, Mor V, Hiris J. Clinical symptoms and length of survival in patients with terminal cancer. *Arch Intern Med* 1988; 148:1586–1591.
41. Allard P, Dionne A, Patvin D: Factors associated with length of survival among 1081 terminally ill cancer patients. *J Palliat Care* 1985; 11(3):20–24.
42. Schonwetter RS, Robinson BE, Ramirez G. Prognostic factors for survival in terminal lung cancer patients. *J Gen Intern Med* 1994; 9:366–371.
43. Anderson F. Downing GM, Hill J, et al. Palliative Performance Scale (PPS): a new tool. *J Palliat Care* 1996; 12(1):5–11.
44. Escalante CP, Martin CG, Elting LS, et al. Dyspnea in cancer patients. Etiology, resource utilization, and survival-implications in a managed care world. *Cancer* 1996; 78:1314–1319.
45. DeWys W. Management of cancer cachexia. *Semin Oncol* 1985; 12:452–460.
46. Heyse-Moore LH, Ross V, Mullee MA. How much of a problem is dyspnea in advanced cancer? *Palliat Med* 1991; 5:20–26.
47. Krech RL, Walsh D. Symptoms of pancreatic cancer. *J Pain Symptom Manage* 1991; 6:360–367.
48. Kaasa S, Mastekaasa A, Lund E. Prognostic factors for patients with inoperable non-small cell lung cancer, limited disease: the importance of patients' subjective experience of disease and psychosocial well-being. *Radiother Oncol* 1989; 15:235–242.
49. Ventafridda V, Ripamonti C, Tamburini M, et al. Unendurable symptoms as prognostic indicators of impending death in terminal cancer patients. *Eur J Cancer* 1990; 26:1000–1001.
50. Morita T, Tsumoda J, Inoue S, et al. Prediction of survival of terminally ill cancer patients. A prospective study. *Gan Kagaku Ryoho* 1998; 25(8):1203–1211.
51. Schonwetter RS, Teasdale TA, Storey P. The terminal cancer syndrome. *Arch Intern Med* 1989; 149:965–966.
52. Wachtel T, Masterson SA, Reuben D, et al. The end stage cancer patient: terminal common pathway. *Hospice J* 1988; 4:43–80.
53. Viganò A, Bruera E, Suarez-Almarzor ME. Terminal cancer syndrome: myth or reality? *J Palliat Care* 1998: 16(3):127. Abstract 56.
54. Nelson KA, Walsh D, Sheehan FB. The cancer anorexia-cachexia syndrome. *J Clin Oncol* 1994; 12:213–225.
55. Bruera E. Pharmacological treatment of cachexia: any progress? *Support Care Cancer* 1998; 6:109–113.

56. Fulop T, Hermann F, Rapin CH. Prognostic role of serum albumin and prealbumin levels in elderly patients at admission to a geriatric hospital. *Arch Gerontol Geriatr* 1991; 12:31–39.

57. Romagnoli A, Rapin CH: Valeur prognostique de certains parametres biologiques chez des sujets agés hospitalisés. *Age Nutr* 1991; 2(3):130–136.

58. Constans T, Bruyere A, Grab B, et al. PINI as mortality index in hospitalized elderly patient: research note. *Int J Vitam Nutr Res* 1992; 62(2):191.

59. Hermann FR, Safran C, Levkoff SF, et al. Serum albumin level on admission as a predictor of death, length of stay and readmission. *Arch Intern Med* 1992; 152(1): 125–130.

60. Salamagne ME, Vinant-Binam P. Valeur prognostique de parametres biologiques de denutrition chez des patients hospitalises en unité de soins palliatifs. *InfoKara* 1996; 44:21–32.

61. Forster LE, Lynn J. The use of physiologic measures and demographic variables to predict longevity among impatient hospice applicants. *Am J Hospice Care* 1989; 6(2):31–34.

62. Osterlind K, Andersen PK. Prognostic factors in small cell lung cancer; multivariate model based on 778 patients treated with chemotherapy with or without irradiation. *Cancer Res* 1986; 46:4189–4194.

63. Goodwin JS, Samet JM, Hunt WC. Determinants of survival in older cancer patients. *J Natl Cancer Inst* 1996; 88(15):1031–1038.

64. Caraceni A, Maltoni M, Nanni O, et al. The impact of delirium on a Palliative Prognostic Score (PaP Score). *J Pain Symptom Manage* 1998; 15(4):520. Abstract 63.

65. Cassileth BR, Lusk EJ, Miller DS, et al. Psychosocial correlates of survival in advanced malignant disease? *N Engl J Med* 1985; 312:1551–1555.

66. Morris JN, Sherwood S. Quality of life of cancer patients at different stages in the disease trajectory. *J Chronic Dis* 1987; 40(6):545–553.

67. Coates A. Quality of life and supportive care. *Support Care Cancer* 1997; 5(6):435–438.

68. Chang VT, Thader HT, Polyak TA, et al. Quality of life and survival. The role of multidimensional symptom assessment. *Cancer* 1998; 83:173–179.

69. Earlam S, Glover C, Fordy C, et al. Relation between tumor size, quality of life, and survival in patients with colorectal liver metastases. *J Clin Oncol* 1996; 14:171–175.

70. Sorensen JB, Badsberg JH, Olsen J. The prognostic factors in inoperable adenocarcinoma of the lung: a multivariate regression analysis in 259 patients. *Cancer Res* 1989; 49(20):5748–5754.

71. Paesmans M, Sculier JP, Libert P, et al. Prognostic factors for survival in advanced non-small cell lung cancer: univariate and multivariate analysis including recursive partitioning and amalgamation algorithms in 1052 patients. *J Clin Oncol* 1995; 13:1221–1230

72. Shoenfeld Y, Tal A, Berliner S, et al. Leukocytosis in non haematological malignancies: a possible tumor-associated marker. *J Cancer Res Clin Oncol* 1986; 111:54–58.

73. Ventafridda V, De Conno F, Saita L, et al. Leukocyte-lymphocytes ratio: a prognostic indicator of survival in cachetic cancer patients. *Ann Oncol* 1991; 2:196.

74. Cohen MH, Makuch R, Johnston-Early A, et al. Laboratory parameters as an alternative to performance status in prognostic stratification of patients with small cell lung cancer. *Cancer Treat Rep* 1981; 65:187–195.

75. Ralston SH, Gallacher SJ, Patel U, et al. Cancer-associated hypercalcemia: morbidity and mortality. *Ann Intern Med* 1990; 112:499–504.

76. Schwartz MK. Enzymes as prognostic markers and therapeutic indicators in patients with cancer. *Clin Chim Acta* 1992; 206:77–82.

77. Lassauniere JM, Vinant P. Prognostic factors, survival and advanced cancer. *J Palliat Care* 1992; 8(4):52–54.

78. Den-Daas N. Estimating length of survival in end-stage cancer: a review of the literature. *J Pain Symptom Manage* 1995; 10:548–555.

79. Hoy AM. Clinical pointers to prognosis in terminal disease. *Dev Oncol* 1987; 48:79–88.

80. Viganò A, Bruera E, Buckingham J, et al. Bedside prognostic factors in advanced cancer patients: a systematic review of the literature. *J Palliat Care* 1998; 14(3):126. Abstract 55.

81. Bruera E, Kuehn N, Miller MJ, et al. The Edmonton Symptom Assessment System (ESAS) for the assessment of palliative care patients. *J Palliat Care* 1991; 7(2):6–9.

82. Strause L, Herbst L, Ryndes T, et al. A severity index designed as an indicator of acuity in palliative care. *J Palliat Care* 1993; 9(4):11–15.

83. Headley J, Theriault R, Smith TJ. Independent validation of Apache II severity of illness score for predicting mortality in patients with breast cancer admitted to the intensive care unit. *Cancer* 1992; 70:497–503.

84. Knaus WA, Wagner DP, Draper EA, et al. The APACHE III prognostic system. Risk prediction of hospital mortality for critically ill hospitalized adults. *Chest* 1991; 100:1619–1636.

85. Selker HP, Griffith JL, D'Agostino RB. A time insensitive predictive instrument for acute myocardial infarction mortality: a multicenter study. *Med Care* 1991; 29:1196–1211.

86. Groeger JS, Lemeshow S, Price K, et al. Multicenter outcome study of cancer patients admitted to the intensive care unit. A probability of mortality model. *J Clin Oncol* 1998; 16:761–770.

87. McGuire WT, Tandon AK, Albert DC, et al. How to use prognostic factors in axillary node-negative breast cancer patients. *J Natl Cancer Inst* 1990; 82:1006–1015.

88. Marubini E, Bonfanti G, Bozzetti F, et al. A prognostic score for patients resected for gastric cancer. *Eur J Cancer* 1993; 29A(6):845–850.

89. Graff W, Bergstrom R, Pahòman F, et al. Appraisal of a model for prediction of prognosis in advanced colo-rectal cancer. *Eur J Cancer* 1994; 30A(4):453–457.

90. The SUPPORT Principal Investigators: A controlled trial to improve care for seriously ill hospitalized patients. The study to understand prognoses and preferences for outcomes and risks of treatment. *JAMA* 1995; 274:1591–1598.

91. ASCO: cancer care during the last phase of life. *J Clin Oncol* 1998; 16:1986–1996.

92. Kaplan EL, Meier P. Nonparametric estimation from incomplete observations. *J Am Stat Assoc* 1958; 53:457–481.

93. Mantel N. Evaluation of survival data and two new rank order statistics arising in its considerations. *Cancer Chemother Rep* 1966; 50:163–170.

94. Cox DR. Regression models and life-tables (with discussion). *J Royal Stat Soc* 1972; 34:187–220.

95. Lawless JS (ed). *Statistical Model and Methods for Lifetime Data*. New York: Wiley, 1982.

96. Marubini E, Valsecchi MG. Analysing survival data from clinical trials and observational studies. In *Statistics in Practice*. Wiley, 1995:295–329.

97. Harrell FE Jr, Lee KL, Califf RM, et al. Regression modelling strategies for improved prognostic prediction. *Stat Med* 1984; 3:143–152.

98. Lausen B, Schumacher M. Maximally selected rank statistics. *Biometrics* 1992; 48:73–85.

99. Henderson R. Problems and prediction in survival-data analysis. *Stat Med* 1995; 14:161–184.

100. Nagelkerke NJD. Miscellanea. A note on a general definition of the coefficient of determination. *Biometrika* 1991; 78(3):691–692.

101. Korn ED, Simon R. Measures of explained variation for survival data. *Stat Med* 1990; 9:487–503.

102. Schemper M. The explained variation in proportional hazards regression. *Biometrika* 1990; 77(1):216–218.

103. Van Houwelingen JC, Le Cassie S. Predictive value of statistical models. *Stat Med* 1990; 9:1303–1325.

104. Harrell FE, Lee KL, Mark DB. Tutorial in biostatistics. Multivariable prognostic models: issues in developing models, evaluating assumptions and adequacy, and measuring and reducing errors. *Stat Med* 1996; 15:361–387.

105. Harrell FE, Califf RM, Pryor DB, et al. Evaluating the field of medical tests. *JAMA* 1982; 247(18):2543–2546.

2

The Value of Symptoms in Prognosis
of Cancer Patients

VICTOR T. CHANG

The ability to make prognostic assessments has practical implications in planning care and in counseling a patient's family and friends. One example of its clinical application is the timing of hospice referral, which usually occurs 1–2 months before death even though 6 months of benefits are available.[1,2] Although many reasons are possible, the difficulty of predicting survival in cancer patients is a contributing factor.[3–9,9a] Significant variation exists among health professionals in their ability to predict survival. In one study, a panel consisting of a community oncologist, university oncologist, social worker, nurse, and general internist was asked to estimate the survival of 108 potential hospice patients on the basis of case summaries presented in a 10-page packet. Correlations of estimates with actual survival ranged from .02 for the community oncologist to .41 for the nurse. These results suggest that different ways of perceiving and processing clinical information exist, leading to differing estimates.[10]

Recognition of impending death is well known in folk cultures around the world. Predicting survival may also be important. In the holy Indian city of Benares, elderly poor persons are brought in by their families from the country-side to die in charity hospices, as dying in Benares is believed to confer salvation. A 14-day length of stay is allowed. In one series of patients, 10% of arrivals died on the date of admission and 84% were dead at 1 week. All patients were dead by 17 days. When the families and priests were asked how they knew when to bring the patient in, they answered that the patient no longer wanted to eat or drink. These results may not apply to cancer patients, as persons who have an illness such as infection or cancer are not eligible to die in these hospices.[11]

At the time of diagnosis of cancer, assessments of prognosis are based on the stage of disease, the histologic diagnosis and anatomical extent of disease, and the patient's performance status. However, many clinical observers have noted a range of survival times for patients with the same histologic diagnosis. In 1958, Morgan proposed the theory of biologic predeterminism to explain the finding that patients with the same histology might have different survival periods. He believed that biologic features of the tumor might help account for these differences, but he was unable to specify what these differences might be.[12] In patients with incurable disease, the prognosis is usually based on the extent of disease and the patient's performance status (see below)

The enumeration and description of symptoms is a basic clinical skill and common practice. The availability of time to obtain good histories of symptoms has always been a challenge, and symptom checklists have been developed to expedite this process.[13,14] However, symptoms have traditionally been considered a guide to diagnosis and follow-up rather than to the prediction of survival. This belief may be related to the availability of therapy for many conditions. The prognosis is important when there is no control over the outcome. Where effective treatments are available, interest in prognosis has diminished. By this line of reasoning, symptoms and prognosis will always be of interest in the field of palliative medicine.[15]

Evidence from a variety of studies shows that measures of symptoms status convey independent prognostic information in cancer patients at different points of their illness.

Methodology

To review these data, searches by MEDLINE, and hand searches through reference lists, were conducted to identify articles that included symptoms as part of a prognostic analysis. Anything other than TNM staging for prognostic purposes was considered to be related to symptoms for the purpose of this review. It should be noted that definitions of physical functioning and symptom assessments vary from article to article. A review of psychological distress as a prognosticator of survival was beyond the scope of this analysis and is presented elsewhere.[16]

B Symptoms and Hematologic Malignancies

The first studies focused on lymphomas, for which the prognostic value of night sweats, fever, and weight loss (B symptoms) continues to be an area of active research. Early series of patients with Hodgkins lymphoma suggested that the presence of constitutional symptoms before the start of radiation therapy had a correlation with survival.[17,18] The potential importance of B symptoms was recognized in the Ann Arbor classification[19] and continues in the Cotswold classification (see Table 2.1).[20]

Tubiana et al.[21] examined survival data on 454 patients with Hodgkin disease who had been treated at the Institute Gustav Roussy between 1922 and 1963 before the advent of modern therapeutic techniques. They performed univariate analyses on clinical stage, age, sex, histological subtype, presence or absence of systemic symptoms (fever, night sweats, pruritus, asthenia, anorexia, weight loss), and biologic indicators such as erythrocyte sedimentation rate (ESR), granulocyte count, lymphocyte count, and anemia. Fever, weight loss, asthenia, and anorexia were highly correlated with survival, and all six symptoms mentioned above were correlated with each other. Night sweats and pruritus did not contribute prognostic information. In early-stage Hodgkin disease, the presence of B symptoms has been correlated with elevated ESR, but these symptoms remain independent prognostic indicators of survival. In another study of 180 patients, the presence of both fevers and weight loss, but not night sweats, was associated with decreased survival and freedom from relapse at 7 years.[22] With the advent of more effective therapy, B symptoms all no longer significant predictors in multivariate models for patients with nodular sclerosis subtype[23] or advanced Hodgkin disease.[24,25] B symptoms may have prognostic value in patients with relapsed Hodgkin's Disease.[25a]

Bloomfield et al.[26] studied prognostic factors in a retrospective series of 128 patients with non-Hodgkin lymphoma seen at University of Minnesota hospitals. Variables in the models were age, sex, histology, bone marrow involvement, extranodal involvement, treatment, and presence of symptoms (fever, weight loss, or night sweats). A multiple linear regression was performed and it was found that histology, the presence of symptoms, and the clinical stage of the disease were the most important prognostic factors. In another survey of 199 patients with non-Hodgkin lymphoma classified by the Kiel system,[27] the presence of B symptoms and the disease stage were the two independent predictors of survival; performance status was not assessed. B symptoms were not predictors of survival in the model underlying the International Non-Hodgkin Lymphoma Prognostic Index.[28]

More recent analyses have also focused on specific types of hematologic malignancies. B symptoms have remained independent prognostic factors in patients with small lymphocytic lymphoma and leukocytosis,[29] diffuse large B-cell lymphoma,[30,31] and advanced follicular lymphoma.[32] In a study of 347 patients with mycosis fungoides, chills and malaise, but not pruritus or burning, were independent prognostic factors for survival after adjustment for stage.[33] Facon et al. performed a retrospective analysis of survival in 167 patients with Waldenstrom's macroglobulinemia seen at a single institution. Seventeen variables were examined in a Cox multivariate regression analysis. One of these variables, general symptoms, was significant on univariate analysis but not in the multivariate model.[34]

Performance Status

The Karnofsky Performance Status (KPS) represents one of the first attempts to systematize clinical assessment. Although this score is a functional index, it was also considered a form of symptom assessment.[35] It is an ordinal 11-point scale ranging from 0% (death) to 100% (normal function). The Zubrod Performance Status,[36] adopted by the Eastern Cooperative Oncology Group (ECOG), is another widely used 5-point measure in which 0 is normal function and 4 represents death. Correspondences between these two systems have been proposed.[37,38]

Studies on survival in lung cancer patients showed how prognosis could be related to performance status. Lanzotti et al.[39] studied the records of 428 patients with inoperable lung cancer seen in 1972 at the MD Anderson Hospital and performed a Cox regression survival analysis to identify prognostic factors. In their model, age, staging (limited or extensive), ECOG performance status, weight loss, site of metastatic disease, and treatment with radiation or chemotherapy were the variables. They found that weight loss, performance status, and age were the major predictors of survival in patients with limited disease, and performance status and age were the predominant predictors for survival in patients with extensive disease.

Stanley[40] analyzed 77 potential prognostic factors retrospectively on a database of 5138 patients who had participated in seven Veterans Administration Lung Cancer Study Group protocols from 1968 to 1978. His model included 14 symptoms, as well as categories of metastatic and systemic symptoms, but only their presence or absence was considered. After performing a Cox regression analysis, he found that only performance status, weight loss, and extent of disease were independent additive prognostic factors. He commented that weight loss was a surrogate way of representing (or indicating) prior physical status, and that an index combining a more comprehensive weight loss measure and systemic symptoms might prove to be a better variable in future prognostic studies.

The concept of performance status has been criticized.[41] Reasons include inability to predict early death,[42] a conceptually unclear delineation of what is being measured, and low physician interrater reliability, with ratings of 29–34% in a population of hemodialysis patients.[43]

Mor et al.[44] reported on experience with the KPS in the National Hospice Study. They noted statistically significant correlations among 47 interviewers asked to assign KPS scores to a series of 17 vignettes. The KPS correlated strongly with performance activity concurrently measured by the Katz Activity Daily Living index[45] and with the Physical Quality of Life score, an index designed specifically for use in the National Hospice Study. There was no significant relationship between pain and other symptoms or the number of symptoms with the KPS. This was attributed to the very debilitated state of the study patients. A significant relationship between KPS and survival was also demonstrated by analysis of variance and linear regression analyses.[45]

Schag et al.[46,47] evaluated the interrater reliability of the KPS in 75 patients and studied the relationship between KPS ratings and concurrent answers by 293 patients to the Cancer Inventory of Problem Situations (CIPS),[46] an index of patient-rated problem severity. They found a Pearson correlation coefficient of 0.89 and a kappa statistic of 0.53. Seven items on the CIPS were related to the KPS: daily activity, continuing weight loss or gain, self-care, ability to work, difficulty driving, and decreased energy. Interestingly, mental health professionals who interviewed patients consistently gave lower KPS ratings than did physicians who observed and examined patients.[47]

Loprinzi et al. assessed the prognostic value of patient-rated performance status. In this study, 1115 patients with advanced lung or colorectal cancer were asked to rate their KPS and ECOG performance status and answer questions about their nutritional status before receiving chemotherapy in protocols of the North Central Cancer Treatment Group. Physicians also rated the patients' performance status. In a Cox multivariate analysis, the physician-judged ECOG performance status, the physician estimate of survival, patient-judged ECOG performance status, and patient-judged appetite were independent significant predictors of survival. Physicians tended to give a higher rating of performance status than did the patients themselves.[48] This disparity between physician and patient ratings were confirmed in another study of patients with advanced lung cancer.[49]

Neurologic performance status has been defined by the Radiation Therapy Oncology Group in patients with brain metastases. An index of neurologic function has been shown to correlate with survival.[50,50a]

The performance of KPS as a predictor of survival has been shown to be either better than[51] or worse than[52] clinicians' estimates. Nevertheless, because of its simplicity, it remains important in prognostic assessments and has become the standard against which other predictors of prognosis are compared.

New instruments to define functional status have been developed, such as the Palliative Performance Scale[53] and the Edmonton Functional Assessment Tool.[54] The Palliative Performance Scale is based on the KPS but presents a more explicit description of ambulation, activity of disease, self-care abilities, nutritional intake, and mentation. In a study of hospice patients, the Palliative Performance Scale was highly correlated with the KPS. The Edmonton Functional Assessment Tool assesses 10 functional activities that are important to terminally ill patients and is intended to serve as a possible functional outcome measure.

Weight Loss

The prognostic effect of weight loss was most thoroughly examined in a study of 3047 patients who had been enrolled in 12 chemotherapy protocols of the ECOG. These patients represented nine primary sites of cancer (leukemia, non-Hodgkin lymphoma, lung, prostate, breast, stomach, pancreas, sarcoma, colorectum). Information on weight loss and ECOG performance status was collected before registration. Weight loss was significantly correlated with performance status, and was significantly correlated with tumor extent in breast cancer alone.

After stratification for performance status, comparison of median survivals showed a significant effect in patients with non-Hodgkin lymphoma and with breast, sarcoma, colon, or lung cancers who had good performance status (ECOG 0–1), as well as in patients with non-small cell lung cancer who had poor performance status.[55]

Symptom Status

In 1966, Feinstein proposed that symptoms reported by the patient could serve as a guide to the biologic behavior of the symptom. He developed a classification of symptoms: primary symptoms related to the primary site, systemic symptoms (e.g., cachexia, fatigue, weight loss, joint pain), and symptoms related to the presence of metastatic disease (hoarseness, dysphagia, swelling, palpable mass) (Table 2.1). Combinations of symptoms were further defined with the use of Venn diagrams, and symptom stages were specified. Symptom Stage I represented asymptomatic patients, Stage II patients with symptoms of 6 months' or greater duration, Stage III patients with symptoms of less than 6 months' duration, Stage IV patients with systemic symptoms, and Stage V patients with metastatic symptoms. Stage I and II patients were considered to have had indolent symptoms, Stage III and IV patients had obtrusive symptoms, and Stage V patients had deleterious symptoms. Feinstein applied this staging system retrospectively to a series of patients diagnosed with lung cancer[56] at the Yale-New Haven and West Haven Veterans Administration hospitals and showed correlation with 5-year survival rates, as well as with survival after surgical resection when the histology and lymph node status could be assessed.[57] A clinicoanatomic staging system was then proposed whereby symptom and anatomic staging could be combined to define a new staging system with four categories.[58]

The correlation of Feinstein symptom stage with survival was confirmed in a retrospective review of another group of 646 lung cancer patients seen at Walter Reed General Hospital by Senior and Adamson.[59] Green et al. were unable to confirm the usefulness of this system in a retrospective review of 617 patients with lung cancer, although they did note that within each stage, dyspnea, anorexia, asthenia, and weight loss were powerful prognostic findings.[60] Coy et al. reviewed a series of 1839 patients with unresected lung cancer in British Columbia and concluded that either the number of symptoms or Feinstein's index provided prognostic information independent of histology and stage. The presence of four or more symptoms at assessment predicted worsened survival.[61] Pater and Loeb performed a retrospective analysis on a series of 651 patients with bronchogenic carcinoma and analyzed survival with a Cox regression model that included the variables TNM status, performance status, weight loss, symptom type, symptom duration, histology, and age, and found that only weight loss and performance status added to anatomic stage as a predictor of survival.[62] Many of these studies were done with simple analytical approaches.

Table 2.1. Studies of symptoms

First Author	N	Disease	Population	Symptom measure	Model	Result
Green et al.	347	Mycosis fungoides	Multicenter study	Four symptoms	Weibull	Chills, malaise
Facon et al.	167	Waldenstrom's	Case series	General symptoms	Cox	Not significant
Crnkovich et al.	180	Hodgkin I–IIB	RT or Chemo	B symptoms	Cox	B symptoms significant
Ferry et al.	79	Hodgkin NS	RT series	B symptoms	Cox	B symptoms not significant
Fabian et al.	278	Hodgkin, advanced	Protocol	B symptoms	Cox	B symptoms not significant
Hasenclever et al.	5141	Hodgkin, advanced	Chemotherapy	B symptoms	Cox	B symptoms not significant
Leonard et al.	199	Non-Hodgkin	Case series	B symptoms	Log rank test	B symptoms significant
Ben Ezra et al.	268	Small lymphocytic	Protocol	B symptoms	Cox	B symptoms significant in pts with leukocytosis
Wood et al.	157	Follicular lymphoma, adv.	Case series	B symptoms	Cox	B symptoms significant
Armitage et al.	75	Diffuse large cell	Chemotherapy	B symptoms	Cox	B symptoms significant
Nakamine et al.	114	Diffuse large cell, I–IV	Protocol	B symptoms	Cox	B symptoms significant
Intl Group	3273	Non-Hodgkin's I–IV, intermediate to high grade	Chemotherapy	B symptoms	Cox	KPS
Coy et al.	1839	All lung	Retrospective	Feinstein	Log rank test	Number of symptoms: more than four
Lanzotti et al.	316	All lung	Retrospective	Feinstein	Multiple regression	Symptom status of patients with limited disease
Senior et al.	646	NSCLC	Retrospective	Feinstein	Life tables	Symptom status significant
Green et al.	617	NSCLC	Retrospective	List	Chi square	Not significant
Pater et al	651	NSCLC	Lung cancer/RT	Feinstein	Cox	KPS, weight loss
Stanley et al	5138	NSCLC	VA Lung Group	List	Cox	KPS, weight loss
Kaasa et al	102	NSCLC	RT/CT protocol	Own measure	Multiple regress	General symptoms (tiredness, appetite, difficulty sleeping, pain)
Furuta et al	240	NSCLC	RT	Feinstein-like	Cox	Weight loss
Wigren et al	502	NSCLC	RT patients, retrospective	Feinstein	Cox	Metastatic symptoms significant
Wigren	210	NSCLC	RT patients	Feinstein	Validation of index	Symptom stage of index

(continued)

Table 2.1. Studies of symptoms—Continued

First Author	N	Disease	Population	Symptom measure	Model	Result
Kukull et al	53	NSCLC	Case series	SDS	Cox	Symptom distress
Degner et al	84	NSCLC	Outpatients	SDS	Wilcoxon correlations	Symptom distress
Feinstein et al	192	Larynx	Retrospective	Feinstein	Graphic	Symptom stage
Piccirillo et al	193	Larynx	Retrospective	Feinstein	Cox	Age, symptom stage, comorbidity
Pugliano et al	265	Oral cavity	Retrospective	Feinstein	Various	Symptom stage
Pugliano et al	1032	Head and neck	Retrospective	Feinstein	Cox	Dysphagia, otalgia, weight loss, neck lump
Neel et al	182	Nasopharyngeal	Prospective	List	Cox	Number of symptoms: more than seven
Earlam et al	50	Colorectal	Prospective	Rotterdam	Multiple regression	PWB Physical Well Being
Feinstein et al	318	Rectal	Retrospective	Feinstein		Symptom stage practical
Peipert et al	134	Gyn. (cervical, IB)	Retrospective	Feinstein	Cox	Symptom stage significant
Wells et al	142	Gyn. (endometrial)	Retrospective	Feinstein	Five-year survival	Symptom stage practical
DiSilvestro et al	137	Gyn. (ovarian)	Retrospective	Feinstein	Cox	Symptom stage significant
Clemens et al	280	Prostate	Retrospective	Feinstein	Logistic reg	Symptom stage significant
Rana A et al	279	Prostate, metastatic	Retrospective	List	Log rank test	Bladder outflow and bone pain
Bruera et al	47	Mixed	Prospective	ESAS	Logistic reg	Cognitive failure, weight loss, dysphagia
Reuben et al	1592	Mixed	Natl. Hospice	Survey	Logistic reg	Dry mouth, dyspnea, difficulty swallowing, weight loss
Chang et al	240	Mixed	Inpt/output	MSAS	Wilcoxon	MSAS Physical symptom distress (PHYS) subscale
Maltoni et al	530	Mixed	Hospice	Survey	Exponential	Loss of appetite, KPS, dyspnea
Tamburini et al	115	Mixed	Hospice	TIQ	Cox	Global health status, cognition
Morita et al	150	Mixed	Hospice	Survey	Cox	Performance status (PS), dyspnea, loss of appetite, delirium, edema

The Feinstein[63] approach has since evolved toward summarizing both symptom status and comorbidity and incorporating both of them into an anatomic staging system. Symptoms have been divided into primary symptoms due to local disease, systemic symptoms such as weight loss and fatigue, and symptoms resulting from metastases. Comorbid conditions have been defined, and a functional severity stage has been proposed: alpha (no symptoms or comorbidity), beta (moderate symptoms and no comorbidity), and gamma (presence of a comorbidity). The functional severity stage was cross-tabulated against the anatomic staging of the tumor. Patients who had Stage I disease and alpha status were called A; patients who had Stage II disease and alpha status were called B; patients who were Stage III alpha, I beta, II beta, and III beta were called C; and all Stage IV or gamma patients were called D.

These general ideas have been applied successfully to survival analysis of patients with a large variety of cancers (larynx,[64,65] oral cavity,[66] head and neck,[67] lung,[68] prostate,[69] rectal,[70,71] cervical,[72] endometrium,[73] ovary,[74] Hodgkin disease[75]). This model also has been tested for robustness in patients with lung cancer[76] and has proved to be successful.

Wigren et al.[77] developed a prognostic model in a retrospective series of 502 inoperable lung cancer patients treated with radiation therapy. The model has five variables: disease extent, Feinstein clinical score, performance status, tumor size, and hemoglobin level.[77] In a validation study performed on a second group of 210 patients, Wigren reported that each variable contributed independently to survival.[78]

A shortcoming of the Feinstein model is that most studies were retrospective, and the presence of symptoms was determined from chart review. Difficulties encountered with this approach have been the ability to classify the patients' symptoms in a category and the need to attribute symptoms to equally plausible comorbid conditions (e.g., dyspnea and cough; patient with lung cancer and COPD ??). The KPS has not been included in these analyses. These factors may have hindered the acceptance of this approach.

Studies of the Prognostic Significance of Symptoms in Patients with Other Cancers

As noted, the importance of the presence or absence of symptoms has been difficult to prove conclusively. This has also been true in studies of patients with other cancers.

Neel et al. prospectively studied symptoms at presentation and 5-year survival in 182 patients with nasopharyngeal carcinoma. Symptoms were grouped into nasal, ear, throat, neck, and general symptoms; duration of symptoms prior to arrival; and number of symptoms on arrival. Patients with fewer than seven symptoms had a 58% 5-year survival, whereas those with seven or more symptoms had 25% 5-year survival. In a Cox regression analysis, Neel et al. found that the presence of seven or more symptoms was an independent risk factor for survival.[79]

Graf et al.[80] reported a retrospective study of 340 patients with advanced colorectal cancer who participated in three chemotherapy trials. In addition to hemoglobin level, performance status, and treatment, the number of symptoms (pain, nausea, fatigue, bleeding) present were independent predictors of survival.[80] However, in a subsequent prospective validation study of this model in 198 patients undergoing a chemotherapy trial, the number of symptoms was no longer predictive.[81]

In a series of 279 consecutive patients with metastatic prostate cancer, the effect on survival of six symptoms (bladder outflow, bone pain, anemia, weight loss, paraplegia, and change in bowel habits) was studied.[82] Cox regression analysis was performed to control for the amount of bone disease. The presence of bone pain, bladder symptoms, and anemia had independent prognostic value. Performance status was not included in this model.

Furuta et al.[83] examined the presence of symptoms in combination with anatomic stage in 240 patients with non-small cell lung cancer who underwent definitive radiation therapy. They found that symptoms were related to clinical stage and performance status but, except for weight loss, were not independent prognostic factors. Chest pain, weight loss, and breathlessness were correlated with poor outcomes, whereas cough, hemoptysis, and fever were correlated with good outcomes.[83]

The presence of symptoms may be an independent prognostic factor in patients with brain tumors. The presence of mental changes was a prognostic factor independent of performance status in a retrospective series of 379 patients with low-grade glioma.[84] In a sample of 103 patients with brain metastases from lung cancer, the presence of chest symptoms at the time of diagnosis was an independent prognostic factor.[85] In another series of 159 patients with lung cancer and brain metastases, urine incontinence, and stool incontinence, but not weakness, headache, vomiting, or disturbance of consciousness, were independent predictors of survival.[86]

Studies of hospice patients

Forster and Lynn[87] examined the prognostic value of physiologic and demographic variables in a logistic regression model of survival at 3 and 6 months in a heterogeneous sample of 111 hospice patients. Their 14-variable model for death within 3 months included two significant symptoms: pain and disorientation. Weakness and KPS were not independent predictors. For death within 6 months, pain, weakness, and disorientation were all independent predictors. These results suggest that different symptoms may be important in predicting short- and long-term survival.[88] In contrast to these results, performance status was predictive in another large survey of hospice patients.[88]

Table 2.2. Quality of life (QOL) measures

Author	N	Disease	Population	QOL measure	Statistics	Result
Coates et al	152	Melanoma	DTIC ± IFN	LASA	Linear regression	LASA for mood, appetite, overall QOL and QOL index
Coates et al	308	Breast, IV	Chemotherapy	LASA	Linear regression	PWB, QOL index change in QOL
Seidman et al	49	Breast, IV	Chemotherapy	FLIC	Regression	FLIC, MSAS Global Distress Index
Ruckdeschel et al	437	NSCLC	LCSG protocols	FLIC	Cox	QL score
Ganz et al	40	NSCLC	Best supportive	FLIC	Cox	FLIC score, marital status
Herndon et al	206	NSCLC	CALGB study CT ± hydralazine	QLQC30	Cox	Pain
Ringdal et al	253	Mixed	Hospital inpts	QLQ-C30	Cox	Physical function
Dancey et al	474	Mixed	Chemotherapy	QLQ-C30	Cox	Global QOL, absence of dyspnea, low emotional function
Coates et al	735	Mixed	Palliative	QLQ-C30	Cox	Physical, General QOL, global functioning, PS, age
Wisloff et al	581	Multiple myeloma	Chemotherapy	QLQ-C30	Cox	Physical function
Cella et al	571	NSCLC	Chemotherapy	FACT-L	Cox	Physical, functional, lung cancer subscales
Hwang et al	54	Mixed	Palliative care	FACT-G	Mixed effects	Sum QOL, change in QOL

CALGB, cancer leukemia Group B; CT, chemotherapy; DTIC, dacarbazine; IFN, Interferon; LASA, linear analogue self assessment; LCSG hung cancer study group; Phys-EORTC, Physical functioning subscale; PS, performance status; PWB, physical well being (LASA).

Dyspnea is highly prevalent in hospice populations. In the National Hospice Study, the presence of dyspnea was associated with low performance status, with pulmonary and cardiac disease, and with decreased survival.[89] Severe dyspnea was associated with decreased survival in a group of 303 patients admitted to a hospice.[90] In a retrospective sample of cancer patients who presented with dyspnea to the emergency room of a major cancer center, the median survival was 12 weeks; patients with lung cancer had a median survival of 4 weeks.[91] However, in a retrospective Cox regression study of survival of 405 patients who were admitted to an outpatient hospice and survived for a median period of 29 days, Christakis found that dyspnea was not associated with shorter survival; decreased activity and disorientation were associated with shorter survival, and other symptoms were not assessed.[92] The absence of dyspnea also has been associated with improved survival (see below).

Pain has been identified as a prognostic factor in only a handful of studies.[93] Clee et al.[94] performed a retrospective survey of 337 patients who had a resection for bronchial carcinoma between 1963 and 1977 and studied the effects of 14 preoperative variables and 2 operative variables on survival. Patients with small cell lung cancer were included. A multivariate log-logistic regression model was developed to predict survival at 2 years; tumor size, pain, and weight loss were identified as independent prognostic factors. Schonwetter et al.[95] studied a group of 310 consecutive lung cancer patients admitted to a hospice and developed an accelerated failure time survival model to estimate short-term survival. The model incorporated multiple factors; among the symptoms, severe pain and dry mouth were independent prognostic factors, while disorientation, KPS, and appetite status were not.[95]

Herndon et al.[96] evaluated survival in a group of 206 patients with advanced non-small cell lung carcinoma who enrolled in CALGB 8931, a randomized trial of chemotherapy. With Cox regression analyses, only the pain subscale in the EORTC QLQ-C30[97] was found to have prognostic importance.

Brescia et al.[98] examined survival in 1103 patients with advanced cancer admitted to Calvary Hospital. This institution is an acute care facility that specializes in the management of patients with advanced cancer. Patients were assessed at admission for pain, performance status, and mental status, in addition to demographic and laboratory variables. In a Cox survival analysis, neither pain on admission nor mental status contributed to the risk of death.

Other symptoms, such as fatigue, need to be considered in future studies. Fatigue has been a significant predictor of survival in univariate analyses by Wisloff, Tamburini, Ringdal, Dancey (see below), and Hwang et al.[99] but not in multivariate analyses. Fatigue may be a predictor of the KPS.

Groups of symptoms

Reuben et al.[100] examined the survival of 1592 patients who were enrolled in the National Hospice Study. At the time of enrollment at a hospice, patients were interviewed about their symptoms and their performance status was assessed. A log-normal accelerated time survival model, which incorporated KPS and the presence or absence of 14 symptoms, was developed. KPS ratings of 10–20 and 30–40, as well as the symptoms of dry mouth, shortness of breath, problems eating, recent weight loss, and trouble swallowing, predicted decreased survival. Within each KPS rating, an increasing number of symptoms correlated with a decreased range of survival times.[100] The primary site of disease was not important.

The importance of cognitive dysfunction was highlighted by Bruera and coworkers, who prospectively evaluated 47 consecutive patients admitted to the Palliative Care Unit at Edmonton General Hospital.[101] Patients were evaluated for performance status, eight symptoms (pain, nausea, depression, anxiety, anorexia, dry mouth, dysphagia, and dyspnea), weight loss, and cognitive status. The endpoint was survival for more than or less than 4 weeks. On logistic regression analysis, dysphagia, cognitive failure, and weight loss were associated with survival for less than 4 weeks. Dyspnea was not a predictor.[101]

Rosenthal et al.[102] studied 19 parameters in 148 consecutive patients admitted to the Victoria Hospice in Australia. These parameters included symptoms, physical findings, laboratory findings, and disease status (number of metastatic sites). Survival times were converted into ordinal variables and analyzed by ordinal regression analysis. In this model, performance status was predictive factors, but confusion and weight loss were not.[102]

Hardy et al.[103] collected data on 107 patients admitted to the Royal Marsden Hospital Palliative Care Unit during a 6-month period. Symptoms were categorized as pain, other symptoms, and pain and other. In a multivariate analysis of survival, the original cancer site and the presence of dyspnea and decubiti were predictive factors. In an analysis of symptoms alone, dyspnea, constipation, immobility, and weakness were important predictors of decreased survival. It is not clear how systematically symptom assessment was performed.[103]

Maltoni et al.[104] studied survival in 530 hospice patients throughout Italy. Patients were assessed at intake for the presence of fever, anorexia, dry mouth, dysphagia, dyspnea, and pain, as well as other factors. Multivariate analysis with an exponential regression model identified six predictive factors, three of which could be considered symptoms: anorexia, dyspnea, and KPS. The others were clinical predictors of survival, palliative steroid use, and hospitalization status.[104]

Tamburini et al.[105] studied 115 hospice patients in Italy. In a multicenter home-care unit study, the patients completed the Therapy Impact Questionnaire,[105] which included questions on the severity of fatigue (insomnia, sleeping problems, weakness, feeling tired), gastrointestinal symptoms, pain, loss of appetite, drowsiness, dry mouth, and difficulty breathing. Analysis of data from 100 patients using a Cox survival model suggested that confusion, weakness, and loss of appetite were significantly related to the risk of dying. The cumulative number of symptoms, as well as a combination of global health status and cognitive status, showed a strong association with survival. Performance status was not an independent predictive factor in this analysis[106]

Morita et al.[107] prospectively studied 150 patients admitted to Japanese hospice inpatient units to identify prognostic factors. Of 11 factors, 5 were found to be significant by multivariate Cox analysis: performance status, dyspnea at rest, loss of appetite, edema, and delirium. Death rattle, dysphagia, dry mouth, malaise, stomatitis, and fever were not significant.

Symptom attributes

In addition to their presence, descriptive or qualitative aspects of symptoms may have prognostic significance. These aspects may include symptom duration, symptom distress, and impact on quality of life.

The duration of symptoms may have prognostic significance, an issue with implications for the value of screening for early detection of cancer. In an analysis of symptom duration in 385 patients presenting with head and neck cancer, there was no correlation, and perhaps a negative correlation, between duration of symptoms and stage at presentation.[108]

One study of patients with colon cancer suggested that a duration of symptoms of less than 3 months may be associated with a worse prognosis;[109] other studies have found no relation between symptom duration and survival.[110–112] In a population-based sample of 154 colorectal cancer patients,[113] symptom duration of up to 1 year before diagnosis did not affect survival, but the total number of symptoms (up to six) was a significant predictor; performance status was not included in the model.[113] In a recent series of 777 consecutive patients with colorectal cancer, duration of symptoms was not a significant predictor of survival after tumor stage and the presence of obstruction were included.[114] In general, patients who were asymptomatic had lower stages of disease and better survival, but for symptomatic patients, duration of symptoms did not correlate closely with stage of disease or survival.

In patients with primary brain tumors, duration of symptoms has been a significant predictor in studies of patients with supratentorial tumors,[115] diffuse low-grade astrocytoma,[116] and malignant glioma.[117] Although different cutoff periods were used, longer symptom duration was associated with improved survival.

In a retrospective series of 187 patients with osteosarcoma, symptom duration of less than 6 months was a poor prognostic sign.[118] In a larger study of 1887 patients with seven primary sites of disease, only lung and rectal cancer showed some relationship between the interval of presenting symptoms and diagnosis and survival.[119]

Symptom duration may be important for patients with rapidly growing tumors. For patients with germ cell tumors, increasing symptomatic intervals from 10 to 19 weeks correspond to a more advanced stage of disease.[120] A more recent analysis over an 18-year period[121] suggested that symptom duration of greater

than 16 weeks is associated with decreased survival in patients with nonsemi-
nomatous germ cell tumors.

These studies suggest that patients who are asymptomatic at diagnosis have
better prognoses than symptomatic patients. Among symptomatic patients, duration of symptoms does not correlate closely with stage for many classes of solid
tumors. The data suggest that rapidity of onset may be a significant predictor in
rapidly growing tumors.

Patient-rated symptom attributes
A newer approach to the measurement and assessment of symptoms has been to
ask the patient to rate attributes, such as frequency, severity or distress, and
impact of the symptom on specific aspects of life.[122] Clinicians do this frequently
when interviewing patients. Interest in this approach may have been stimulated
by studies of cancer pain, in which patients have been shown to be able to rate
and quantify their pain in a reproducible and consistent manner.

Symptom distress is an attribute that may have prognostic features. Symptom
distress has been defined by McCorkle and Young[123] as "the degree of discomfort
reported by the patient[s] in relation to their perception of the symptoms being
experienced." The concept and its applications have been recently reviewed.[124]

Kukull et al.[125] reported a prospective study of 65 lung cancer patients who
were assessed at diagnosis in a radiation therapy clinic. Patients were interviewed
twice using the Symptom Distress Scale (SDS)[123] and other instruments. Of 53
evaluable patients who were followed for survival, 45 had died at the time of
analysis. A multivariate Cox regression analysis was performed. Only the SDS was
a predictor of survival ($p < .02$) in models constructed from each interview, and
patients with higher scores of distress (above 24) had a shorter survival than
patients with lower scores. The symptoms measured by the SDS were nausea,
appetite, insomnia, pain, fatigue, changes in bowels, concentration, breathing,
outlook, and cough. This study was one of the first to attempt to measure
symptom intensity. However, other prognostic variables, such as performance
status and weight loss, were not included in the analysis.

Degner and Sloan[126] subsequently reported on symptom distress in a sample
of 434 newly diagnosed ambulatory cancer patients seen in tertiary care referral
clinics. In a subsample of 82 lung cancer patients, symptom distress was independent of age and stage as a predictor of survival, and high symptom distress
scores were associated with early death. The performance status of these
patients was not examined. The most troubling symptoms were fatigue and
insomnia.

Emotional distress may be related to the meaning of a symptom to the
patient, but physical distress may be related to the severity of illness. Severe
physical distress in one series of hospice patients was linked to impending
death.[127] The concept of symptom distress has been an important component of
more recent symptom instruments, such as the Rotterdam Symptom Checklist[128]

and the Memorial Symptom Assessment Scale.[129] Symptom distress is conceptually attractive as a way to link symptoms with quality of life.

Quality of life

Quality of life measurements have been found to be predictive of survival in patients undergoing treatment in institutional and cooperative group trials. Coates et al.[130] analyzed data from a randomized clinical trial of chemotherapy for patients with metastatic or measurable breast cancer. Patients rated physical well-being, mood, pain, nausea and vomiting, appetite, and overall quality of life with a Linear Analog Self Assessment scale.[131] Their physicians completed the Spitzer Quality of Life (QL) Index.[132] Because the assumptions underlying the proportional hazards model did not hold, these workers adopted a multiple linear regression model; the cube root of the survival time was used as a dependent variable because this transformation had a normal distribution. In multivariate analyses that added the QL Index, or the patient-rated Physical Well Being linear analogue scale score to the model, ECOG performance status was no longer a significant predictor of survival.[130] Similar findings were reported from a randomized trial in melanoma.[133]

Kaasa et al.[134] prospectively studied 102 patients with inoperable Stage II or Stage III non-small cell lung cancer who were randomized to chemotherapy or chemotherapy with radiation treatment groups. Median survival in both arms was the same at 10 months. At enrollment, the patients answered questions about fatigue, lack of appetite, difficulty sleeping, and pain in the past 30 days using a 5-point Likert scale ranging from "none" to "very much." Physical functioning was measured by assessment of dyspnea, and psychosocial well-being was assessed with questions about strength, tiredness, mood, depression, meaninglessness, self-satisfaction, self-confidence, and whether life was worth living. In a stepwise multiple regression analysis, only the presence of general symptoms and psychosocial well-being were independent predictors of survival. Physical well-being (dyspnea) and performance status were not independent predictors. Good psychosocial well-being correlated with few symptoms and poor World Health Organization performance status.

Addington-Hall et al.[135] studied survival in 1128 cancer patients and assessed whether the Spitzer QL Index could predict death better than doctors and nurses. They found that patients with a low QL Index were more likely to be dead at 6 months but that this finding could not be used to make predictions on an individual basis. They suggested that the QL Index should be combined with symptoms to determine the prognosis.

Ruckdeschel et al.[136] studied 439 patients who enrolled in eight Lung Cancer Study Group trials and who completed the Functional Living Index of Cancer (FLIC)[137] before starting treatment and at regular intervals afterward. A multivariate proportional hazards model for survival stratified by cell type demonstrated that quality of life scores, T1 or N2 status, and KPS were independent predictors of survival.

Ganz et al.[138] studied a series of 40 patients with metastatic lung cancer who completed the FLIC at baseline and had been randomized to the supportive care arm in a trial that compared supportive care to supportive care with combination chemotherapy. Most subjects had a KPS above 80%. In the survival model, it was found that patients with a baseline FLIC score greater than the median score had significantly increased survival after examination for other covariates, such as performance status, weight loss, number of metastatic sites, age, and KPS. Marital status was also a significant predictor.[138]

Wisloff et al.[139] obtained baseline quality of life assessments with the European Organization for Research & Treatment of Cancer Core Quality of Life Questionnaire (EORTC QLQ-C30) in 581 patients with multiple myeloma who participated in a randomized trial of melphalan/prednisone compared to melphalan/prednisone and interferon alpha 2b. In a multivariate analysis of clinical predictors for overall survival, World Health Organization performance status and the physical functioning subscale were significant. Similar results were obtained in a landmark analysis for survival exceeding 12 months. Fatigue, pain, and cognitive functioning were significant predictors in univariate analyses but not in the multivariate analysis.

Dancey et al.[140] examined the prognostic value of baseline scores on the QLQ-C30 of 474 cancer patients who had enrolled in trials of anti-emetic therapy before receiving chemotherapy. In a Cox multivariate analysis, dyspnea, global quality of life, and emotional functioning domains had predictive value independent of performance status.

Convenience populations

Chang et al.[141] examined the relationship between quality of life scores and survival in a heterogeneous population of 240 cancer patients with one of four tumor types—ovarian, breast, prostate, and colon—who completed the Memorial Symptom Assessment Scale (MSAS), the FLIC, the Symptom Distress Scale, and the Rand Mental Health Inventory.[142] While all of these measures were predictors of survival in univariate analyses, the multivariate survival model revealed that only extent of disease, inpatient status, an increased score on the physical symptom distress subscale of the MSAS, and a decreased KPS rating independently predicted survival.[142]

Ringdal et al.[143] studied responses to a variety of instruments, including the EORTC QLQ-C30 and the Hospital Anxiety and Depression Scale,[144] in 352 hospitalized cancer patients in Norway. On univariate analysis, pain, fatigue, and cognitive functioning items on the QLQ-C30 significantly affected survival. However, in the multivariate analysis, only treatment intent and physical functioning were independently predictive. KPS was not included in the model.

Palliative medicine patients

Coates et al.[145] analyzed items on the EORTC QLQ-C30 for their relation to survival in a group of 735 patients with advanced cancer. Single-item QL scores on physical condition, overall quality of life, and global and social functioning scales carried independent prognostic information.[145]

Earlam et al.[146] followed 50 patients with colorectal liver metastases prospectively with monthly administration of the Sickness Impact Profile,[147] the Rotterdam Symptom Checklist, and the Hospital Anxiety and Depression Scale. In a stepwise multivariate survival analysis model that included the physical score of the Rotterdam Symptom Checklist, anxiety and depression scores from the Hospital Anxiety and Depression Scale, the Sickness Impact Profile Score, and the KPS, only the physical score of the Rotterdam Symptom Checklist was significantly associated with survival. Size of metastases was not related to survival. Further analysis of each of the questions in these instruments suggested that the items diarrhea, feeling restless, lack of appetite, cheerfulness, vomiting, and ability to work were most predictive of survival.

Changes in quality of life: possible predictors of survival

In a trial comparing intermittent to continuous chemotherapy in patients with metastatic breast cancer, Coates et al.[148] reported that changes in physical well-being (measured with a linear analogue scale) and in the QL Index before 180 days were predictors of survival beyond 180 days.[148]

Seidman et al.[149] reported on a trial of 49 advanced breast cancer patients with metastatic disease who underwent chemotherapy with paclitaxel in a phase II study. Baseline scores on the FLIC and the MSAS Global Distress Index independently predicted overall survival in a univariate analysis. On multivariate analysis, either the FLIC or the MSAS Global Distress Index combined with the KPS described survival better than the KPS alone.[149]

Cella et al.[150] reported on the prognostic significance of quality of life data gathered in a chemotherapy trial in 571 patients with advanced non-small cell lung cancer. QOL was measured with the Functional Assessment of Cancer Therapy-Lung (FACT-L)[151] at baseline, 6 weeks, 12 weeks, and 6 months. The Trial Outcome Index (TOI), a combination of the physical, functional, and lung cancer subscales, was defined. In a multivariate survival model, the TOI was the most significant predictor, followed by symptoms, ECOG performance status, stage, and the presence of paclitaxel-containing chemotherapy arms. Both baseline and change from baseline on subsequent assessment with the TOI were significant, and change from baseline had a higher relationship to survival than did the baseline TOI.

Hwang et al.[152] reported a longitudinal study of 54 cancer patients with terminal disease followed at 3- to 6-week intervals with the Functional Assessment of Cancer Therapy-General (FACT-G).[153] Both baseline quality of life and

Table 2.3. Symptoms studied by hospices

First author	N	Population	Median survival	Pain	Dyspnea	Swallowing	KPS	Cognition	Sleeping	Wt loss	Dry mouth	Weakness
Allard et al	1014	Hospice	11 days	°	°	°	Sig	°	°	°	°	°
Rosenthal et al	148	Hospice	14 days	°	°	°	Sig	NS	°	NS	°	°
Portenoy et al	1103	Hospital	26 days	NS	°	°	NS	NS	°	°	°	°
Bruera et al	47	Hospice	28 days	NS	NS	Sig	NS	Sig	°	Sig	NS	°
Christakis et al	405	Hospice output	29 days	°	NS	°	Sig	Sig	°	°	°	°
Maltoni et al	530	Hospice	32 days	NS	Sig	NS	Sig	°	°	°	NS	°
Reuben et al	1592	Hospice	35 days	°	Sig	Sig	Sig	NS	°	Sig	Sig	°
Hardy et al	107	Pall. care unit	42 days	NS	Sig	°	Sig	°	°	°	°	Sig
Schonwetter et al	310	Lung	51 days	Sig	°	°	Sig	NS	°	°	Sig	°
Morita et al	150	Hospice	152	NS	Sig	NS	Sig	Sig	°	°	NS	°
Earlam et al	50	Advanced	200+	NS	NS	°		°	NS	°	°	NS
Coates et al	735	Advanced CA	234+	°	°	°	Sig	°	°	Sig	°	°
Forster et al	111	Hospice	NA	Sig	°	°	NS	Sig	°	°	°	NS (3 mo)
			NA	Sig	°	°	Sig	Sig	°	°	°	Sig (6 mo)
Tamburini et al	150	Home care unit	NA	°	NS	NS	NS	Sig	NS	°	°	Sig

NA, not available; NS, not significant; °, not evaluated.

the rate of change in quality of life predicted survival, but the rate of change in quality of life demonstrated a much stronger association with survival than did the baseline quality of life.

The common threads in quality of life assessment are multidimensionality and patient-rated assessments. Physical symptoms are a well-recognized component of quality of life. Where well-defined physical symptom subscales are present, these have often been the predictive subscale in quality of life measures.[152a] However, a measure for overall quality of life is also prognostic. The meaning of this finding is still unclear. Global quality of life may reflect the sum of physical and psychological distress. Possibly, where physical symptoms are not carefully assessed, global quality of life may become an important and independent predictor of survival. A conclusion that emerges is that aspects of patient-rated information may help refine estimates of the prognosis independent of the performance status.

Research Aspects and Caveats

A number of methodological problems are present in many of the articles reviewed.

1. Symptom reporting. In many studies, symptom assessment has been retrospective or unsystematic. The dangers of this problem are illustrated in one study of 294 colorectal cancer patients, in which patient reports were compared to a symptom checklist and only 54% of the total number of symptoms were verbally reported.[154] The best predictors of symptom reporting were symptoms that were severe, unusual, or developed quickly. Symptom reporting may be affected by perceived stigmatization, and the rating of symptoms may be affected by emotional distress.[155] The role of comorbidity as an independent predictor of survival is becoming increasingly recognized, especially in elderly patients. How comorbidity affects the number, severity, and prognostic importance of symptoms needs to be studied. In future work of this type, validated symptom assessment instruments can be used prospectively, especially if patient-rated symptom severity or distress is the key feature. This can help eliminate the issue of ascertainment bias. A related issue is ascertainment of all articles bearing on this subject.

2. Models of survival. Shortcomings and pitfalls of current modeling approaches in cancer patients have been the subject of excellent reviews.[156–158] First, the selection of variables has varied from one series of patients to another. Many symptoms may share the same underlying pathophysiology, and combining these variables in the same model causes redundancy. For similar reasons, the prognostic importance of specific symptoms may be confounded by laboratory values when put in the same model, such as fatigue and hemoglobin level. Second, there may be significant differences between populations in terms of underlying distributions of diseases or survival, which affects the generalizability of the predictive model. However, it is striking that similar conclusions concerning the prognostic importance of symptoms have been reached in the wide variety of populations studied, including case series and retrospective and prospective cohorts of patients undergoing therapy or receiving palliative care alone. It should be noted that as therapy improves, the value of symptoms at presentation may diminish in cohorts of treated patients.

3. Interactions among KPS, symptom status, and quality of life constructs. Patients with lower performance status have more severe symptoms,[159] a poorer quality of life,[160] and more emotional distress.[161] Symptom scales generally correlate well with the KPS. Symptom attributes may interact with quality of life. For example, the number of symptoms has been shown to correlate directly with quality of life measured by the FACT.[162,163] In an analysis of the MSAS instrument, which assesses symptom frequency, severity, and distress, physical symptom–related distress and psychological symptom frequency on the MSAS were the most informative measures of impact on quality of life measured by the FLIC.[164] Interference by symptoms can also affect quality of life. In cancer patients with moderate to severe pain, interference by pain has a clear inverse relationship with quality of life measured by the Medical Outcomes Study Short Form-36 (SF-36)[165] and by the FACT.[166] These relationships challenge simplistic interpretations of how quality of life or symptoms may predict survival.

Conclusions and Future Directions

Symptoms have long been considered soft data and unreliable in developing a staging system.[167] The development of validated symptom assessment instruments, and of patient-rated items in quality of life instruments, is important in reassuring investigators that such data can contribute to analyses of survival. Clinicians often use the presence or severity of symptoms to guide treatment decisions. Interest in the prognostic value of symptoms will continue for the same reason that performance status measures are used: convenience and relevance to physician–patient communication.

What is it about symptoms that could make them useful for predicting survival? The absence of a clear relationship between symptom duration and survival, and the variable relationship between size of metastases and survival, suggest that symptoms may reflect both a local and a systemic host response to disease. The magnitude of the response may be deleterious to the host and may be reflected in patient-rated symptom severity or distress, as well as by markers of inflammation.[168] Severe symptoms interfere with functional status and with measures of functional status.

Further studies can help us better understand the meaning of performance status from the patient's standpoint. What does the KPS represent? The KPS has a mystical aura, representing the sum of the disease process and the untouchable hand of fate. A low KPS is associated with severe symptoms and with psychological distress. If a large part of the KPS is determined by specific symptoms, such as fatigue, then addressing these symptoms may improve the KPS and the patient's quality of life. A low KPS may serve as a guide to the need for symptom assessment and management. We can imagine a future in which a symptom status score will have as much, if not more, prognostic validity than the KPS and will point to more therapeutic options for symptom relief. Further studies may also help physicians improve their bedside clinical assessments by helping them to observe patients and listen to patients' reports of symptoms in a more informed way.

Perhaps researchers should agree on a common core group of symptoms to study in future efforts to allow comparability and pooling of results. Preliminary analysis of responses by 479 patients to the MSAS Short Form[169] and the FACT, as well as patient survival, suggests that approximately 10–15 symptoms may convey most of the information needed for both prognostic and quality of life assessment.[170] One approach might be the consolidation of symptoms into prognostic complexes with a common underlying pathophysiology. Another possibility is that some symptoms may be more helpful in predicting longer-term survival (e.g., 3 months) and others in predicting shorter-term survival (1–2 weeks). Perhaps symptom data can identify patients with good performance status who are likely to deteriorate rapidly. Future approaches may include groupings of symptoms and the application of newer techniques such as recursive partitioning or neural network analysis to develop prognostic models. Finally, we may wish to combine prospective measures of symptom distress with anatomic staging and measures of comorbidity in future studies. As the use of quality of life and symptom assessment instruments increases in clinical trials and prospective studies, we will be better able to understand the prognostic value of symptoms.

References

1. Christakis NA, Escarce JJ. Survival of Medicare patients after enrollment in hospice programs. *N Engl J Med* 1996; 335:172–178.
2. Kinzbrunner BM. Utilization of hospice services by terminally ill cancer patients. *Proc ASCO* 1999; 18:577a, abstract 2226.
3. Murray Parkes C. Accuracy of predictions of survival in later stages of cancer. *Br Med J* 1972; 2:29–31.
4. Heyse-Moore LH. Can doctors accurately predict the life expectancy of patients with terminal cancer? *Palliat Med* 1987; 1:165–166.
5. Miller RJ. Predicting survival in the advanced cancer patient. *Henry Ford Hosp Med J* 1991; 39:81–84.
6. Mackillop WJ, Quirt CF. Measuring the accuracy of prognostic judgments in oncology. *J Clin Epidemiol* 1997; 50:21–29.
7. Muers MF, Shevlin P, Brown J. Prognosis in lung cancer: physicians opinions compared with outcome and a predictive model. *Thorax* 1996; 51:894–902.

8. Laussaniere J, Vinant P. Prognostic factors, survival and advanced cancer. *J Palliat Care* 1992; 8(4):52–54.

9. den Daas N. Estimating length of survival in end-stage cancer: a review of the literature. *J Pain Symptom Manage* 1995; 10:548–555.

9a. Viganò A, Dorgan M, Bruera E, et al. The relative accuracy of the chemical estimation of the duration of life for patients with end of life cancer. *Cancer* 1999; 86:170–176.

10. Forster LE, Lynn J. Predicting life span for applicants to inpatient hospice. *Arch Intern Med* 1988; 148:2540–2543.

11. Justice C. The "natural death" while not eating: a type of palliative care in Banaras, India. *J Palliat Care* 1995; 11(1):38–42.

12. MacDonald I. Individual basis of biologic variability in cancer. *Surg Gynecol Obstet* 1958; 106:227–229.

13. Osoba D. Self-rating symptom checklists: a simple method for recording and evaluating symptom control in oncology. *Cancer Treat Rev* 1993; 19 (suppl A):43–51.

14. Brodman K, Erdmann AJ, Lorge I, et al. The Cornell Medical Index, an adjunct to the medical interview. *JAMA* 1949; 140:530–534.

15. Christakis NA. The ellipsis of prognosis in modern medical thought. *Soc Sci Med* 1997; 44:301–315.

16. Fox BH. Psychosocial factors in cancer incidence and prognosis. In: Holland JC (ed). *Psycho-Oncology,* 2nd ed. New York: Oxford University Press, 1998: 110–124.

17. Peters VM. A study of survival in Hodgkin's disease treated radiologically. *Am J Roentgenol* 1950; 63:299–311.

18. Westling P. Studies of the prognosis in Hodgkin's disease. *Acta Radiol Suppl* 1965; 245.

19. Carbone PP, Kaplan HS, Musshoff K, et al. Report of the committee on Hodgkin's disease staging classification. *Cancer Res* 1971; 31:1860.

20. Lister TA, Crowther D, Sutcliffe SB, et al. Report of a committee convened to discuss the evaluation and staging of patients with Hodgkin's disease: Cotswold's meeting. *J Clin Oncol* 1989; 7:1630–1636.

21. Tubiana M, Attie E, Flamant R, et al. Prognostic factors in 454 patients with Hodgkin's disease. *Cancer Res* 1971; 31:1801–1810.

22. Crnkovich MJ, Leopold K, Hoppe RT, et al. Stage I to IIB Hodgkin's disease: the combined experience at Stanford University and the Joint Center for Radiation Therapy. *J Clin Oncol* 1987; 5:1041–1049.

23. Ferry JA, Linggood RM, Convery KM, et al. Hodgkin disease, nodular sclerosis type. Implications of histologic subclassification. *Cancer* 1993; 71:457–463.

24. Hasenclever D, Diehl V, for the International Prognostic Factors Project on Advanced Hodgkin's Disease. A prognostic score for advanced Hodgkin's disease. *N Engl J Med* 1998; 339:1506–1514.

25. Fabian CJ, Mansfield CM, Dahlberg S, et al. Low dose involved field radiation after chemotherapy in advanced Hodgkin's Disease. A Southwest Oncology Group randomized study. *Ann Intern Med* 1994; 120:903–912.

25a. Specht LK, Hasenclever D. Prognostic factors in Hodgkin's Disease. In: Mauch PM, Armitage JO, Diehl V, Hoppe RT, Weiss LM (eds). *Hodgkin's Disease.* Philadelphia, PA: Lippincott Williams and Wilkins, 1999:295–325.

26. Bloomfield CD, Goldman A, Dick F, et al. Multivariate analysis of prognostic factors in the non-Hodgkin's malignant lymphomas. *Cancer* 1974; 33:870–879.

27. Leonard RCF, Cuzick J, MacLennan ICM, et al. Prognostic factors in non-Hodgkin's lymphoma: the importance of symptomatic stage as an adjunct to the Kiel histopathological classification *Br J Cancer* 1983; 47:91–102.

28. International Non-Hodgkin's Lymphoma Prognostic Factors Project. A predictive model for aggressive non-Hodgkin's lymphoma. *N Engl J Med* 1993; 329:987–994.

29. Ben-Ezra J, Burke JS, Swartz WG, et al. Small lymphocytic lymphoma: a clinicopathologic analysis of 268 cases. *Blood* 1989; 73:579–587.

30. Armitage JO, Dick FR, Corder MP, et al. Predicting therapeutic outcome in patients with diffuse histiocytic lymphoma treated with cyclophosphamide, adriamycin, vincristine and prednisone (CHOP). *Cancer* 1982; 50:1695–1702.

31. Nakamine H, Bagin RG, Vose JM, et al. Prognostic significance of clinical and pathologic features in diffuse large B cell lymphoma. *Cancer* 1993; 71:3130–3137.

32. Wood LA, Coupland RW, North SA, et al. Outcome of advanced stage low grade follicular lymphomas in a population-based retrospective cohort. *Cancer* 1999; 85:1361–1368.

33. Green SB, Byar DB, Lamberg SI. Prognostic variables in mycosis fungoides. *Cancer* 1981; 47:2671–2677.

34. Facon T, Brouillard M, Duhamel A, et al. Prognostic factors in Waldenstrom's macroglobulinemia: a report of 167 cases. *J Clin Oncol* 1993; 11:1553–1558.

35. Karnofsky DA, Burchenal JH. The clinical evaluation of chemotherapeutic agents in cancer. In: MacLeod CM, ed. *Evaluation of Chemotherapeutic Agents.* New York: Columbia University Press, 1949: 191–205.

36. Zubrod CG, Scheiderman M, Frei E, et al. Appraisal of methods for the study of chemotherapy of cancer in man: comparative therapeutic trial of nitrogen mustard and triethylene thiophosphoramide. *J Chronic Dis* 1960; 11:7–33.

37. Verger E, Salamero M, Conill C. Can Karnofsky performance status be transformed to the Eastern Cooperative Oncology Group scoring scale and vice versa? *Eur J Cancer* 1992; 28A:1328–1330.

38. Buccheri G, Ferrigno D, Tamburini M. Karnofsky and ECOG performance status scoring in lung cancer: a prospective, longitudinal study of 536 patients from a single institution. *Eur J Cancer* 1996; 32A:1135–1141.

39. Lanzotti VJ, Thomas DR, Boyle LE, et al. Survival with inoperable lung cancer. An integration of prognostic variables based on simple clinical criteria. *Cancer* 1977; 39:303–313.

40. Stanley KE. Prognostic factors for survival in patients with inoperable lung cancer. *J Natl Cancer Inst* 1980; 65:25–32.

41. Orr ST, Aisner J. Performance status assessment among oncology patients: a review. *Cancer Treat Rep* 1986; 70:1423–1429.

42. Yates JW, Chalmer B, McKegney FP. Evaluation of patients with advanced cancer using the Karnofsky Performance Status. *Cancer* 1980; 45:2220–2224.

43. Hutchinson TA, Boyd NF, Feinstein AR. Scientific problems in the Karnofsky Index of performance status. *J Chronic Dis* 1979; 32:661–666.

44. Mor V, Laliberte L, Morris JN, et al. The Karnofsky Performance Status scale. An examination of its reliability and validity in a research setting. *Cancer* 1984; 53:2002–2007.

45. Katz S, Ford AB, Moskowitz RW, et al. Studies of illness in the aged. The Index of ADL: a standardized measure of biological function. *JAMA* 1963; 185:914–919.

46. Schag CC, Heinrich RL, Ganz PA. The Cancer Inventory of Problem Situations: an instrument for assessing cancer patients' rehabilitation needs. *J Psychosoc Oncol* 1983; 1:11–24.

47. Schag CC, Heinrich RL, Ganz PA. Karnofsky Performance Status revisited: reliability, validity, and guidelines. *J Clin Oncol* 1984; 2:187–193.

48. Loprinzi CL, Laurie JA, Wieand HS, et al. Prospective evaluation of prognostic variables from patient-completed questionnaires. *J Clin Oncol* 1994; 12:601–607.

49. Ando M, Ando Y, Sakai S, et al. Discrepancy in assessment of performance status of patients with lung cancer between patients themselves and health professionals. *Proc ASCO* 1999; 18:481a, Abstract 1857.

50. Hendrickson FR. The optimum schedule for palliative radiotherapy for metastatic brain cancer. *Int J Radiat Oncol Biol Phys* 1977; 2:165.

50a. Kramer S, Hendrickson F, Zelen M, et al. Therapeutic trends in the management of metastatic brain tumors by different time/dose fraction schemes of radiation therapy. *Natl Cancer Inst Monogr* 1977; 46:213–221.

51. Evans C, McCarthy M. Prognostic uncertainty in terminal care: can the Karnofsky index help? *Lancet* 1985; 1:1204–1206.

52. Maltoni M, Nanni O, Derni S, et al. Clinical prediction of survival is more accurate than the Karnofsky Performance Status in estimating life span of terminally ill cancer patients. *Eur J Cancer* 1994; 30A:764–766.

53. Anderson F, Downing GM, Hill J, et al. Palliative Performance Scale (PPS), a new tool. *J Palliat Care* 1996; 12(1):5–11.

54. Kaasa T, Loomis J, Gillis K, et al. The Edmonton Functional Assessment Tool: preliminary development and evaluation for use in palliative care. *J Pain Symptom Manage* 1997; 13:10–19.

55. Dewys WD, Begg C, Lavin PT, et al. Prognostic effect of weight loss prior to chemotherapy in cancer patients. *Am J Med* 1980; 69:491–497.

56. Feinstein AR. Symptomatic patterns, biologic behavior, and prognosis in cancer of the lung. Practical application of Boolean algebra and clinical taxonomy. *Ann Intern Med* 1964; 61:27–43.

57. Feinstein AR. Symptoms as an index of biological behavior and prognosis in human cancer. *Nature* 1966; 209:241–245.

58. Feinstein AR. A new staging system for cancer and reappraisal of "early" treatment and "cure" by radical surgery. *N Engl J Med* 1968; 279:747–753.

59. Senior RM, Adamson JS. Survival in patients with lung cancer. An appraisal of Feinstein's symptom classification. *Arch Intern Med* 1970; 125:975–980.

60. Green N, Kurohara SS, George FW III. Cancer of the lung. An in-depth analysis of prognostic factors. *Cancer* 1971; 28:1229–1233.

61. Coy P, Elwood JM, Coldman AJ. Clinical indicators of prognosis in lung cancer. *Chest* 1981; 80:453–458.

62. Pater JL, Loeb M. Nonanatomic prognostic factors in carcinoma of the lung. A multivariate analysis. *Cancer* 1982; 50:326–331.

63. Kaplan M, Feinstein AR. The importance of classifying initial co-morbidity in evaluating the outcome of diabetes mellitus. *J Chronic Dis* 1974; 27:387–404.

64. Feinstein AR, Schimpff CR, Andrews JF, et al. Cancer of the larynx: a new staging system and a re-appraisal of prognosis and treatment. *J Chronic Dis* 1977; 30:277–305.

65. Piccirillo JF, Wells CK, Sasaki CT, et al. New clinical severity staging system for cancer of the larynx. Five year survival rates. *Ann Otol Rhinol Laryngol* 1994; 103:83–92.

66. Pugliano FA, Piccirillo JF, Zequiera MR, et al. Clinical-severity stating system for oral cavity cancer: five-year survival rates. *Otolaryngol Head Neck Surg* 1999; 120:38–45.

67. Pugliano FA, Piccirillo JF, Zequeira MR, et al. Symptoms as an index of biologic behavior in head and neck cancer. *Otolaryngol Head Neck Surg* 1999; 120:380–386.

68. Feinstein AR, Wells CK. A clinical-severity staging system for patients with lung cancer. *Medicine* 1990; 69:1–33.

69. Clemens JD, Feinstein AR, Holabird N, et al. A new clinical-anatomic staging system for evaluating prognosis and treatment of prostatic cancer. *J Chronic Dis* 1986; 39:913–928.

70. Feinstein AR, Schimpff CR, Hull EW. A reappraisal of staging and therapy for patients with cancer of the rectum. I. Development of two new systems of staging. *Arch Intern Med* 1975; 135:1441–1453.

71. Feinstein AR, Schimpff CR, Hull EW. A reappraisal of staging and therapy for patients with cancer of the rectum. II. Patterns of presentation and outcome of treatment. *Arch Intern Med* 1975; 135:1454–1462.

72. Peipert JF, Wells CK, Schwartz PE, et al. Prognostic value of clinical variables in invasive cervical cancer. *Obstet Gynecol* 1994; 84:746–751.

73. Wells CK, Stoller JK, Feinstein AR, et al. Comorbid and clinical determinants of prognosis in endometrial cancer. *Arch Intern Med* 1984; 144:2004–2009.

74. DiSilvestro P, Peipert JF, Hogan JW, et al. Prognostic value of clinical variables in ovarian cancer. *J Clin Epidemiol* 1997; 50:501–505.

75. Boyd NF, Feinstein AR. Symptoms as an index of growth rates and prognosis in Hodgkin's disease. *Clin Invest Med* 1978; 1:25–31.

76. Walter SD, Feinstein AR, Wells CK. A comparison of multivariable mathematical models for predicting survival—II. Statistical selection of prognostic variables. *J Clin Epidemiol* 1990; 43:349–359.

77. Wigren T, Oksanen H, Kellokumpu-Lehtinen P. A practical prognostic index for inoperable non-small cell lung cancer. *J Cancer Res Clin Oncol* 1997; 123:259–266.

78. Wigren T. Confirmation of a prognostic index for patients with inoperable non-small cell lung cancer. Radiother Oncol 1997; 44:9–15.

79. Neel HB, Taylor WF, Pearson GR. Prognostic determinants and a new view of staging for patients with nasopharyngeal carcinoma. *Ann Otol Rhinol Laryngol* 1985; 94:529–537.

80. Graf W, Glimelius B, Pahlman L, et al. Determinants of prognosis in advanced colorectal cancer. *Eur J Cancer* 1991; 27:1119–1123.

81. Graf W, Bergstrom R, Pahlman L, et al. Appraisal of a model for prediction of prognosis in advanced colorectal cancer. *Eur J Cancer* 1994; 30A:453–457.

82. Rana A, Chisholm GD, Rashwan HM, et al. Symptomatology of metastatic prostate cancer: prognostic significance. *Br J Urol* 1994; 73:683–686.

83. Furuta M, Hayakawa K, Saito Y, et al. Clinical implication of symptoms in patients with non-small cell lung cancer treated with definitive radiation therapy. *Lung Cancer* 1995; 13:275–283.

84. Lote K, Egeland T, Hager B, et al. Survival, prognostic factors, and therapeutic

efficacy in low-grade glioma: a retrospective study in 379 patients. *J Clin Oncol* 1997; 15:3129–3140.

85. Sen M, Demiral AS, Cetingoz R, et al. Prognostic factors in lung cancer with brain metastasis. *Radiother Oncol* 1996; 46:33–38.

86. Hsiung CY, Leung SW, Wang CJ, et al. The prognostic factors of lung cancer patients with brain metastases treated with radiotherapy. *J Neuro-Oncol* 1998; 36:71–77.

87. Forster LE, Lynn J. The use of physiologic measures and demographic variables to predict longevity among inpatient hospice applicants. *Am J Hospice Care* 1989; 6:31–34.

88. Allard P, Dionne A, Potvin D. Factors associated with length of survival among 1081 terminally ill cancer patients. *J Palliat Care* 1995; 11(3):20–24.

89. Reuben DB, Mor V. Dyspnea in terminally ill cancer patients. *Chest* 1986; 89: 234–236.

90. Heyse-Moore LH, Ross V, Mullee MA. How much of a problem is dyspnoea in advanced cancer? *Palliat Med* 1991; 5:20–26.

91. Escalante CP, Martin CG, Elting LS, et al. Dyspnea in cancer patients. Etiology, resource utilization, and survival—implications in a managed care world. *Cancer* 1996; 78:1314–1319.

92. Christakis NA. Timing of referral of terminally ill patients to an outpatient hospice. *J Gen Intern Med* 1994; 9:314–320.

93. Staats PS. The pain-mortality link. In: Payne R, Patt RB, Hill CS, eds. *Assessment and Treatment of Cancer Pain: Progress in Pain Research and Management.* Seattle: IASP Press, 1998: 145–156.

94. Clee MD, Hockings NF, Johnston RN. Bronchial carcinoma: factors influencing postoperative survival. *Br J Dis Chest* 1984; 78:225–235.

95. Schonwetter RS, Robinson BE, Ramirez G. Prognostic factors for survival in terminal lung cancer patients. *J Gen Intern Med* 1994; 9:366–371.

96. Herndon JE II, Fleishman S, Kornblith AB, et al. Is quality of life predictive of the survival of patients with advanced nonsmall cell lung carcinoma? *Cancer* 1999; 85:333–340.

97. Aaronson NK, Ahmedzai S, Bergman B, et al. The European Organization for Research and Treatment of Cancer QLQ-C30: a quality-of-life instrument for use in international clinical trials in oncology. *J Natl Cancer Inst* 1993; 85:365–376.

98. Brescia FJ, Portenoy RK, Ryan M, et al Pain, opioid use, and survival in hospitalized patients with advanced cancer. *J Clin Oncol* 1992; 10:149–155.

99. Hwang SS, Chang VT, Cogswell J, O et al. Fatigue, depression, symptom distress, quality of life and survival in male cancer patients at a VA medical center. *Proc ASCO* 1999; 18:594a, Abstract 2294.

100. Reuben DB, Mor V, Hiris J. Clinical symptoms and length of survival in patients with terminal cancer. *Arch Intern Med* 1988; 148:1586–1591.

101. Bruera E, Miller MJ, Kuehn N, et al. Estimate of survival of patients admitted to a palliative care unit: a prospective study. *J Pain Symptom Manage* 1992; 7:82–86.

102. Rosenthal MA, Gebski VJ, Kefford RF, et al. Prediction of life expectancy in hospice patients: identification of novel prognostic factors. *Palliat Med* 1993; 7:199–204.

103. Hardy JR, Turner R, Saunders M, et al. Prediction of survival in a hospital-based continuing care unit. *Eur J Cancer* 1994; 30A:284–288.

104. Maltoni M, Pirovano M, Scarpi E, et al. Prediction of survival of patients terminally

ill with cancer. Results of an Italian prospective multicenter study. *Cancer* 1995; 75:2613–2622.

105. Tamburini M, Rosso S, Gamba A, et al. A therapy impact questionnaire for quality-of-life assessment in advanced cancer research. *Ann Oncol* 1992; 3:565–570.

106. Tamburini M, Brunelli C, Rosso S, et al. Prognostic value of quality of life scores in terminal cancer patients. *J Pain Symptom Manage* 1996; 11:32–41.

107. Morita T, Tsunoda J, Inoue S, et al. Prediction of survival of terminally ill cancer patients—a prospective study. *Jpn J Cancer Chemother* 1998; 25:1203–1211.

108. Kaufman S, Grabau JC, Lore JM. Symptomatology in head and neck cancer. A quantitative review of 385 cases. *Am J Public Health* 1980; 70:520–522.

109. McDermott FT, Hughes S, Pihl E, et al. Prognosis in relation to symptom duration in colon cancer. *Br J Surg* 1981; 68:846–849.

110. Schillaci A, Cavallaro A, Nicolanti V, et al. The importance of symptom duration in relation to prognosis of carcinoma of the large intestine. *Surg Gyncol Obstet* 1984; 158:423–426.

111. Khubchandani M. Relationship of symptom duration and survival in patients with carcinoma of the colon and rectum. *Dis Colon Rectum* 1985; 28:585–587.

112. Barillari P, de Angelis R, Valabrega S, et al. Relationship of symptom duration and survival in patients with colorectal carcinoma. *Eur J Surg Oncol* 1989; 15:441–445.

113. Polissar L, Sim D, Francis A. Survival of colorectal cancer patients in relation to duration of symptoms and other prognostic factors. *Dis Colon Rectum* 1981; 24: 364–369.

114. Mulcahy HE, O-Donoghue DP. Duration of colorectal cancer symptoms and survival: the effect of confounding clinical and pathological variables. *Eur J Cancer* 1997; 33:1461–1467.

115. Hutton JL, Smith DF, Sandemann D, et al. Development of a prognostic index for primary supratentorial intracerebral tumors. *J Neurol Neurosurg Psychiatry* 1992; 55:271–274.

116. Schuurman PR, Troost D, Verbeeten B Jr, et al. Five year survival and clinical prognostic factors in progressive supratentorial diffuse "low-grade" astrocytoma: a retrospective analysis of 46 cases. *Acta Neurochir* 1997; 139:2–7.

117. Salminen E, Nuutinen JM, Huhtula S. Multivariate analysis of prognostic factors in 106 patients with malignant glioma. *Eur J Cancer* 1996; 32A:1918–1923.

118. Bentzen SM, Poulsen HS, Kaae S, et al. Prognostic factors in osteosarcomas. A regression analysis. *Cancer* 1988; 62:194–202.

119. Maguire A, Porta M, Malats N, et al. Cancer survival and the duration of symptoms. An analysis of possible forms of the risk function. *Eur J Cancer* 1994; 30A:785–792.

120. Bosl GJ, Vogelzang NJ, Goldman A, et al. Impact of delay in diagnosis on clinical stage of testicular cancer. *Lancet* 1981; 2:970–973.

121. Moul JW, Paulson DF, Dodge RK, et al. Delay in diagnosis and survival in testicular cancer: impact of effective therapy and changes during 18 years. *J Urol* 1990; 143:520–523.

122. Ingham J, Portenoy RK. The measurement of pain and other symptoms. In: Doyle D, Hanks GWC, MacDonald N, eds. *Oxford Textbook of Palliative Medicine.* 2nd ed. New York Oxford University Press, 1998: 203–219.

123. McCorkle R, Young K. Development of a symptom distress scale. *Cancer Nurs* 1978; 1:373–378.

124. McClement SE, Woodgate RL, Degner L. Symptom distress in adult patients with cancer. *Cancer Nurs* 1997; 20:236–243.

125. Kukull WA, McCorkle R, Driever M. Symptom distress, psychosocial variables, and survival from lung cancer. *J Psychosoc Oncol* 1986; 4:91–104.

126. Degner LF, Sloan JA. Symptom distress in newly diagnosed ambulatory cancer patients as a predictor of survival in lung cancer. *J Pain Symptom Manage* 1995; 10:423–431.

127. Ventafridda V, Ripamonti C, Tamburini M, et al. Unendurable symptoms as prognostic indicators of impending death in terminal cancer patients. *Eur J Cancer* 1990; 26:1000–1001.

128. De Haes JCJM, van Knippenburg FCE, Nejit JP. Measuring psychological and physical distress in cancer patients: structure and application of the Rotterdam Symptom Checklist. *Br J Cancer* 1990; 62:1034–1038.

129. Portenoy RK, Thaler HT, Kornblith AB, et al. The Memorial Symptom Assessment Scale: an instrument for the evaluation of symptom prevalence, characteristics and distress. *Eur J Cancer* 1994; 30A:1326–1336.

130. Coates A, Gebski V, Signorini D, et al. Prognostic value of quality of life scores during chemotherapy for advanced breast cancer. *J Clin Oncol* 1992; 10:1833–1838.

131. Selby PJ, Chapman JAW, Etazadi-Amoli J, et al. The development of a method for assessing the quality of life of cancer patients. *Br J Cancer* 1984; 50:13–22.

132. Spitzer WO, Dobson AJ, Hall J, et al. Measuring the quality of life of cancer patients: a concise QL index for use by physicians. *J Chronic Dis* 1981; 34:585–597.

133. Coates A, Thomson D, McLeod GRM, et al. Prognostic value of quality of life scores in a trial of chemotherapy with or without interferon in patients with metastatic malignant melanoma. *Eur J Cancer* 1993; 29A:1731–1734.

134. Kaasa S, Mastekaasa A, Lund E. Prognostic factors for patients with inoperable non-small cell lung cancer, limited disease. *Radiother Oncol* 1989; 15:235–242.

135. Addington-Hall JM, MacDonald LD, Anderson HR. Can the Spitzer Quality of Life Index help to reduce uncertainty in terminal care? *Br J Cancer* 1990; 62:695–699.

136. Ruckdeschel JC, Piantadosi S, Lung Cancer Study Group. Quality of life assessment in lung surgery for bronchogenic carcinoma. *Theor Surg* 1991; 6:201–206.

137. Schipper H, Clinch J, McMurray A, et al. Measuring the quality of life of cancer patients: the Functional Living Index—Cancer: development and validation. *J Clin Oncol* 1984; 2:472–483.

138. Ganz PA, Lee JJ, Siau MS. Quality of life assessment: an independent prognostic variable for survival in lung cancer. *Cancer* 1991; 67:3131–3135.

139. Wisloff F, Hjorth M, Nordic Myeloma Study Group. Health-related quality of life assessed before and during chemotherapy predicts for survival in multiple myeloma. *Br J Haematol* 1997; 97:29–37.

140. Dancey J, Zee B, Osoba D, et al. Quality of life scores: an independent prognostic variable in a general population of cancer patients receiving chemotherapy. *Qual Life Res* 1997; 6:151–158.

141. Chang VT, Thaler HT, Polyak TA, et al. Quality of life and survival. The role of multidimensional symptom assessment. *Cancer* 1998; 83:173–179.

142. Ware JE Jr, Johnston SA, Davies-Avery A, et al. *Conceptualization and Measurement of Health for Adults. The Health Insurance Study: Mental health,* vol III. Santa Monica, Calif.: RAND; 1979.

143. Ringdal GI, Gotestam KG, Kaasa S, et al. Prognostic factors and survival in a hetero-geneous sample of cancer patients. *Br J Cancer* 1996; 73:1594–1599.

144. Zigmond AS, Snaith RP. The Hospital Anxiety and Depression Scale. *Acta Psychol Scand* 1983; 67:361–370.

145. Coates A, Porzsolt F, Osoba D. Quality of life in oncology practice: prognostic value of EORTC QLQ-C30 scores in patients with advanced malignancy. *Eur J Cancer* 1997; 33:1025–1030.

146. Earlam S, Glover C, Fordy C, et al. Relation between tumor size, quality of life, and survival in patients with colorectal liver metastases. *J Clin Oncol* 1996; 14:171–175.

147. Bergner M, Bobbitt RA, Carter WB, et al. The Sickness Impact Profile: development and final revision of a health status measure. *Med Care* 1981; 19:787–805.

148. Coates A, Gebski V, Bishop JF, et al. Improving the quality of life during chemother-apy for advanced breast cancer. A comparison of intermittent and continuous treatment strategies. *N Engl J Med* 1987; 317:1490–1495.

149. Seidman AD, Portenoy R, Yao TJ, et al. Quality of life in phase II trials: a study of methodology and predictive value in patients with advanced breast cancer treated with paclitaxel plus granulocyte colony-stimulating factor. *J Natl Cancer Inst* 1995; 87:1316–1322.

150. Cella D, Fairclough DL, Bonomi PB, et al. Quality of life (QOL) in advanced non-small cell lung cancer (NSCLC): results from Eastern Cooperative Oncology Group (ECOG) study E5592. *Proc Am Soc Clin Oncol* 1997; 16:2a (abstr 4).

151. Cella DF, Bonomi AE, Lloyd SR, et al. Reliability and validity of the Functional Assessment of Cancer Therapy-Lung (FACT-L) quality of life instrument. *Lung Cancer* 1995; 12:199–220.

152. Hwang SS, Chang VT, Fairclough DL, et al. Longitudinal measurements of quality of life and symptom distress in terminal cancer patients. Submitted for publication. Proc ASCO 1996; 15:536 Abstract 1737.

152a. Coates A, Gebski V. On the receiving end. VI. Which dimensions of quality-of-life scores carry prognostic information? *Cancer Treat Rev* 1996; 22 (suppl A):63–67.

153. Cella DF, Tulsky DS, Gray G, et al. The Functional Assessment of Cancer Therapy Scale: development and validation of the general measure. *J Clin Oncol* 1993; 11:570–579.

154. Funch DP. Predictors and consequences of symptom reporting behaviors in colorec-tal cancer patients. *Med Care* 1988; 26:1000–1008.

155. Koller M, Kussman J, Lorenz W, et al. Symptom reporting in cancer patients. The role of negative affect and experienced social stigma. *Cancer* 1996; 77:983–995.

156. Simon R, Altman DG. Statistical aspects of prognostic factor studies in oncology. *Br J Cancer* 1994; 69:979–985.

157. Harrell FE Jr, Lee KL, Mark DB. Multivariable prognostic models: issues in devel-oping models, evaluating assumptions and adequacy, and measuring and reducing errors. Tutorial in biostatistics. *Stat Med* 1996; 15:361–387.

158. Justice AC, Covinsky KE, Berlin JA. Assessing the generalizability of prognostic information. *Ann Intern Med* 1999; 130:515–524.

159. Hopwood P, Stephens RJ, Girling DJ. Symptoms at presentation for treatment in patients with lung cancer: implications for the evaluation of palliative treatment. *Br J Cancer* 1995; 71:633–636.

160. Kornblith AB, Thaler HT, Wong G, et al. Quality of life of women with ovarian cancer. *Gynecol Oncol* 1995; 59:231–242.

161. Cella DF, Orofiamma B, Holland JC, et al. The relationship of psychological distress, extent of disease, and performance status in patients with lung cancer. *Cancer* 1987; 60:1661–1667.

162. Chang CH, Peterman A, Cella D, et al. Relationship between symptoms and overall quality of life. *Qual Life Res* 1997; 6:631, abstract 62.

163. Chang VT, Hwang SS, Kasimis BS. Symptom and Quality of Life Survey of Oncology Patients at a VA Medical Center. *Proc ASCO* 1995; 14:525a:abstract 1726.

164. Portenoy RK, Thaler HT, Kornblith AB, et al. Symptom prevalence, characteristics and distress in a cancer population. *Qual Life Res* 1994; 3:183–189.

165. Wang SX, Cleeland CS, Mendoza TR, et al. The effects of pain severity on health-related quality of life: a study with Chinese patients. *Cancer* 1999:86;1848–1855.

166. Chang VT, Hwang SS, Fairclough D, et al. Outcomes of cancer pain management. *Am Pain Soc* 1998; Proc 17th Annual Scientific Meeting, Abstract 622, p. 88.

167. Piccirillo JF, Feinstein AR. Clinical symptoms and comorbidity: significance for the prognostic classification of cancer. *Cancer* 1996; 77:834–842.

168. Gabay C, Kushner I. Acute phase proteins and other systemic responses to inflammation. *N Engl J Med* 1999; 340:448–454.

169. Chang VT, Hwang SS, Feuerman M. Validation of the Memorial Symptom Assessment Scale Short Form (MSAS-SF). *Proc ASCO* 1997; 16:47a abstract 165.

170. Chang VT, Hwang SS, Kasimis B, et al. Shorter symptom assessment instruments. *Proc ASCO* 1999; 18:583a, Abstract 2250.

3

Survival Estimation in Noncancer Patients with Advanced Disease

RONALD S. SCHONWETTER AND CHIRAG R. JANI

The distribution of the population has shifted in both the number and proportion of older persons. This proportion will continue to grow at a more rapid rate well into the next century, and a larger number of patients will have chronic illnesses. The leading causes of death in the United States are heart disease, cancer, cerebrovascular disease, and chronic obstructive pulmonary disease, which are responsible for 32.1%, 23.4%, 6.7%, and 4.5% of all (2,278,994) deaths, respectively.[1] Many individuals with heart disease die suddenly rather than living with the manifestations of their disease for an extended period of time. As our population ages, however, increasing numbers of patients with advanced illnesses such as cancer, heart disease, lung disease, cerebrovascular disease, and dementias will require high-quality care for prolonged periods of time.

Many treatment goals and decisions related to the care of patients with chronic illnesses are dependent on the severity of their illness. During the early stages of a chronic illness, treatment is generally aggressive and its goal may be cure, remission, or control of the disease. As the illness progresses and the patient's condition changes, the burdens of traditional medical therapies may begin to outweigh their benefits. When cure or remission is not possible, treatment goals may change appropriately from prolonging life to controlling symptoms and maximizing the quality of life so that patients can remain as comfortable as possible. The transition from traditional to palliative care can be one of the most difficult aspects of caring for patients with life-limiting illnesses. More specifically, decisions concerning patients with advanced disease involving life-sustaining treatment and do-not-resuscitate orders ought to be based on both the likely outcomes of treatment and the patient's informed preferences.[2–4] These topics have and can, at times, mark the first official discussion of disease severity with patients who have very advanced disease. Therefore, the determination of the prognosis is complex and critical to the discussion of care for patients with advanced disease and those near the end of life.

Current incentives in the health care market generally favor maximal treatment unless the patient and/or family request limitation of treatment. In the years ahead, these incentives may change and less aggressive care may be provided. Therefore, the timing of the transitions discussed above plays an important role in the care provided for those near the end of life. Very often in the United States, the transitions in goals of care occur late in the patient's illness.

Palliative care refers to the comprehensive management of the physical, social, spiritual, and existential needs of patients—in particular, those with incurable, progressive illness.[5] The goal of palliative care is to achieve the best quality of life through relief of suffering, control of symptoms, and restoration of functional capacity while remaining sensitive to the patient's personal, cultural, and religious values, beliefs, and practices. Palliative care can complement other therapies that are available and appropriate to the identified goals of care. The intensity and range of palliative interventions generally increase for patients as their illness progresses and as the complexity of care and needs of the patients and their families increase. In the United States, much of the palliative care provided is for patients who receive hospice care. Hospices provide multidisciplinary care for terminally ill patients, with one of their major goals being improvement of the patient's quality of life during the terminal phase of life. The most common diagnoses of patients admitted to hospices in the United States are cancer, heart disease, lung disease, and dementia. Inadvertently, however, access to hospice care has been limited by its reimbursement system. Medicare, which provides the majority of reimbursement for hospice care under the Medicare Hospice Benefit (MHB), limits eligible beneficiaries to those who have a life expectancy of 6 months or less should the disease take its usual course. Unfortunately, relatively little scientific information is available on the prognosis of patients with these diseases near the end of life. Medicare reimbursement for hospice care is based on a per diem amount, regardless of the specific care and treatment provided on particular days. It is therefore important for medical practitioners to be able to provide a reasonably accurate prognosis for patients with life-limiting illnesses in order to support their decision that hospice care is an appropriate choice for the patient and family.

To prevent potential fraud and abuse of the MHB, the Office of the Inspector General, as well as Medicare and its fiscal intermediaries, continue to provide regulatory oversight by auditing charts and supportive documentation of the limited life expectancies of hospice patients. In some states, Medicaid also reviews patient appropriateness for hospice care to prevent potential abuse of the reimbursement system. Because of this increased regulatory concern, it is even more important for practitioners to make an accurate prognosis.

Most studies of mortality have been performed with patients who received standard curative medical therapy when they became acutely ill. Few studies have looked at the natural course of end-stage illness when palliative care principles are used. Thus, it is possible that the medical literature may suggest a prognosis that is longer than that of patients who are receiving palliative care.

Survival time measurements can also be misleading, depending on the group of subjects described. For example, survival may vary, depending on the severity of illness of a particular cohort, the socioeconomic class, or the place of residence.

There are several instruments that can be used to assess the prognosis of seriously ill patients: the Apache III Prognostic System,[6] the Simplified Acute Physiology Score II,[7] and the SUPPORT Prognostic Model.[8] The Apache III is the most widely used prognostic tool for patients hospitalized in an intensive care unit, which obtains prognostic data from chart abstraction. Outcomes based on the use of this tool have been validated for survival of hospitalization. The Simplified Acute Physiology Score also predicts hospital survival for patients in an intensive care unit. The SUPPORT model predicts survival time for seriously ill hospitalized patients with certain diagnoses.

Both the SUPPORT and Apache III prognostic models generated multivariable prognostic estimates of survival for hospitalized patients.[9] The relationship between median survival estimates and time to death has been examined for each source of data, for different diseases, and for intensive care unit settings of care. In the SUPPORT model, median prognoses varied substantially among diseases: the median for congestive heart failure patients was a .62 chance of surviving for 2 months on the day before death, while lung cancer patients had a .17 chance and coma patients a .11 chance. Median prognosis estimates were not very different when given by physicians and were only a little more pessimistic using the Apache model (the median estimate for hospital survival on the day before death was .14, and 7 days before death it was .45). Based on these analyses and their poor prognostic abilities, it is unreasonable to use these statistical models of prognosis to designate a category of "terminally ill" patients for policy purposes.

It is important to understand that prognoses may sometimes be difficult to determine, as patients with chronic diseases may develop an acute illness (e.g., pulmonary embolus, myocardial infarction, sepsis) that will result in unexpected death. The National Hospice Organization (NHO), however, has developed a set of medical guidelines to assist practitioners in assessing the prognosis of patients in the advanced stages of multiple noncancer illnesses. The second edition of the NHO's *Medical Guidelines for Determining Prognosis in Patients with Selected Non-cancer Diseases*[10] later led Medicare fiscal intermediaries to develop their own policies about appropriate admissions to hospice services.[11] Some of these policies may have been developed prematurely without evidence-based supportive information. They may not be very sensitive instruments and may thus limit eligibility for hospice admission to patients with extremely short survival times.[12] Shortened lengths of stay in hospices have been associated with increased suicidal ideations[13] experienced by patients, as well as more difficult bereavements of caregivers.[14] In addition, it has been reported that although the timing of patient admission to a hospice varies substantially, most patients who enroll in a hospice do so late in the course of their disease, when they may not benefit from all the services the hospice has to offer.[15,16] These studies emphasize the importance of continued research in this area to predict survival more accurately in patients near the end of life.

To date, assessing prognoses for patients with advanced disease has been a relatively inaccurate science. A recent study reported that physicians commonly encounter clinical situations that require prognostication and are poorly prepared for this task.[17] This study also reported that most physicians believe that patients expect too much certainty and might judge them adversely for making prognostic errors, as well as having varied interpretations of what constitutes terminal illness. Many studies report health professionals' typical overestimation of the prognosis in patients near the end of life.[18,19] Clinicians, however, appear to be more comfortable with assessing prognoses in patients with most cancer diagnoses compared to those with noncancer diagnoses. Most studies assessing the prognosis in patients with advanced disease include specific yet limited factors affecting survival. Realizing the limitations in the literature, and understanding that applying population-based studies to specific patients is difficult due to individual variations in survival, we will describe general factors that can assist practitioners in determining prognoses for patients with advanced disease and, more specifically, for those with advanced heart disease, lung disease, and dementia.

General Considerations

Prognostication is a complex and challenging task that relies on clinical judgment to a great degree. To determine a terminal prognosis, the clinician must take into account not only the advanced disease state, but also the comorbid conditions of the patient and the mental and emotional condition of the patient and family.[20] Nevertheless, some general indicators of mortality are helpful in determining a terminal prognosis:

1. The reported mortality rate for a disease is one component of the prognosis for an individual patient. Comorbid conditions may profoundly affect the course of the illness.
2. Assessment of the patient's performance and nutritional status is a useful global measure of illness in that patient. The rate of disease progression may be related to the rate of decline in performance and/or nutritional status.
3. Directives to limit medical interventions may have profound effects on the prognosis. In addition, the emotional state of the patient and/or family may be related to the prognosis.

Functional impairment in activities of daily living (ADLs) is due to the pathophysiologic and psychosocial effects of illness. Typically, the greater the functional impairment, the more advanced the illness and the closer the patient is to death. The Karnofsky Performance Status (KPS)[21] scale is one of several scales that has been used to quantify the concept of functional impairment for the purposes of research and prognostication. The KPS scale has 11 different classifications ranging in 10-point increments from 0 (death) to 100 (normal; fully functional, with no evidence of disease). In the National Hospice Study, the validity and reliability of the KPS scale were assessed in 685 cancer patients admitted to a hospice program who had a KPS score below 50. Each increase of 10 in the KPS between 0 and 50 roughly correlated with an increase in survival of 2 weeks.[22]

Several studies have attempted to identify specific prognostic factors for patients near the end of life.[23-26] Many of these studies have been carried out in cancer patients, as these patients may have more readily available predictors of a short-term prognosis. One study of patients with advanced cancer admitted to an inpatient palliative care unit reported that three simple determinations (weight loss of 10 kg or more, cognitive failure with a Mini-Mental Status Examination score below 24 or dysphagia to solids or liquids) can predict survival of more or less than 4 weeks as accurately as two skilled physicians.[23] Two additional studies involving patients newly admitted to a hospice described prognostic factors associated with significantly shortened survival, including low performance status,[24,25] elevated serum bilirubin,[24] hypotension,[24] tachycardia,[25] and impaired appetite.[25] However, although these factors appeared significant in the samples studied, they factors were not validated in additional populations. Studies of nursing home patients revealed that weight loss exceeding 10% of body weight from the time of admission was significantly associated with death.[26,27] A decreased serum albumin concentration has also correlated with a high mortality rate. This may be due in part to the fact that serum albumin concentration serves as a measure of overall nutritional status. One study including 4116 patients above 70 years of age demonstrated that the serum albumin concentration was linearly and continuously related to all causes of mortality in this population.[28] Functional impairment was independently related to mortality in this study as well. While many of the studies on general guidelines for prognostication have been conducted in cancer patients and may not have been validated in other populations, it appears that certain measures of impaired nutrition and functional status may be used as predictors of shortened prognoses in many types of patients with advanced disease.

Specific Noncancer Diseases

Heart disease

Heart disease is the leading cause of death in the United States, responsible for almost 800,000 deaths in 1994.[1] It is estimated that over 10% of the population over the age of 75 have congestive heart failure (CHF).[29,30] Heart failure is now the single most common diagnosis for hospital patients over 65 years of age and continues to increase.[31] CHF is most commonly due to ischemic heart disease, but it may result from other cardiomyopathies as well. Many patients with CHF experience a chronic, progressive illness related to their underlying disease, with periodic exacerbations that may result in lower functional status levels. While sudden death associated with acute myocardial infarction or a malignant arrhythmia are feared consequences of advanced cardiac disease, CHF is responsible for significant morbidity in patients with cardiac disease.

Understanding the severity of the syndrome of heart failure in terms of its prognosis can be very important for medical management and in counseling the patient. Studies generally evaluate the prognosis in patients with advanced cardiac disease to determine the appropriate use of aggressive interventions such as active hemodynamic support with ventricular assistive devices or heart transplantation. However, it is also important to understand the prognoses in these patients to guide patients and families appropriately during the patients' terminal period.

Physician estimates of prognoses in patients with CHF continue to be inaccurate. A recent study of emergency room physicians reported that these physicians identified only 15/90 (17%) patients admitted to a Veterans Administration hospital with an acute exacerbation of CHF and thought to have less than a 10% chance of surviving for 90 days.[32] The actual mortality rate was 67%. Some believe that determination of prognoses in patients with heart failure remains an art form.[31]

The prognosis in heart failure depends primarily on the nature of the underlying disease and the presence or absence of a precipitating factor that can be treated. When this factor can be identified and removed, the outlook for immediate survival is far better than if heart failure occurs without any obvious precipitating factor. In the latter scenario, survival usually ranges from 6 months to 4 years, depending on the severity of the heart failure. The long-term prognosis for heart failure is most favorable when the underlying heart disease can be treated. The prognosis can also be estimated by observing the patient's response to treatment.

The most widely used functional classification for patients with heart failure is the New York Heart Association (NYHA) Classification (see Table 3.1). Patients who demonstrate persistent Class IV heart disease despite optimal medical therapy typically have a very limited prognosis. A recent prospective multicenter study of 1390 adult hospitalized patients with NYHA Class III–IV CHF found a 38.5% mortality rate at 1 year.[33] Patients with more impaired functional status were more likely to die.

In addition to impaired function secondary to advanced cardiac disease, several factors appear to contribute to poorer prognoses in these patients, including impaired ventricular function, impaired cardiac functional status, impaired nutritional status, reduced oxygen consumption, elevated norepinephrine and renin levels, and arrhythmias identified on Holter monitors. Relationships between survival and serum sodium levels, as well as heart size on chest radiographs, have also been reported in these patients. The precise contribution of each of these factors to survival remains unclear.

Table 3.1. NYHA classification system

Class	Description
I	No limitation of physical activity.
II	Comfortable at rest. Slight limitation of physical activity. Ordinary physical activity results in fatigue, palpitation, dyspnea, or anginal pain.
III	Comfortable at rest. Marked limitation of physical activity. Less than ordinary physical activity results in fatigue, palpitation, dyspnea, or anginal pain.
IV	Symptoms of fatigue, palpitations, dyspnea, or anginal pain at rest. Unable to carry on any physical activity without discomfort. Physical activity increases discomfort.

In more advanced disease, NYHA Class IV heart failure generally correlates with a resting left ventricular ejection fraction of 20% or less. In a prospective study of 170 patients with ischemic cardiac disease, the presence of CHF was independent of the ejection fraction in predicting mortality.[34] In that study, each 1% increase in left ventricular ejection fraction was associated with a 2% decrease in mortality. Other factors that were predictive of mortality in that study included dilated cardiomyopathy, uncontrolled arrhythmia, and the NYHA class level. Another study reported that patients with a left ventricular ejection fraction below 20% exhibited annual mortality rates exceeding 30%.[35] An additional study confirmed the relationship between left ventricular ejection fraction and survival but also reported heart size and exercise tolerance as reliable measures of prognosis.[31]

With impaired left ventricular function in heart failure, some believe that an initiating event results in an intrinsic morphologic alteration in the cardiac wall that changes over time. Contractile dysfunction, rather than a primary deficiency in contractility, may be a manifestation of this ongoing remodeling process in the left ventricle.[30] It has also been suggested that the manner in which contractility changes over time may be even more important than the absolute left ventricular ejection fraction in determining mortality.[36]

Short-term prognoses were studied in a retrospective analysis of 142 ambulatory patients with advanced heart failure (NYHA Class III–IV) being evaluated for a heart transplant.[37] This study suggested that right ventricular function was a crucial determinant of the short-term prognosis in severe chronic heart failure, with short-term survival (<10 months) being significantly different in patients with a right ventricular ejection fraction exceeding, equaling, or less than 24%. It was also noted that the cardiothoracic ratio, as measured on a standard posteroanterior chest radiograph, assesses the size of the cardiac chambers, in particular the atria and the right ventricle. The cardiothoracic ratio may have potential for providing data on cardiac enlargement and insight into the severity of right ventricular dysfunction, which may be an independent determinant of prognosis.[38]

Impaired nutritional status and decreased oxygen consumption are reported to be related to survival in patients with advanced CHF. One study prospectively evaluated potential prognostic factors (exercise capacity, functional status, left ventricular ejection fraction, and nutritional status) in patients with CHF.[39] This study reported that cachexia (weight loss of 7.5% of normal body weight in 6 months) was a strong independent risk factor for mortality in patients with CHF. Combined with low peak oxygen consumption, it identified a subset of patients at extremely high risk of death. Another study verified that the cachectic state is a strong independent risk factor for survival in patients with CHF.[40] An additional study showed that 52% of ambulatory heart failure patients who had a peak oxygen consumption less than or equal to 14 ml/kg/min either died or underwent emergent cardiac transplantation.[41]

Decreased left ventricular function usually results in inadequate blood flow to peripheral tissues. A series of neurohumoral changes occur consequent to the two principal hemodynamic changes in heart failure (reduction in cardiac function and atrial hypertension). Release of norepinephrine by adrenergic cardiac cells augments cardiac contractility, and the activation of the renin-angiotensin-aldosterone system maintains arterial pressure and perfusion of vital organs. Patients with heart failure demonstrate increased adrenergic nerve outflow. Concentrations of norepinephrine in endomyocardial biopsy specimens correlate directly with ejection fractions and inversely with plasma epinephrine concentrations. A relationship has been found between plasma norepinephrine levels and survival.[42] In addition, an inverse linear relationship exists between plasma renin activity and serum sodium concentration in patients with CHF, and the renin-angiotensin system is activated in proportion to the clinical severity of the syndrome. Survival is also related directly to plasma renin activity in patients with CHF and inversely with serum sodium concentration.[43]

Ventricular arrhythmias are a common manifestation of heart failure. Mechanisms contributing to these arrhythmias include myocardial scarring, left ventricular stretching, subendocardial ischemia, and increased sympathetic activity. The frequency of premature ventricular beats and the incidence of runs of ventricular tachycardia on Holter monitoring are directly related to the severity of left ventricular dysfunction.[44] The presence of nonsustained ventricular tachycardia carries a poor prognosis.[35]

A retrospective chart review of 231 elderly patients (>80 year old) evaluated demographic, clinical, and electrocardiographic data to determine prognostic factors in those hospitalized with CHF.[45] This study found that very elderly patients with CHF had a poor long-term prognosis, with 63% dead at 1 year. Patients who died during that first year were more likely to be nursing home residents, have NYHA Class IV heart failure, have impaired left ventricular function on an echocardiogram, and have renal insufficiency.

With the advent of relatively new treatments (angiotensin-converting enzyme [ACE] inhibitors and vasodilators) for CHF, mortality has decreased in symptomatic patients treated with these medications.[46] However, the effect of some of these newer medications on prognosis is unclear in patients with asymptomatic disease. At this time, the most important prognostic markers in patients with advanced CHF are ventricular function, cardiac functional status, nutritional status, oxygen consumption, and possibly serum norepinephrine and renin levels, as well as the presence of ventricular arrhythmias and heart size.[30]

Lung disease

Chronic obstructive pulmonary disease (COPD) is a constellation of clinical and pathologic findings that produce chronic progressive airflow obstruction, disability, and sometimes death. Chronic bronchitis and emphysema are two types of COPD that often present in combination. Currently, more than 14 million Americans are affected by COPD.[47] Between 1972 and 1992, deaths due to COPD increased by 48%, while deaths due to all other causes decreased by 12%.

Patients with COPD typically have a slow, relentless decrease in ventilatory function, typically exceeding the rate of change found with normal aging. In a study of patients with COPD requiring hospitalization, reported 5-year survival was 45%.[48]

Presently, there is no widely accepted staging system for patients with COPD. Such a stratification system could have several potential applications, including clinical recommendations, prognostication, and health resource planning, as well as facilitating communication. Ideally, a staging system would provide a composite picture of disease severity based on the interrelationships among the sensation of breathlessness (dyspnea), the impairment in airflow, and the derangement in gas exchange (arterial blood gas). Unfortunately, no staging system has been developed that can integrate these factors into a single parameter. However, the American Thoracic Society has proposed dividing COPD into three stages according to disease severity (see Table 3.2).[49] These stages were defined according to the overall impact of the disease and the complexity of care required. Refinements of this staging system may further incorporate information on dyspnea, hypoxemia, and hypercarbnea directly.

Determining the prognosis in patients with COPD is very difficult. There is marked variability in survival in these patients. Applying the results of population-based epidemiologic studies or limited clinical trials to specific patients is hazardous because of the marked individual variation in survival even when patients are

Table 3.2. Clinical characteristics of patients with COPD

	COPD stage		
	I	*II*	*III*
FEV_1, predicted (postbronchodilator)	>50%	34–50%	<34%
Dyspnea	Mild	Moderate	Severe
Hypoxemia	Very rare	Infrequent	Common
Hypercarbnea	Very rare	Very rare	May be present

close to death. Predicting survival is difficult even when patients have respiratory failure and require intubation and mechanical ventilation.[50] One study evaluating physicians' estimates of survival for a hypothetical COPD patient with respiratory failure revealed marked variability in survival estimates.[51] Shorter estimates of survival were associated with the acquisition of select case information: (1) subjective information from family members and a professional colleague and (2) physiologic and functional data previously demonstrated to be predictive of survival.

Prognostic evaluation of patients with advanced pulmonary disease is dependent on the pathophysiology of progressive respiratory failure in these patients. Although there are many types of COPD, the mechanisms of the end-stage events are limited to a few pathways. Patients die of either respiratory failure (hypoxemia or hypercarbnea), CHF (right heart failure due to pulmonary hypertension or left heart failure due to ischemic heart disease), or infection.[52]

In view of the marked variability in survival among COPD patients, the most powerful predictor of prognosis and survival is the forced expiratory volume at 1 sec (FEV_1).[48,53–55] Most studies conducted in this area, however, have included patients who are in the early stages of the disease. Patients with initial FEV_1 measurements of 30–50% of the normal predicted values have a mortality rate of 25–35% in 3 years.[54] As the FEV_1 falls below the 50th percentile of the predicted value in normal patients, ADLs become impaired. In addition, it has been reported that decreases in the FEV_1 over time on serial testing are associated with a poorer prognosis.[56]

Respiratory failure is a significant predictor of poor survival in patients with advanced COPD. The likelihood of acute respiratory failure increases when the FEV_1 falls below 25% of the predicted normal value. One study reported a 1-year mortality of 66% in patients with respiratory failure,[57] while another study showed a 1-year mortality exceeding 60% only when the episode of respiratory failure requires endotracheal intubation.[58] Still another study showed a similar mortality rate at 2 years.[59] Although in-hospital mortality rates for patients with a single episode of respiratory failure approach 30%, the 5-year survival rate after an initial episode of respiratory failure averages 15–20%.[54] Some investigators believe that a single episode of respiratory failure has no effect on the prognosis of patients with COPD; however, most believe that there is a consistent increase in mortality after the second episode.[58] Patients with predominant emphysema have a poorer prognosis after the onset of respiratory failure than those with predominant bronchitis.

Cor pulmonale arises as a result of pulmonary hypertension secondary to hypoxemia. It is common in patients with COPD and results in reduced exercise tolerance, increased dyspnea, and decreased overall functional status. A study of patients with advanced COPD revealed a 60% prevalence of cor pulmonale.[57] In these patients, an episode of right heart failure secondary to cor pulmonale had a deleterious effect on survival. An additional study reported a relationship between right ventricular ejection fraction and survival, but the association was weaker than the relationship between arterial oxygen and carbon dioxide tensions and survival.[60] This study concluded that although right ventricular function is predictive of survival in patients with COPD, it is probably a reflection of the severity of disease rather than having a direct affect on prognosis.

Nutritional status also affects the prognosis of patients with chronic lung disease.[55] The National Institute of Health's IPPB Trial found that low body weight, expressed as a percentage of ideal body weight, was an independent prognostic factor in patients with COPD.[61] Two mechanisms contribute to weight loss in COPD patients: (1) hypermetabolism due to the increased work of breathing and (2) reduced caloric intake resulting from dyspnea and fatigue.[62]

Several other factors have been reported as prognostic factors in patients with COPD. Age has been repeatedly reported to affect survival in these patients.[55,63,64] One study assessing the relationship between personality, clinical factors, and survival in patients with advanced COPD reported that overall psychological distress and difficulty in coping with the disease were important prognostic indicators irrespective of the results of pulmonary function tests.[65] Other conditions reported to be negative prognostic factors in patients with COPD include hypoxemia,[52] polycythemia,[52] resting tachycardia,[10] decreased vital capacity,[55] and continued smoking.[55]

The value of long-term oxygen supplementation in increasing survival for patients with severe COPD with hypoxemia has been demonstrated in large trials.[55] In the National Heart, Lung, and Blood Institute's Nocturnal Oxygen Therapy Trial, at 26 months, mortality in the continuous oxygen group was one-half that in the nocturnal oxygen group.[66] These findings, along with those reported in a study by the British Medical Research Council,[67] serve as the basis for current recommendations regarding supplemental oxygen in patients with COPD. One recent report supports supplemental oxygen as a better predictor of survival than the FEV_1 or the degree of hypoxemia or hypercarbnea.[67] In one study evaluating prognostic factors in COPD patients receiving oxygen therapy, the best prognostic factor was the pulmonary artery pressure.[68]

One large ($n = 1016$) prospective study of hospitalized patients with an acute exacerbation of COPD and an arterial carbon dioxide tension ($PaCO_2$) of 50 mm Hg or more evaluated multiple prognostic factors.[69] Although only 11% of the patients died during the hospitalization period, 33% and 49% died within 6 months and 1 year, respectively. Survival time in this study was independently related to severity of illness, body mass index, age, prior functional status, arterial oxygen pressure/inspired flow of oxygen ($PaO_2/FI(O_2)$), CHF, serum albumin concentration, and the presence of cor pulmonale.

Due to the variability in survival in patients with advanced COPD, caution must be used when discussing the prognosis with these patients and their families. However, several factors have consistently been associated with limited survival in these patients: decreased FEV_1, the presence of cor pulmonale, repeated episodes of respiratory failure, and poor nutritional status. Other variables that may be related to survival in these patients include poor functional status, hypoxemia, psychological distress, polycythemia, resting tachycardia, decreased vital capacity, and continued smoking.

Dementia

Dementia is a major health problem that will continue to grow as the U.S. population ages. It is a clinical syndrome characterized by acquired losses of cognitive abilities severe enough to interfere with daily functioning. There are many causes of dementing illnesses, this chapter focuses on the chronic, progressive, degenerative types. Alzheimer's disease is the most common type of chronic degenerative dementia. Patients with Alzheimer's disease and vascular (multi-infarct) dementia follow a similar clinical course, although those with vascular dementia usually progress in a stepwise manner.

Dementing illnesses are estimated to affect more than 2 million Americans.[70] One recent study estimated that 7.1% of all deaths in the United States are due to Alzheimer's disease, placing it on par with cerebrovascular disease as the third leading cause of death.[71] The prevalence of dementia is higher in nursing home facilities and other institutional or residential settings than in the community home setting. One study, however, reported a very high prevalence of dementia among community-dwelling elderly persons, with almost 50% of those over 85 years of age affected.[72]

Although most research on the prognosis in dementia has focused on patients with Alzheimer's disease, patients with vascular dementia appear to progress to death more rapidly.[73,74] Although dementia shortens life independent of culture or ethnicity,[75] prediction of 6-month mortality is challenging. The mean survival in dementia patients is reported to range from 5 to 8 years.[73,76,77] Survival of patients with dementia is decreased in institutional settings[78]; however, some patients with advanced dementia survive for long periods with meticulous care when no life-threatening complications arise.

The affect of changes in treatment on survival in patients with dementia is unclear. One study has shown a shortened survival time in dementia patients after an episode of fever when treated with a palliative care approach rather than a more traditional approach.[79] Nonetheless, shifts in reimbursement policy and regulatory expectations may affect decisions about treatments and services. In addition, comparison of the benefits and burdens associated with aggressive medical interventions in patients with advanced Alzheimer's disease and attention to life values have led to the consideration of alternative approaches for the care of these patients. The routine use of aggressive medical interventions, which may decrease patients' comfort without altering the underlying disease, may not be appropriate.[80] The use of hospice services for dementia patients suggests that this approach is feasible as well as ethical. In one survey, 90% of family members and professional caregivers for dementia patients viewed hospice care as appropriate for the end stages of the disease.[81] However, only 13% were aware that hospices serve dementia patients compared with 87% who knew that they serve cancer patients. Dementia patients in hospices also survive significantly longer than those with other diagnoses; 35% survive for more that 6 months.[15] Difficulty in predicting survival in dementia patients has been documented as one of the barriers for hospices in serving dementia patients.[82] As such, little research has been conducted on the development of empirically based standards for enrolling patients with end-stage dementia in hospices. The importance of accurate prognostication for these patients emphasizes the need for additional research in this area.

Studies in patients with early dementia examining factors associated with survival have been limited, and the findings are inconsistent.[83] Identifying prognostic factors in dementia patients with far advanced disease is difficult as well, as these patients may have a life expectancy of up to 2 years. However, many studies have identified multiple factors significantly related to survival in dementia patients, including dementia type, age, gender, severity of the dementing illness, functional status, and nutritional status.

Prognostic factors appear to differ, depending on the type of dementing illness. While one study identified older age, male gender, lower educational level, presence of comorbidities, and functional dependency as related to survival in patients having all types of dementia, it also showed that predictors of death for those having vascular dementia were only age and functional dependency.[84]

Functional status appears to be related to survival in dementia patients. The Functional Assessment Staging (FAST) Scale[85] (see Table 3.3), a scale of functional impairment, has been used as a research tool to classify patients with dementia. Scores on the FAST Scale and the Global Deterioration Scale (a measure of global impairment) have been shown to be associated with survival in patients with dementia.[86] One restriction of the use of the FAST Scale is that the patient's disease should progress in an ordinal fashion throughout the stages of the scale, rather than progress while skipping a stage or two secondary to a comorbid condition. The median survival and mean survival of hospice dementia patients who could be scored ordinally and had reached Stage 7C on the FAST Scale were 4 and 6.9 months, respectively.[87] Another study confirmed the importance of functional loss in predicting death but also reported that severe language disability (aphasia), a measure of disease severity, was the best predictor of death among patients with Alzheimer's disease.[88]

Nutritional status is probably related to survival in dementia patients. One longitudinal study of 666 patients with Alzheimer's disease reported that weight loss is a predictor of mortality; weight loss of 5% or more in any year is a significant predictor of mortality.[89] Severe cachexia and severe cognitive impairment were associated with significantly higher mortality in another study of patients with probable Alzheimer's disease.[90] An additional study evaluated the value of enteral feedings in patients with advanced dementia. This study reported that marked weight loss and dysphagia occurring in a specific clinical pattern were found to be associated with death and probably implied the failure of basic

Table 3.3. Functional Assessment Staging (FAST) scale
(check highest level of disability)

Stage	Description
1	No difficulty either subjectively or objectively.
2	Complains of forgetting location of objects. Subjective work difficulties.
3	Decreased job functioning evident to co-workers. Difficulty in traveling to new locations. Decreased organizational capacity.°
4	Decreased ability to perform complex tasks, e.g., planning dinner for guests, handling personal finances (such as forgetting to pay bills), difficulty marketing, etc.
5	Requires assistance in choosing proper clothing to wear for the day, season or occasion, e.g., patient may wear the same clothing repeatedly unless supervised.°
6	A. Improperly putting on clothes without assistance or occasional cueing (e.g., may put street clothes on over night clothes, or put shoes on wrong feet, or have difficulty buttoning clothing) occasionally or more frequently over the past weeks.°
	B. Unable to bathe properly (e.g., difficulty adjusting bath-water temperature) occasionally or more frequently over the past weeks.°
	C. Inability to handle mechanics of toileting (e.g., forgets to flush the toilet, does not wipe properly or properly dispose of toilet tissue) occasionally or more frequently over the past few weeks.°
	D. Urinary incontinence (occasionally or more frequently over the past weeks).°
	E. Fecal incontinence (occasionally or more frequently over the past weeks).°
7	A. Ability to speak limited to approximately a half dozen intelligible different words or fewer in the course of an average day or in the course of an intensive interview.
	B. Speech ability is limited to the use of a single intelligible word in an average day or in the course of an intensive interview (the person may repeat the word over with assistance).
	C. Cannot sit up without assistance (e.g., the individual will fall over if there are not lateral arms on the chair).
	D. Loss of ability to smile.
	E. Loss of ability to hold up head independently.

°Scored primarily on the basis of acknowledgeable information.

homeostatic mechanisms. This study suggested that patients with this clinical pattern may be less likely to benefit from enteral feedings.[91]

Behavioral factors in both the patient and the caregiver may be related to survival in dementia patients. One study of community-dwelling patients with Alzheimer's disease reported that the severity of disease, the combination of wandering and falling, and behavioral problems were related to shorter survival.[92] Another study reported that select neurologic and psychiatric symptoms were associated with poorer survival only in men.[93] An additional study reported that several factors were associated with earlier death in patients with Alzheimer's-type dementia, including severity of disease, rate of deterioration, and age, as well as greater psychological morbidity in caregivers. One other study identified significant prognostic factors, including male gender, presence of extrapyramidal signs, lower score on the modified Mini-Mental State Examination, and a shorter duration of illness.[95]

Brain perfusion studies are sometimes used in the evaluation and/or management of dementia patients. One study evaluated the use of brain perfusion imaging in assessing prognosis and demonstrated that brain perfusion in the right parietal lobe is a significant predictor of survival in patients with Alzheimer's disease even when controlling for known prognostic factors.[96]

While most of the prognostic studies involving dementia patients include those with early stages of the disease, it appears that age, gender, severity of disease, and type of dementia, as well as functional and nutritional status, are related to survival even with advanced disease. Additional research is needed to confirm these relationships.

Conclusion

Accurate estimation of survival in patients with advanced noncancer illnesses remains very difficult. Most studies on mortality use samples of patients who receive traditional medical care. Survival time measurements vary according to the selection of a particular cohort. In addition, applying the results of population-based epidemiologic studies to specific patients is difficult because of marked individual variation in survival even in patients with very advanced disease. It appears, however, that certain measures of disease severity, functional and nutritional status, and potential comorbidities all have a significant effect on the survival of most patients with advanced noncancer diseases. Additional research is needed to improve the clinician's ability to assess the prognosis in this complex and critical area of patient care.

References

1. National Center for Health Statistics. *Vital Statistics of the United States, 1994.* Washington, D.C.: Public Health Service, 1997.
2. Teno JM. Indicators for medical care at the end of life and survival time. Center to Improve Care of the Dying. *http://www.gwu.edu/ficicd/toolkit/survive.htm*
3. President's Commission for the Study of Ethical Problems in Medicine and Biomedical and Behavioral Research: *Deciding to Forego Life-Sustaining Treatment: A Report on the Ethical, Medical, and Legal Issues in Treatment Decisions.* Washington, D.C.: Government Printing Office, 1983.
4. Hakim RB, Teno JM, Harrell FE. Factors associated with the Do-Not-Resuscitate Orders: Patients' preferences, prognoses, and physicians' judgments. *Ann Intern Med.* 1996; 125:284–293.
5. Task Force on Palliative Care, Last Acts Campaign, Robert Wood Johnson Foundation. Precepts of palliative care. *J Palliat Med* 1998; 1(2):109–112.

6. Knaus WA, Wagner DP, Draper EA. The Apache III Prognostic System: risk prediction of hospital mortality for critically ill hospitalized adults. *Chest* 1991; 100:1619–1636.

7. LeGall JR, Lemeshow S, Saulnier F. A new simplified acute physiology score (SAPS II) based on a European/North American multicenter study. *JAMA* 1993; 270: 2957–2963.

8. Knaus WA, Harrell FE Jr, Lynn, J, et al. The SUPPORT prognostic model. Objective estimates of survival for seriously ill hospitalized adults. Study to Understand Prognoses and Preferences for Outcomes and Risks of Treatments. *Ann Intern Med* 1996; 122:191–203.

9. Lynn J, Harrell F Jr, Cohn F, et al. Prognoses of seriously ill patients on the days before death: implications for patient care and public policy. *New Horizons* 1977; 5(1):56–61.

10. Standards and Accreditation Committee, Medical Guidelines Task Force of the National Hospice Organization. *Medical Guidelines for Determining Prognosis in Selected Non-cancer Diseases,* 2nd ed. Arlington, Va.: National Hospice Organization, 1996.

11. Palmetto Government Benefits Administrators: Medicare Advisory Hospice 97-11. Hospice provisions enacted by the Balanced Budget Act (BBA) of 1997. September 1997.

12. Schonwetter RS, Soendker S, Perron V, et al. Review of Medicare's proposed hospice eligibility criteria for select noncancer patients. *Am J Hospice Palliat Care* May–June 1998; 155–158.

13. Walker RM. Personal communication, January 1999.

14. Speer DC, Robinson BE, Reed MP. The relationship between hospice length of stay and caregiver adjustment. *Hospice J* 1995; 10:45–58.

15. Christakis NA, Escarce JJ. Survival of Medicare patients after enrollment in hospice programs. *N Engl J Med* 1996; 335(3):172–178.

16. Christakis NA. Predicting survival before and after hospice enrollment. *Hospice J* 1998; 13(1–2):71–78.

17. Christakis NA, Iwashyna TJ. Attitude and self-reported practice regarding prognostication in a national sample of internists. *Arch Intern Med* 1998; 158(21):2389–2395.

18. Parkes CM. Accuracy of predictions of survival in later stages of cancer. *Br Med J* 1972; 2:29–31.

19. Evans C, McCarthy M. Prognostic uncertainty in terminal care: can the Karnofsky index help? *Lancet* 1985; 1:1204–1205.

20. von Gunten CF, Twaddle ML. Terminal care for noncancer patients. In Schonwetter RS, ed. *Clinics in Geriatric Medicine.* 1996; 12(2):349–358.

21. Karnofsky DA, Burchenal JH. The clinical evaluation of chemotherapeutic agents in cancer. In: Macleod CM, ed. *Evaluation of Chemotherapeutic Agents.* New York: Columbia University Press, 1949:191–205.

22. Mor V, Laliberte L, Morris JN, et al. The Karnofsky Performance Status Scale: an examination of its reliability and validity in a research setting. *Cancer* 1984; 53: 2002–2007.

23. Bruera E, Miller MJ, Kuehn N, et al. Estimate of survival of patients admitted to a palliative care unit: a prospective study. *J Pain Symptom Manage* 1992; 7(2):82–86.

24. Rosenthal MA, Gebski VJ, Kefford RF, et al. Prediction of life-expectancy in hospice patients: identification of novel prognostic factors. *Palliat Med* 1993; 7(3):199–204.
25. Schonwetter RS, Teasdale TA, Storey P, et al. Estimation of survival time in terminal cancer patients: an impedance to hospice admissions. *Hospice J* 1990; 6(4):65–79.
26. Chang JI, Katz PR, Ambrose P. Weight loss in nursing home patients: prognostic implications. *J Fam Pract* 1990; 30(6):671–674.
27. Dwyer JT, Coleman A, Krall E, et al. Changes in relative weight among institutionalized elderly adults. *J Gerontol* 1987; 42:246–252.
28. Corti MC, Guralnik JM, Saline ME, et al. Serum albumin level and physical disability as predictors of mortality in older persons. *JAMA* 1994; 272:1036–1042.
29. Kannel WB, Belanger AJ. Epidemiology of heart failure. *Am Heart J* 1991; 121:951–957.
30. Vranckx P, Van Cleemput J. Prognostic assessment of end-stage cardiac failure. *Acta Cardiol* 1998; 53(2):121–125.
31. Francis GS. Determinants of prognosis in patients with heart failure. *J Heart Lung Transplant* 1994; 13(4):S113–S116.
32. Poses RM, Smith WR, McClish DK, et al. Physicians' survival predictions for patients with acute congestive heart failure. *Arch Intern Med* 1997; 157(9):1001–1007.
33. Jaagosild P, Dawson NV, Thomas C, et al. Outcomes of acute exacerbation of severe congestive heart failure: quality of life, resource use, and survival. SUPPORT Investigators. The Study to Understand Prognosis and Preferences for Outcomes and Risks of Treatment. *Arch Intern Med* 1998; 158(10):1081–1089.
34. Marantz PR, Tobin JN, Wassertheil-Smoller S, et al. Prognosis in ischemic heart disease: can you tell as much at the bedside as in the nuclear laboratory? *Arch Intern Med* 1992; 152:2433–2437.
35. Cohn JN, Johnson GR, Shabetai R, et al. Ejection fraction, peak exercise oxygen consumption, cardiothoracic ratio, ventricular arrhythmias and plasma norepinephrine as determinants of prognosis in heart failure. *Circulation* 1993; 87:VI-5–VI-16.
36. Cintron G, Johnson G, Francis G, et al. Prognostic significance of serial changes in left ventricular ejection fraction in patients with congestive heart failure. *Circulation* 1993; 87(suppl VI):VI-17–VI-23
37. Gavazzi A, Berzuini C, Campana C, et al. Value of right ventricular ejection fraction in predicting short-term prognosis of patients with severe chronic heart failure. *J Heart Lung Transplant* 1997; 16(7):774–785.
38. Polack JF, Holman BL, Wynne J, et al. Right ventricular ejection fraction: an indicator of increased mortality in patients with congestive heart failure associated with coronary artery disease. *J Am Coll Cardiol* 1983; 2:217–234.
39. Anker SD, Ponikowski P, Varney S. Wasting as an independent risk factor for mortality in chronic heart failure. *Lancet* 1997; 349(9058):1050–1053.
40. Anker SD, Chua TP, Ponikowski P, et al. Hormonal changes and catabolic/anabolic imbalance in chronic heart failure and their importance for cardiac cachexia. *Circulation* 1997; 96:526–534.
41. Mancini DM, Eisen H, Kussmaul W, et al. Value of peak exercise oxygen consumption for optimal timing of cardiac transplantation in ambulatory patients with heart failure. *Circulation* 1991; 83(3):778–786.
42. Cohn JN, Levine TB, Olivari MT, et al. Plasma norepinephrine as a guide to prognosis in patients with chronic congestive heart failure. *N Engl J Med* 1984; 311:819–823.

43. Francis GS, Benedict C, Johnstone DE, et al. Comparison of the neuroendocrine activation in patients with left ventricular dysfunction with and without heart failure. A substudy of the studies of left ventricular dysfunction (SOLVD). *Circulation* 1990; 82:1724–1729.

44. Franciosa JA, Park M, Levine TB. Lack of correlation between exercise capacity and indices of resting left ventricular performance in heart failure. *Am J Cardiol* 1981; 47:33–39.

45. Wang R, Mouliswar M, Denman S, et al. Mortality of institutionalized old-old hospitalized with congestive heart failure. *Arch Intern Med* 1998; 158:2464–2468.

46. Pitt B, Cohn JN, Francis, GS, et al. The effect of treatment on survival in congestive heart failure. *Clin Cardiol* 1992; 15(5):323–329.

47. *Statistical Compendium on Adult Lung Disease.* New York: American Lung Association, 1987.

48. Vestbo J, Prescott E, Lange P, et al. Vital prognosis after hospitalization for COPD: a random population sample. *Respir Med* 1998; 92(5):772–776.

49. Standards for the diagnosis and care of patients with chronic obstructive pulmonary disease. American Thoracic Society. *Am J Respir Crit Care Med* 1995; 152:S77–S121.

50. Kaelin RM, Assimacopoulos A, Chevrolet JC. Failure to predict six-month survival of patients with COPD requiring mechanical ventilation by analysis of simple indices. *Chest* 1987; 92(6):971–978.

51. Pearlman RA. Variability in physician estimates of survival for acute respiratory failure in chronic obstructive pulmonary disease. *Chest* 1987; 91(4):516–521.

52. Herbst LH. Prognosis in advanced pulmonary disease. *J Palliat Care* 1996; 12(2):54–56.

53. Kanner R. Predictors of survival in subjects with chronic airflow limitation. *Am J Med* 1983; 74:249–255.

54. Anthonisen NR, Wright EC, Hodgkin JE. Prognosis in chronic obstructive pulmonary disease. *Am Rev Respir Dis* 1986; 33(1):14–20.

55. Hodgkin JE. Prognosis in chronic obstructive pulmonary disease. *Clin Chest Med* 1990; 11(3):555–569.

56. Postma DS, Sluiter, HJ. Prognosis of chronic obstructive pulmonary disease: the Dutch experience. *Am Rev Respir Dis* 1989; 140:S100–S105.

57. Gottlieb L, Balchum O. Course of chronic obstructive pulmonary disease following first onset of respiratory failure. *Chest* 1973; 63(1):5–8.

58. Braghiroli A, Zaccaria S, Ioli F, et al. Pulmonary failure as a cause of death in COPD. *Monaldi Arch Chest Dis* 1997; 52(2):170–175.

59. Martin T, Lewis S, Albert R. The prognosis of patients with chronic obstructive pulmonary disease after hospitalization for acute respiratory failure. *Chest* 1982; 82:310–314.

60. France AJ, Prescott RJ, Biernacki W, et al. Does right ventricular function predict survival in patients with chronic obstructive lung disease? *Thorax* 1988; 43(8):621–626.

61. Wilson D, Rogers R, Wright E, et al. Body weight in chronic obstructive pulmonary disease; the NIH IPPB Trial. *Am Rev Respir Dis* 1989; 139:1435–1438.

62. Muers MF, Green JH. Weight loss in chronic obstructive pulmonary disease. *Eur Respir J* 1993; 6:729–734.

63. Dallari R, Barozzi G, Pinelli G, et al. Predictors of survival in subjects with chronic obstructive pulmonary disease treated with long-term oxygen therapy. *Respiration* 1994; 61(1):8–13.

64. Quality of life and predictions of survival in patients with advanced emphysema. *Chest Surg Clin North Am* 1995; 5(4):659–671.

65. Ashutosh K, Haldipur C, Boucher ML. Clinical and personality profiles and survival in patients with COPD. *Chest* 1997; 111(1):95–98.

66. Nocturnal Oxygen Therapy Trial Group. Continuous or nocturnal oxygen therapy in hypoxemic chronic obstructive lung disease: a clinical trial. *Ann Intern Med.* 1980; 93:391–398.

67. Medical Research Council Working Party. Long term domiciliary oxygen therapy in chronic hypoxic cor pulmonale complicating chronic bronchitis and emphysema. *Lancet* 1981; 1:681–686.

68. Oswald-Mammosser M, Weitzenblum E, Quiox E, et al. Prognostic factors in COPD patients receiving long-term oxygen therapy. Importance of pulmonary artery pressure. *Chest* 1995; 107(5):1193–1198.

69. Connors AF Jr, Dawson NV, Thomas C, et al. Outcomes following acute exacerbation of chronic obstructive lung disease. The SUPPORT investigators. *Am J Respir Crit Care Med* 1996; 154(4Pt 1):959–967.

70. Katzman R. Medical progress—Alzheimer's disease. *N Engl J Med* 1986; 314:964–973.

71. Ewbank DC. Deaths attributable to Alzheimer's disease in the United States. *Am J Public Health* 1999; 89(1):90–92.

72. Evans DA, Funkenstein HH, Albert MS, et al. Prevalence of Alzheimer's disease in a community population of older persons. Higher than previously reported. *JAMA* 1989; 262(18):2551–2556.

73. Barclay LL, Zemcov A, Class JP, et al. Survival in Alzheimer's disease and vascular dementia's. *Neurology* 1985; 35:834–840.

74. Molsa PK, Marttila RJ, Rinne UK. Long term survival and predictors of mortality in Alzheimer's disease and multi-infarct dementia. *Acta Neurol of Scand* 1995; 91(3): 159–164.

75. Katzman R, Hill LR, Yu E, et al. The malignancy of dementia: predictors of mortality in clinically diagnosed dementia in a population survey of Shanghai, China. *Arch Neurol* 1994; 51(12):1220–1225.

76. Reding MJ, Haycox J, Wigforss K, et al. Follow-up of patients referred to a dementia service. *J Am Geriatr Soc* 1984; 32:265–268.

77. Molsa PK, Marttila RJ, Rinne UK. Survival and cause of death in Alzheimer's disease and multi-infarct dementia. *Acta Neurol Scand* 1986; 74:103–107.

78. Drachman DA, O Donnell BF, Lew RA, et al. The prognosis in Alzheimer's disease: "how far" rather than "how fast" best predicts the outcome." *Arch Neurol* 1990; 47(8):851–856.

79. Volicer BJ, Hurley A, Fabiszewski KJ, et al. Predicting short-term survival for patients with advanced Alzheimer's disease. *J Am Geriatr Soc* 1993; 41:535–540.

80. Volicer L, Rheaume Y, Brown J. Hospice approach to the treatment of patients with advanced dementia of the Alzheimer's type. *JAMA* 1986; 256(16):2210–2213.

81. Luchins DJ, Hanrahan P. What is the appropriate level of health care for end-stage dementia patients? *J Am Geriatr Soc* 1993; 41:25–30.

82. Hanrahan P, Luchins DJ. Access to hospice programs in end-stage dementia: a national survey of hospice programs. *J Am Geriatr Soc* 1995; 43:56–59.

83. Walsh JS, Welch G, Larson EB. Survival of outpatients with Alzheimer's-type dementia. *Ann Intern Med* 1990; 113:429–434.

84. Aguero-Torres H, Fratiglioni L, Guo Z, et al. Prognostic factors in very old demented adults: a seven year follow-up from a population-based survey in Stolkholm. *J Am Geriatr Soc* 1998; 46(4):444–452.

85. Reisberg, B. Functional assessment staging (FAST). *Psychopharmacol Bull* 1988; 24:653–659.

86. Reisberg B, Ferris SH, Franssen EH. Mortality and temporal course of probable Alzheimer's disease: a 5-year prospective study. *Int Psychogeriatri* 1996; 8(2):291–311.

87. Luchins DJ, Hanrahan P, Murphy K. Criteria for enrolling dementia patients in hospice. *J Am Geriatr Soc* 1997; 45(9):1054–1059.

88. Bracco L, Gallato R, Grigoletto F, et al. Factors affecting course and survival in Alzheimer's disease. A 9-year longitudinal study. *Arch Neurol* 1994; 51(12):1213–1219.

89. White H, Piper C, Schmader K. The association of weight change in Alzheimer's disease with severity of disease and mortality: a longitudinal study. *J Am Geriatr Soc* 1998; 46(10):1223–1227.

90. Evans DA, Smith LA, Scherr PA. Risk of death from Alzheimer's disease in a community population of older persons. *Am J Epidemiol* 1991; 134(4):403–412.

91. Chouinard J, Lavigne E, Villeneuve C. Weight loss, dysphagia, and outcome in advanced dementia. *Dysphagia* 1998; 13(3):151–155.

92. Kaszniak AW, Fox J, Gandell DL, et al. Predictors of mortality in presenile and senile dementia. *Ann Neurol* 1978; 3:246–252.

93. Moritz DJ, Fox PJ, Luscombe FA. Neurologic and psychiatric predictors of mortality in patients with Alzheimer's disease in California. *Arch Neurol* 1997; 54(7):878–885.

94. Brodaty H, McGilchrist C, Harris L, et al. Time until institutionalization and death in patients with dementia. *Neurology* 1993; 50:643–650.

95. Stern Y, Tang M, Albert M, et al. Predicting time to nursing home care and death in individuals with Alzheimer's disease. *JAMA* 1997; 277(10):806–812.

96. Jagust WJ, Haan MN, Reed BR. Brain perfusion imaging predicts survival in Alzheimer's disease. *Neurology* 1998; 51(4):1009–1013.

4

Communicating a Poor Prognosis

GARY S. FISCHER, JAMES A. TULSKY,
AND ROBERT M. ARNOLD

One of the most essential tasks in caring for a dying patient is communicating the prognosis accurately to the patient. Not only do patients need accurate prognostic information to make informed, rational decisions about their medical treatment,[1-3] but they also need the opportunity to prepare for the expected course of their illness and eventual death. An honest, sensitive, and compassionate discussion about a poor prognosis sets the stage for an exploration of the emotions, fears, and spiritual needs surrounding the dying process.[4] Furthermore, the quality of the prognostic discussion has an important influence on the patient's emotional and physical well-being.[5-8]

The goal of this chapter is to present a framework for discussing the prognosis with patients who have a potentially terminal illness. With diagnoses such as cancer, patients often assume (correctly or incorrectly) that the prognosis is poor.[9] On the other hand, there are other diagnoses, such as severe cardiomyopathy, for which patients may not recognize the gravity of their condition until the physician describes the prognosis. In either case, these discussions are stressful for patients and physicians because of their emotional import. Therefore, much of this chapter will focus on how to provide news of a limited life span in a sensitive, compassionate, and honest manner, regardless of whether this information is conveyed in the diagnosis itself or in explanatory prognostic information provided along with the diagnosis.

The chapter will begin by exploring the barriers to discussions about poor prognoses, with attention to emotional barriers and the discomfort most physicians feel. We will then turn to patients' reactions to discussions conveying bad news and end by summarizing expert opinions about how to discuss bad news, emphasizing comparisons between discussions in which the poor prognosis is inferred from the diagnosis and those in which a patient, who already knows the diagnosis, needs to be informed of its poor prognosis.

Barriers to Revealing a Poor Prognosis

Communicating a poor prognosis is one of the most difficult tasks facing physicians. Physicians avoid telling patients about their poor prognosis for a variety of reasons (Table 4.1). In general, physicians want to make patients feel better, and delivering bad news, no matter how skillfully, will inevitably make patients feel bad. Furthermore, informing patients of a terminal illness often evokes feelings of inadequacy and personal blame regarding the physician's medical skills.[10] Finally, physicians may be uncomfortable dealing with patients' strong emotions or may be afraid of unleashing emotions that they cannot control and do not know how to handle.[11-14]

Along with these emotional concerns, there are practical constraints on physicians' ability to deliver prognostic information. When physicians think about providing information about a prognosis, they often think that they need to tell the patient how long he or she has to live or how many people in the patient's situation will die. Indeed, patients may ask for this information.

Nevertheless, providing this sort of detailed information is problematic. Many physicians find it stressful to give prognostic information and wait to be asked before providing it.[15] Little attention is given to the subject of prognosticating in medical training or in textbooks.[16] When they do attempt to prognosticate, physicians are frequently inaccurate, often tending to be overly optimistic in their assessments.[17,18] There are little good prognostic data on most illnesses, and existing data are often difficult to apply to an individual patient. Often, the most doctors can do is to explain what happens to a population of patients with certain characteristics similar to the patient's.[19] The SUPPORT study, which focused on a cohort of seriously ill patients, found that many patients would have been predicted to survive for a mean period of 6 months even up to the day before they died.[20]

Despite these concerns, it is now accepted practice in the United States that patients who desire to know about their condition be told their diagnosis and prognosis.[21] The concern that telling patients the truth about their diagnosis will harm them does not seem to have been well founded. For example, cancer patients who have been told their diagnosis appreciate having been told.[22] Since it is necessary to tell patients the truth about their diagnosis and prognosis, despite

Table 4.1. Barriers to clearly communicating a bad prognosis

The physician's concerns that:
Acknowledgment of a poor prognosis is an admission of failure
The patient will feel abandoned
The patient will be harmed by anxiety or despair
The physician's own unresolved issues about mortality
The physician's discomfort with the patient's anticipated emotional response

the fact that it is uncomfortable for physicians and patients, physicians must learn how to communicate this information in a clear and compassionate manner in order to minimize patient and physician discomfort as much as possible.

Patient Experiences of Hearing Bad News

Most patients who receive bad news are generally satisfied with the way the news is presented.[9,23] Patients with lung cancer feel "more reassured" after hearing about their condition,[22] and parents of children with cleft palate feel that the physicians allowed them to talk, allowed them to show their feelings, tried to make them feel better, and demonstrated caring and confidence.[13] These parents prefer these qualities and prefer physicians to "quickly get to the point." Parents who are informed by a physician whom they know well are more satisfied than those who are not.[13]

A substantial minority of patients have criticized the manner in which they were told of a poor prognosis. One-quarter of patients with advanced cancer felt that they were not told about their diagnosis in a "clear and caring manner."[23] The number of patients receiving news about a poor prognosis who feel the need for more information ranges from 22% to 26%.[9,22] Patients who are informed by telephone or in the recovery room after a diagnostic procedure are more likely to have a negative reaction to the discussion than are patients told in the office or in their hospital rooms.[6]

Krahn and colleagues interviewed the parents of 24 infants diagnosed with disabilities about the prognostic conversation.[24] These parents agreed that bad news should be told in person in a private setting whenever possible. They felt it was important that the information be given by someone whom they knew well, but they also felt that the person giving the information should be knowledgeable about the condition and should speak clearly and directly, avoiding medical terminology. They emphasized the need to be caring and compassionate, and to communicate a position of equality and connectedness (by sitting down, for example). Information should be provided gradually, allowing those present to ask questions before proceeding. Finally, they preferred to have someone with them for support. A study of patients with cancer confirms the importance of receiving adequate information, related in a caring and hopeful way, with a supportive person present.[25]

Recommendations for Delivering News of a Bad Diagnosis or Prognosis

There are two general circumstances in which physicians need to inform the patient of a poor prognosis. In one, there is a new and often unexpected diagnosis that implies a poor prognosis, such as when a physician has discovered metastatic cancer. There are also situations in which the patient knows the diagnosis but does not realize the poor prognosis. There are a number of variations on this scenario. There may be new information about the patient's condition, such as a computed tomography (CT) scan that reveals metastatic disease in a patient with known cancer. The condition may not be responding well to treatment or the patient may be entering a phase of progressive deterioration. Finally, the patient simply may not be aware that the diagnosis carries a grave prognosis. Although the literature is replete with recommendations on how to give bad news in the paradigm case where a patient is receiving a new and perhaps unexpected diagnosis, little attention has been paid to this second setting. Many of the principles of the former situation are applicable to the latter.

There appear to be few, if any, trials of the effectiveness of different strategies in delivering bad news.[11] Given the similarities in findings in the descriptive literature (see above), most expert recommendations on discussing bad news agree on the key features.[26] The recommendations can be organized into five categories: preparation, content of message, dealing with patients' responses, and ending the encounter (Table 4.2).

Preparation

Preparation begins when a physician orders a diagnostic test that is likely to reveal a poor prognosis. If the result turns out to be bad, it will help if the physician has already arranged for a face-to-face meeting with the patient to discuss the results, has assessed the patient's beliefs about his or her illness, and is prepared to deliver the news.

If possible, before a test that is likely to portend a poor prognosis is performed, it is a good idea to arrange a meeting to discuss the result.[27] The physician can make it clear that he or she will not discuss the result over the telephone. Sometimes a routine test will reveal an unexpected problem with a potentially poor prognosis. For example, a routine mammogram might reveal a large, suspicious mass. In these cases, however, the patient should still be asked to come to the office to discuss the results and their implications. The emotional content of bad-news discussions is very difficult to assess and manage over the phone.[26–30] One should remember, however, that the call asking the patient to set up an appointment to discuss test results foreshadows bad news. For this reason, the doctor should make these phone calls, the interval between the call and the visit should be as short as possible, and the doctor should acknowledge the emotional content of the call.

When arranging the meeting to discuss the test results, the physician should also ask the patient to consider having someone present for support.[26,27,29] All agree that bad news should be given in a private setting, where there is ample time to answer questions and deal with emotion.[10,11,26–31] It should not be done when the patient is still recovering from sedation or anesthesia after a procedure.[6,29]

Table 4.2. Summary of recommendations in discussing a poor prognosis

Preparation

Find out what the patient knows and believes

Find out what the patient wants to know

Suggest that a supportive person accompany the patient

Learn about the patient's condition

Arrange the encounter in a private place with enough time

Content

Get to the point quickly

Fire a "warning shot" (e.g., "I have bad news")

State the news clearly, simply, and sensitively

Avoid false reassurance

Make truthful, hopeful statements

Provide information in small chunks

Handle Patient's Reactions

Inquire about the meaning of the condition for the patient

NURSE expressed emotions

Assure continued support

Wrap-Up

Set up a meeting within the next few days

Write down important information

Offer to talk to relatives/friends

Suggest that the patient write down questions

Provide a way to be reached in emergencies

Assess suicidality

There is some disagreement in the literature over who should tell the patient bad news. Often confirmation of bad news comes from information obtained from a diagnostic procedure (endoscopy, bronchoscopy, etc), leading to the question of whether the person who performed the procedure or the primary care physician should reveal the bad news. Although some surgeons suggest that the specialist who will be treating the patient ought to be the one to inform the patient of the news,[32] most authors agree that it is best for the primary care physician to be the bearer of the bad news unless the specialist has a previous relationship with the patient.[28]

Knowledge of what the patient already knows or believes is extremely valuable to have prior to revealing a poor prognosis. This allows the physician to begin the explanation from the patient's perspective, "aligning oneself with the patient," and making communication more efficient and effective.[10,11,26,27,32,33] The time that a test is ordered is a good time to assess this. The physician might ask, "Is there anything that you are particularly concerned about?" If the patient mentions a serious illness that might be present, the physician can follow up by asking what the patient's specific fears and concerns are. Consider, for example, a man in his early 30s who presents with a testicular mass. His family physician finds an enlarged testicle that feels somewhat hard, and the doctor is concerned that it might be testicular cancer. Here is how the physician might approach the patient:

> Physician: Is there anything that you are particularly worried that this might be?
> Patient: I guess anyone would be scared that it is cancer.
> Physician: I'm afraid that it might be cancer. There are other things that it might be too, however. That's why we are going to do the biopsy—to find out. What worries you most about cancer?
> Patient: My grandfather just died of colon cancer. He suffered terribly with it. In the end, he was so weak and thin . . . he had to "do his business" in a bag—you know? And he always seemed to be in pain. . . .

At the end of this exchange, note how the physician begins to find out what the patient's fears are in an effort to anticipate the patient's reactions to the news if the test result does turn out to be bad.[27]

Sometimes a patient will not express any particular beliefs or concerns. In this instance, the physician should consider telling the patient some of the diagnostic possibilities to begin to prepare the patient for the news. For example, the physician might use this approach with the patient who has the testicular mass.

> Physician: I am concerned about the swelling in your testicle and would like to get an ultrasound of your testicles to get a better idea of what it is. Would you like to know some of the different things this could be? Or do you want to wait until we have the result?
> Patient: Do you think it might be cancer?
> Physician: Any time there is a swelling like this, we always worry that it might be cancer. Swelling in the testicle can be due to other things too. It could simply be due to a collection of fluid, something we call a hydrocele, which is nothing to be concerned about.
> Patient: If it is cancer, what does that mean?
> Physician: We would have to remove it, and do special X-rays like a CT scan to see if it spread. Cancer in the testicle can often be cured with chemotherapy.
> Patient: Uh-huh.
> Physician: It's hard to get into the details of everything it might be until we know what the situation is. For now, we should get the ultrasound to get a better idea of what it is.
> Patient: Will the ultrasound tell us if it is cancer?
> Physician: The ultrasound will tell us if it is filled with the fluid. Then it would be a hydrocele and we wouldn't have to worry about it. If the ultrasound tells us that it is solid, you will need to have a biopsy.

In this dialogue, the physician explained the worrisome finding to the patient and asked if he wanted to hear about some of the possibilities of what it might be. The result is that the patient understands the gravity of the situation, knows that the physician is open to answering the patient's questions, and is more prepared to hear bad news if the test result turns out to be cancer.

Although most patients want to be fully informed about their diagnosis and prognosis, there are some patients who would prefer that others, such as family members, be told and make decisions. Korean Americans and Mexican Americans, for example, are less likely than Americans of European or African descent to believe that a patient should be told about a terminal diagnosis.[34] Nevertheless, one cannot be certain, based on a patient's ethnicity, whether that particular patient does or does not want to be told. The best way to respect a patient and his or her culture is to ask the patient directly whether the patient would want to be told if he or she has a condition with a poor prognosis.[27] To avoid an awkward situation in which the physician has to ask whether a patient wants to hear bad news when he or she already knows that the patient's prognosis is poor, physicians should ask patients before they undergo a test whether they would want to be told bad news. Nevertheless, if one has not asked in advance, it is still possible to find out from the patient how much he or she wants to know before giving bad news. A physician might say the following:

> I want to make sure that you and I are on the same wavelength. Some people want to know everything that is going on with them—both good and bad—while others really do not want to hear bad news. What kind of person do you think you are?

If the patient indicates that he or she does not want to know all of the details of the illness, it is important to find out who should be told.

Prior to the visit, the physician may need to do some homework to prepare for the encounter. Inaccurate information given at the first visit may be remembered and may affect future interactions. The physician must become familiar with the implications and prognosis of the illness, as well as the treatment options.[10,27] It may be helpful to make arrangements for a consultation with a specialist in advance.[31] For example, a physician who needs to deliver news of metastatic lung cancer should have a general idea of the prognosis and of treatment options, and might call an oncologist to arrange an appointment for the patient prior to meeting with the patient. The physician will then be in the position of being able to offer the patient a date and time to meet the specialist.

Finally, the physician may need to deal with personal feelings before he or she is ready to deal with the patient's.[27,28] Doctors may experience a variety of emotions related to a patient's prognosis, especially if the patient has been in the doctor's practice for a long time. Physicians may experience grief, guilt, a feeling of inadequacy ("If I had only done a chest X-ray last year"), or dread at having to inform the patient. It often helps to talk to a trusted colleague about these feelings prior to facing the patient.

Content of the message

If a patient is expecting the physician to discuss the results of a test that may reveal a poor prognosis, the physician should get to the point quickly to avoid increasing the patient's anxiety. If many physicians have been involved in a patient's care, it is reasonable to ask, "Have you heard anything yet about the test results?" before launching into an explanation. The physician might learn that the patient already has some inkling about the nature of the diagnosis.[10] On the other hand, when the patient knows the diagnosis and the doctor has decided to have an explicit conversation about the prognosis—because, for example, the illness has not responded as well as was hoped—asking how the patient thinks things are going is a good way to begin.

Before telling news of a new diagnosis, one should begin with a "warning shot" to prepare the patient that bad news will follow.[26,29,32,33] One can say something as simple as "I'm afraid I have bad news." This allows the patient to prepare emotionally for the news to come. The physician should follow with a statement of the diagnosis, using simple language, and then pause to observe the patient's reactions.[10,11,29]

Some authors suggest that the diagnosis should be given gradually, starting with general, perhaps vague, terms and responding to patient's questions to let the patient control how quickly he or she hears the bad news. In this strategy of a "staged delivery," the doctor begins by saying that the test shows that there is a "tumor" and waits for the patient to ask for more details.[32,35] However, vague words may impair patients' ability to think clearly about their illness.[36] Furthermore, a physician's use of euphemisms suggests to patients that these professionals are afraid to speak openly about the condition.[31] This can become a serious impediment to communication. Therefore, physicians should avoid vague terms, euphemisms, and jargon, and should describe the problem clearly and directly in terms the patient can understand.[11,30,31]

After the diagnosis is delivered, there is likely to be a silent interval as the patient reacts. Doctors should avoid the temptation to fill the space with jargon describing the condition, technical information about the prognosis and treatment,[29] or falsely reassuring words.[14,31] If the doctor remains silent, the patient will have time to react and indicate emotional and informational needs.[12,31] At the most, after a long pause, the doctor might ask, "What do you think about this?" or "How are you doing?" or "Tell me about your concerns." It is critically important to give the patient the opportunity to express needs, questions, and emotions.

Once the patient's initial reactions to the news have been dealt with, the physician must continue to monitor the patient constantly while providing more information. Information should be given in small amounts, allowing the patient ample time to respond and ask questions. After each bit of information is given, the doctor should check the patient's understanding and invite comments from the patient before continuing.[10,27]

The goals of the encounter are to inform the patient of the diagnosis, achieve a common perception of the problem, handle the patient's emotional response, answer the patient's questions, and arrange a short-term plan.[27] Patients are unlikely to remember detailed medical information at the first encounter, so this should be provided only if requested.[29] Furthermore, information should be tailored to the patient's own perceptions of the problems and aimed at correcting misperceptions and reinforcing correct perceptions.[27] We believe the physician does well in the first encounter to provide a general outline of the next steps and use the time to deal with the patient's emotions. A return visit, scheduled within 1 to 2 days if possible, can be used to provide more medical information and answer follow-up questions.

Everyone stresses the importance of maintaining hope while remaining truthful.[26,29] Hopeful messages need to be tailored to patients' specific concerns, particularly addressing patients' misconceptions and fears. Once patients' concerns have been explored, they can be reassured more effectively. When effective treatment is available, this fact should be explained. When the treatment options are poor, hope may be found by alleviating patients' worst fears. The doctor may reassure the patient that he or she will not be abandoned during the illness, that he will remain available to consult if things get worse, that he will do his utmost to maintain the patient's comfort, and that he will continue to watch for new treatment developments.[28] Often people find hope and strength from their religious or spiritual beliefs, from having their individuality respected, from meaningful relationships with others, and from finding meaning in their lives.[37] Exploring these with the patient over time may help to foster realistic hope. Although physicians may have a desire to make an overly reassuring statement to the patient right after revealing the diagnosis,[14,32] hopeful statements that are truthful and that are made after taking the time to explore the patient's concerns first are more likely to be accepted by the patient.

One final statement should be made about how specific one needs to be about the prognosis or outcome of the illness. Most doctors have no difficulty bringing this subject up if there is a reasonable chance that medical treatment can cure the illness. It becomes more difficult if treatment is very unlikely to affect the course of the disease or, at best, can slow its progression. Just as it is not necessary to provide complete medical information at first encounter, it is not necessary to give the patient all the prognostic information available at this meeting. Prognostic information can be given in small chunks, like other medical information, and often in response to the patient's questions.

We believe that physicians should rarely try to be very precise when giving prognostic information. Stories abound of patients whose doctors told them they had only "2 months to live" and who, years later, can (fortunately) joke about the story. When giving prognostic information, physicians can be truthful and tell patients what they need to know without destroying all hope.[11,29] For example, in the case of a patient whom the doctor believes has only a few months to live, the doctor could explain: "You need to know that every situation is different, and I can only tell you what usually happens, not what will happen to you. Most people in your situation live only a few months. Of course, some live longer than that." This gives the patient the opportunity to plan for his or her death but maintains some hope at the same time. Notice that the doctor in this example avoids using statistical terminology such as *mean* or *median* (or even *average*) that can be easily misunderstood.

There are times when physicians must provide quantitative prognostic information, either because the patient insists or because it will help the patient make rational treatment decisions. How one frames the prognosis may affect how a patient will perceive his or her status. For example, patients' acceptance of treatment depends in part on whether prognoses are presented as a probability of success or a probability of dying.[38–40] Therefore, physicians should try to frame probabilities in both ways. An example would be to say, "Sixty percent of patients who receive this treatment are alive after five years, and forty percent die."

Discussing a bad prognosis when the diagnosis is known

Much of the discussion above assumes that the patient is receiving a bad diagnosis. Nevertheless, many of the same principles apply if the patient already knows the diagnosis, but events have unfolded such that the physician now must share news of a bad prognosis.

Preparation is still critical. The physician should set up an appointment with the patient to discuss "where things are heading," and should suggest that the patient take along a trusted family member or friend if he or she wishes. The physician should open the discussion by asking the patient how he or she is doing and where the patient thinks things are heading. The physician should take cues from the patient in directing the conversation further. If the patient perceives that he or she is not doing well or may die soon, the physician can express personal concerns about the direction things have taken, explore the patient's emotions about it, and begin to make a plan such as referral for palliative or hospice care.

If the patient believes that he or she is doing well or will get better, the physician is in the awkward position of needing to inform the patient about the condition without destroying the hope that may be allowing the patient to function. One good response might be just to repeat back, "You really think things are getting better?" Often patients' claims that things are getting better are statements of hope rather than statements of belief. The response given above gently assists the patient in distinguishing between the two.

It may be necessary to provide the patient with objective information about the condition while assessing the patient's reaction. For example, the doctor might say, "Unfortunately, the tumor continues to grow despite the chemotherapy" and stop to assess the patient's reaction. The doctor might continue, "I don't think that more chemotherapy will help." A communication technique that helps the physician to remain aligned with the patient while giving unpleasant and unexpected news is to frame statements as "I wish. . . ." For example, the physician might say, "I wish that chemotherapy would help this cancer, but, unfortunately, at this stage, it will only make you sicker." It is important to acknowledge the patient's (and doctor's) sadness about this news.

Dealing with patients' responses

Patients may react to physicians' telling them that they have a poor prognosis in many different ways. Responses have been classified into three categories: psychophysiologic, cognitive, and affective.[10] Psychophysiologic responses include the sympathetic fight or flight response, producing a need to get up and walk around, to flee the room, or to take some immediate action. The parasympathetic, conservation-withdrawal reaction, on the other hand, causes the patient to become quiet, withdrawn, and "numb."[10] The observant physician should recognize these different reactions and tailor his or her approach to the patient's need. The doctor can aid the patient who needs to take immediate action by helping to lay out a precise plan of care, such as referral to a specialist or further testing, making tentative plans, but avoiding irreversible decisions until these patients have time to reflect on their decision. On the other hand, the patient who reacts by shutting down does not need information or a detailed action plan. This patient needs compassionate hand holding, with a plan to get back together in a day or two for more discussion.

The emotional responses patients may exhibit include anger, grief, guilt, fear, and anxiety, to name a few.[10] It is important to let the patient express these feelings and to explore what underlies them.[11,31] Once the emotions are evident, the physician can begin to provide support. Some physicians are afraid of strong emotions because they do not know how to handle them. There may be a strong impulse to try to make the emotion "go away" by providing false reassurance, launching into a biomedical discussion, or referring the patient to counseling. This sends a message to the patient that the physician does not want to hear about his or her emotions, isolating the patient. Doctors need to be able to employ active listening skills, to be comfortable to "sit with the emotion," in order to be able to provide emotional support. The NURSE acronym[41] (Table 4.3) provides a useful mnemonic for physicians trying to improve their skills in this area. It provides a road map for physicians when they confront strong emotions. Not all of the elements always need to be present, and they do not need to be used in

Table 4.3. NURSE-ing an emotion

Name the emotion

Understand the emotion

Respect or praise the patient

Support the patient

Explore what underlies the emotion

any particular order. The acronym reminds physicians to name the emotion that the patient is demonstrating. Physicians should communicate to the patient that they understand how the patient can feel that way. Physicians should make a comment respecting or praising the patient. Physicians should make a statement to support the patient, indicating that they are willing to "hang in there" with the patient. Finally the physician should explore the emotion with the patient. Here is an example of a discussion with a patient with cirrhosis of the liver who is being told that his condition has worsened and that he will probably die soon.

> *Patient becomes tearful.*
> Physician: I see this makes you sad. (Name)
> Patient: Of course I am sad.
> Physician: This is difficult news to hear. I can understand why it would make you sad. (Understand)
> Patient: I don't want to die. *Starts crying.*
> *Physician hands patient a tissues; reaches over and touches her hand.* (Support)
> Patient: I'm sorry. I can't believe I'm crying this way.
> Physician: It's all right. I think you are handling all this very well, all things considered. Take your time. (Respect) *After a few moments.* When different people think about dying, different things make them sad. What makes you sad when you think about dying? (Explore)
> Patient: I wanted to see my grandchildren.
> Physician: I understand. It must be hard to realize that you aren't going to be able to see them. (Understand) I want you to know we will work with you to ensure you have as much quality time with your family as possible. (Support)

One way of exploring the patient's reactions to news of a bad diagnosis or prognosis is to elicit the meaning of the diagnosis for the patient. Patients bring their own beliefs and knowledge about diseases like cancer and heart disease, which they get from reading and from experience with friends and family members. These beliefs, particularly if factually incorrect, can cause unwarranted anxiety and may interfere with rational decision making.[29] Therefore, it is crucial to explore the patient's beliefs and emotions surrounding the diagnosis. Questions like "Has anyone close to you had cancer?" or "Many people with cancer worry about how it will affect their lives or relationships. What questions do you have?" or "What are you most concerned about now?" will help to get at these fears. This is illustrated in the following conversation, in which the doctor is telling his patient that he has prostate cancer.

> Patient: I'm not going to have surgery. I'm telling you that right now!
> Physician: What is it about surgery that bothers you so much?
> Patient: Well, my uncle had surgery for . . . um . . . some cancer down there . . . and after he, well, he had to . . . um . . . well, he couldn't go to the bathroom the normal way . . . he . . . uh . . . had to wear a bag . . .
> Physician: So you're afraid that that will happen to you.
> Patient nods.

Physician: I think that your uncle had colon cancer. You have prostate cancer, which is completely different. We should do surgery to remove your prostate, but you will still be able to have bowel movements the normal way afterward.

Of the various cognitive responses to bad news, including blame, disbelief, and intellectualization,[27] the one that causes the most discomfort for physicians is denial. Denial performs a very important role for patients, defending them against intense and perhaps overpowering anxiety. Denial protects patients from emotional disintegration in the face of severe psychological trauma, allowing them to continue to carry on necessary daily activities while they come to terms with the reality of their illness.[30] Patients in denial are generally aware on some level of their situation but are unable to be explicit about it. The emphasis on truth-telling in our society leads some physicians to believe that if the patient is unable to repeat back, in detail, a grim diagnosis and prognosis, the physician has failed in his or her duty to inform. This is unfortunate. It is true that the physician must truthfully present patients with the facts. Nevertheless, when patients indicate their need to use denial as a defense, physicians may do them great harm by refusing to recognize its value.

If denial is a psychological defense that protects individuals from bad news, one can help the patient by making it safer to talk about the emotions that the illness may raise. One can understand hope without endorsing it ("I understand how badly you want to get better"). One can gently assess whether the patient is ready to talk about the news ("Have you thought about what we will do if things do not go well?"). One can attempt to delineate the patient's possible fears or concerns in a neutral manner ("Some patients with COPD are worried about not being able to breathe"). When giving information, it is safest to give small pieces of information that very gradually inform the patient of the changing prognosis. Over time, especially with attention to the underlying sources of the patient's anxiety, most patients are able to come to terms with their situation.[29]

There are times when denial can interfere with rational decision making, causing the patient who is overly optimistic to seek out care that is not beneficial or perhaps harmful. Therefore, doctors need strategies to help patients make rational decisions without destroying an important defense mechanism. One way is to acknowledge that one can always hope for the best but that one needs to be prepared for the worst. Therefore, a patient can hope to get better, but must still understand that in the event that the illness does cause a cardiac arrest, a resuscitation effort would not be effective. The patient may be able to make other advance, care plans too, using this model, without being forced to give up all hope.

Dealing with difficult questions

Some of the most difficult questions patients ask are related to their prognosis. "How long do I have to live?" is a classic question that makes physicians uncomfortable because it seems to ask for information that is unknowable.[29] There may be many different meanings behind a question like this, so it is important, as always, to elicit the concerns that underlie it. "Gee, that is a difficult question. What are you worried about?" might be a good response. It is impossible for physicians to predict when someone will die. By probing for the concerns underlying the question, the physician may be able to allow the patient to express underlying concerns. Ultimately, many patients who are dying need some estimate of their time left so that they can make plans. Physicians must be clear about the limitations of prognostication for any particular patient.[29] Acknowledging that it is difficult to live with uncertainty may be helpful.

A related question is "What are my chances, doctor?" This question is actually more ambiguous than it sounds. Is the patient referring to the chances of cure, of remission, of a treatment response, or of survival? If the last, is it survival for 6 months, 1 year, or 5 years? The physician will do well to probe further to find out exactly what the patient is asking before endeavoring to answer. The same strategies used for questions about how long one has to live apply to this question.

A frequent question patients have is "Why me?" Physicians confronted with this question must be careful to explore in an open-ended and nonjudgmental manner what the patient thinks may have caused the illness. Patients may believe that they brought their illness on themselves or that they are being punished. It is important to listen carefully to the patient in order to be able to provide appropriate support and comfort. Physicians often can help the patient best by recommending that spiritual and religious concerns such as these be discussed with a member of the clergy or a spiritual advisor.

Wrapping up

There are a few issues that the doctor needs to attend to when wrapping up the visit. Doctors should tell patients that they expect that they will not remember some of the details that were discussed and that they are sure that the patient will have many questions. It helps to give the patient a written summary of the key points that were discussed. If a new diagnosis is involved, doctors should generally set up a follow-up meeting within 24 to 48 hrs to discuss the situation further, make more detailed plans, and answer any questions. The patient should be invited to ask family members or friends to come if necessary.

Doctors also need to consider what will happen to the patient when he or she leaves the office. A patient who has been told about a new diagnosis or has just realized how poor the prognosis is leaves the office fundamentally changed. A person with a new cancer diagnosis, for example, walked into the office essentially healthy and left the office with cancer. Doctors should ask the patient what people are around with whom he or she can talk. They also should offer to speak to significant others about the patient's situation.[11] Information about support services, like support groups and chaplains, should be given.[11] Finally, since there is an increased risk of suicide after receiving bad news, doctors should assess this risk as well.[27]

Conclusion

Discussing a poor prognosis with a patient is a difficult but critical task in caring for dying patients. Physicians must make the proper preparations prior to the encounter during which they will share the information. It helps to find out what the patient is thinking about the situation. This is best done at previous encounters before delivering the news of a poor prognosis. The delivery must be truthful, simple, and clear but sensitive. Information should be presented in small amounts, with ample opportunity for the patient to respond. The physician must pay careful attention to the patient's emotional response, providing emotional support as much as possible. If unexpected news has been given, a follow-up visit should be arranged within a few days to review the information provided and make treatment decisions.

References

1. Weeks JC, Cook EF, O'Day SJ. Relationship between cancer patients' predictions of prognosis and their treatment preferences. *JAMA* 1998; 279:1709–1714.
2. Smith TJ, Swisher K. Telling the truth about terminal cancer. *JAMA* 1998; 279:1746–1748.
3. Christakis NA, Sachs GA. The role of prognosis in clinical decision making. *J Gen Intern Med* 1996; 11:422–425.
4. Weissman DE. Consultation in palliative medicine. *Arch Intern Med* 1997; 157:733–737.
5. McCormick TR, Conley BJ. Patients' perspective on dying and on the care of dying patients. *West J Med* 1995; 163:236–243.
6. Lind SE, Good MD, Seidel S, et al. Telling the diagnosis of cancer. *J Clin Oncol* 1989; 7:583–589.
7. Fallowfield LJ, Hall A, Maguire P, et al. Psychological outcomes of different treatment policies in women with early breast cancer outside a clinical trial. *Br Med J* 1990; 301:575–580.
8. Parle M, Jones B, Maguire P. Maladaptive coping and affective disorders in cancer patients. *Psychol Med* 1996; 26:735–744.
9. Seale C. Communication and awareness about death: A study of a random sample of dying people. *Soc Sci Med* 1991; 32:943–952.
10. Fallowfield LJ. Giving sad and bad news. *Lancet* 1993; 341:476–478.
11. Girgis A, Sanson-Fisher RW. Breaking bad news: consensus guidelines for medical practioners. *J Clin Oncol* 1995; 13:2449–2456.
12. Razavi D, Delvaux N, Hopwood P. Improving communication with cancer patients: a challenge for physicians. *Ann New York Acad Sci* 1997; 809:350–360.
13. Strauss RP, Sharp MC, Lorch SC, et al. Physicians and the communication of "bad news": parent experiences of being informed of their child's cleft lip and/or palate. *Pediatrics* 1995; 96:82–89.
14. Buckman R. Breaking bad news: why is it still so difficult? *Br Med J* 1984; 288:1597–1599.

15. Christakis NA, Iwashyna TJ. Attitude and self-reported practice regarding prognosti-
    cation in a national sample of internists. *Arch Intern Med* 1999; 158:2389–2395.
16. Christakis NA. The ellipses of prognosis in modern medical thought. *Soc Sci Med*
    1997; 44:301–315.
17. Christakis NA. Predicting patient survival before and after hospice enrollment. *Hos-
    pice J* 1998; 13:71–87.
18. Parkes CM. Accuracy of predictions of survival in later stages of cancer. *Br Med J* 1972;
    2:29–31.
19. Lynn J. An 88-year-old woman facing the end of life (clinical crossroads). *JAMA* 1997;
    277:1633–1640.
20. Lynn J, Harrell F Jr, Cohn F, et al. Prognoses of seriously ill hospitalized patients on
    the days before death: implications for patient care and public policy. *New Hori-
    zons* 1997; 5:56–61.
21. Novack DH, Plumer R, Smith RL, et al. Changes in physicians' attitudes toward telling
    the cancer patient. *JAMA* 1979; 241:897–900.
22. Sell L, Devlin B, Bourke SJ, et al. Communicating the diagnosis of lung cancer. *Respir
    Med* 1993; 87:61–63.
23. Chan A, Woodruff RK. Communicating with patients with advanced cancer. *J Palliat
    Care* 1997; 13:29–33.
24. Krahn GI, Hallum A, Kime C. Are there good ways to give "bad news"? *Pediatrics*
    1993; 91:578–582.
25. Peter JR, Abrams HE, Ross DM, et al. Presenting a diagnosis of cancer: patients'
    views. *J Family Pract* 1991; 32:577–581.
26. Ptacek JT, Eberhardt TL. Breaking bad news: a review of the literature. *JAMA* 1996;
    276:496–502.
27. Quill TE, Tounsend P. Bad news: delivery, dialogue, and dilemmas. *Arch Intern Med*
    1991; 151:463–468.
28. Carnes JW, Brownlee, HJ Jr. The disclosure of the diagnosis of cancer. *Med Clin
    North Am* 1996; 80:145–151.
29. Miranda J, Brody RV. Communicating bad news. *West J Med* 1992; 156:83–85.
30. Myers BA. The informing interview: enabling parents to "hear" and cope with bad
    news. *Am J Disabled Children* 1983; 137:572–577.
31. Fallowfield LJ, Clark AW. Delivering bad news in gastroenterology. *Am J Gastroen-
    terol* 1994; 89:473–479.
32. Maguire P. Breaking bad news. *Eur J Surg Oncol* 1998; 24:188–199.
33. Buckman R. Breaking bad news: a six-step protocol. In: *How to Break Bad News: A
    Guide for Health Care Professionals.* Baltimore: Johns Hopkins University Press,
    1992:65–97.
34. Blackhall LJ, Murphy ST, Frank G, et al. Ethnicity and attitudes toward patient
    autonomy. *JAMA* 1995; 274:820–825.
35. Maguire P, Faulkner A. Communicate with cancer patients: 1. Handling bad news and
    difficult questions. *Br Med J* 1988; 297:907–909.
36. Dunn SM, Patterson PU, Butow PN, et al. Cancer by another name: A randomized
    trial of the effects of euphemism and uncertainty in communicating with cancer
    patients. *J Clin Oncol* 1993; 11:989–996.
37. Herth K. Fostering hope in terminally-ill people. *J Adv Nurs* 1990; 15:1250–1259.
38. O'Connor AM, Boyd NF, Tritchler DL, et al. Eliciting preferences for alternative

cancer drug treatments: the influence of framing, medium, and rater variables. *Med Decis Making* 1985; 5:453–463.

39. O'Connor AM. Effects of framing and level of probability on patients' preferences for cancer chemotherapy. *J Clin Epidemiol* 1989; 42:119–126.

40. McNeil BJ, Pauker SG, Sox HC Jr, et al. On the elicitation of preferences for alternative therapies. *N Engl J Med* 1982; 306:1259–1262.

41. Smith RC. Facilitating skills. In: *The Patient's Story: Integrated Patient-Doctor Interviewing.* Boston: Little, Brown and Co. 1996:13–24.

II
EDUCATION AND TRAINING
IN PALLIATIVE CARE

5

Palliative Care Audit: Tools, Objectives, and Models for Training in Assessment, Monitoring, and Review

IRENE J. HIGGINSON AND JULIE HEARN

Palliative care arose out of a desire to improve the quality of care for patients with advancing disease and their families. As a new specialty, and in the face of skepticism or reluctance to support this form of care, evaluations were carried out early in the history of modern palliative care provision to compare hospice services to home and hospital care.[1–4] Hence, palliative care specialists have often led the way in developing methods to examine the quality of care of patients with cancer, and have sought to influence those working in oncology and other professions.[4,5]

The early evaluations were limited to a few exemplary centers, and the methodological difficulties in carrying out effectiveness research in palliative care[6] has so far prevented investigators from obtaining a clear idea of which models of care work best and for which types of disease palliative care is most effective. Those providing care and those purchasing palliative care services will need to know which interventions and in what combination work best, for what kinds of patients and families, and in which type of localities.[4] Hospices and palliative care services bring new therapies to patients, such as advanced symptom control, counseling, or complementary therapies. These new therapies need to be evaluated and audited; otherwise, hospices' resources and patients' time could be wasted.

What Is Audit?

Audit aims to improve care for patients and families by assessing whether we are doing the right thing well.[7] Effective audit is a cyclical activity and includes three key stages (Fig. 5.1). First, standards for the delivery of care are agreed. Second, practice is observed and compared to the standards. In this stage, success is often demonstrated, but so are failings and the need for change. In the third stage, the results are fed back to those providing care so that new or modified standards can be set. The audit cycle is then carried out once again.[8-11] The cycle can be entered at any point. For example, it is possible to begin by implementing new standards and then carry out an audit to determine if these standards are being met.

Audit can assess the structure (the resources, e.g., number and qualifications of staff), the process (use of resources, such as the number of visits or the drugs prescribed), the output (e.g., throughput, discharge rate), or the outcome of care (the change in the patient's quality of life or health status as a result of care, such as pain control).[12]

Audit in palliative care serves not only aims to improve patient care but also to ensure the effective use of resources.[13] Moreover, it provides the opportunity for high-quality education and training of individuals in the field. This chapter will describe the main tools used, or proposed for use, in assessing the outcomes of palliative care and will focus on how these tools can be used in staff education and training, using the Palliative Care Outcome Scale as an example.

Why perform clinical audit?

Clinical audit is the systematic, critical analysis of the quality of clinical care. Clinical audit grew out of separate medical and nursing audits and is most suited to areas where doctors, nurses, and other staff work in teams, sharing decision making. In palliative care, where ideally the patients' concerns are discussed by all

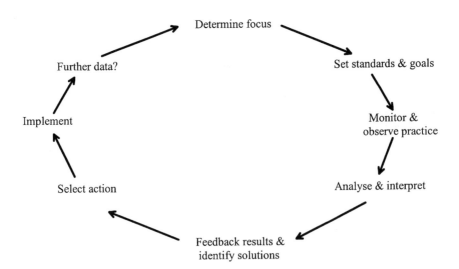

Figure 5.1. The audit cycle.

staff, clinical audit is more appropriate than nursing or medical audit because it reflects the multiprofessional nature of care.[14]

Audit is important for education and training because the structured review allows analysis, comparison, and evaluation of individual performance; promotes adherence to local clinical policies; and offers an opportunity for publication of the results.[15] Educational programs can be constructed to meet the demonstrated needs of individuals or groups. In the future, audit may also be required for the recognition of training posts. Royal colleges and faculties increasingly seek evidence of formally organized review and can withdraw recognition from departments that do not provide this.

What are the benefits and costs of audit in palliative care?

Clinical audit requires the involvement of staff at all levels, and their cooperation is vital if the audit is to be successful.[14] A survey of attitudes toward audit was recently carried out with 68 palliative care staff attending a half-day audit workshop. The study found that those taking part had a positive attitude toward audit, citing its main advantage as a method of evaluating their professional work and highlighting good and bad points.[16] The concerns of the staff were related to the amount of time needed for the audit and whether or not its findings would be acted on. Staff identified several key areas necessary to ensure the continuation of audit, including the need for information and feedback, motivation, assistance, and support.

The persons attending this audit workshop may not accurately reflect the views of other palliative care staff as a result of the bias inherent in using a sample motivated or supported enough to attend a workshop. However, their views were supported by those of the medical or nursing directors of 28 palliative care units in the former North West Thames Regional Health Authority.[17] In this postal survey, the main advantage given for carrying out any audit project was the improvement or maintenance of the quality of care, followed by evaluation and monitoring of current standards of care. The principal disadvantage expressed was the time-consuming nature of audit. These medical and nursing directors reported the fear that the results, may be used against the team as well as the concern that these results are not implemented quickly enough for staff to realize the benefits of doing the audit.

The key issues, therefore, that need to be considered when trying to get all staff involved are:

1. Incorporating audit into routine practice
2. Sharing responsibility
3. Making time for audit

It is extremely difficult for those purchasing services, such as health insurance organizations or other external bodies, to assess the clinical quality of care. Instead, they need to rely on organizational or environmental standards or, when determining whether the professionals are employing proven high-quality treatments, to examine the staff mix and determine whether a clinical audit program is in place. Audit is important for purchasers of health care because it provides tangible evidence that the service is seeking the most effective use of existing clinical resources and wants to improve the quality of care. This is becoming increasingly important when competing for health care contracts.[18] Audit requirements and the implementation of research findings may well be included in such contracts.[19] However, the costs of *not* auditing are as important as the benefits of auditing.[20,21] The costs and benefits of carrying out an audit are summarized in Table 5.1.

Audit takes time and resources. These should not be underestimated and can include:

- time for all staff to prepare for the audit, to agree on the standards or topic, and to review the findings.
- time for some staff to carry out the audit, analyze its results, and document the findings and any recommendations.
- a commitment by *all* staff—managers, nurses, doctors, and so on—to consider the results and act on them.
- resources to pay for the staff time involved, plus any other analytical or computing support needed.

Because of the high costs of audit, it is important to ensure that the audit itself is as effective as possible. What is the purpose of collected audit data if the changes are not acted on? Mechanisms to review the audit and to ensure its effectiveness are discussed below.

Table 5.1. Benefits and costs of audit

Audit of palliative care can help to improve care in the following ways:

1. Reviewing the quality of work and identifying ways to improve means that future patients and families will not suffer the same problems that occur at present.

2. Identifying areas where care is effective or ineffective allows better targeting of services.

3. Prospective audits with systematic assessments of patients and families during care can help to ensure that:

    - Aspects of care are less likely to be overlooked.
    - There is a holistic approach to care.
    - New staff have a clearer understanding of what areas to address.

4. Audit can help most palliative care patients and their families by focusing on routine practice rather than a few special cases.

The costs of not auditing may include:

1. Extra inappropriate treatment or services, wasting the time and resources of patients and their families, and wasting staff time and resources, which could be used elsewhere.

2. Admission to a hospice or hospital or delay of discharge due to uncontrolled symptom causing suffering to the patient, the family, and the staff.

Table 5.2. Organizational commitments required to complete an audit program

1. Training in audit methods should be available to all clinical staff and audit assistants.
2. Session time should be accounted for in staff contracts according to the frequency, duration, and location of meetings, as well as for preparation and follow-up.
3. Technical and clerical assistance should be available for retrieving, tabulating, and presenting the necessary data for an agreed-on audit.
4. Management should make a commitment to ensure that the findings of the audit are acted on.

What are the barriers to involvement?

Shaw[13] asserts that clinical staff should be provided with the time, technical and clerical assistance, and training required to carry out an agreed audit program (Table 5.2). There are resource implications if these suggestions are implemented.

There is often antipathy toward audit by staff in general. This antipathy is based on arguments such as the following:

- There are no problems because palliative care is high in quality and is self-auditing.
- The outcomes of palliative care cannot be measured.
- Resources, information, and time are not available.
- Audit looks past at practices, not at the problems that lie ahead.

In spite of the resource implications of introducing the solutions outlined in Table 5.2 for these arguments, it is clear that for audit to work, organizational systems such as those suggested need to be in place.

Developing an Audit Program

Training and management

Shaw[9] outlined 10 requirements for the successful management of audit: intention, leadership, participation, control, method, resources, guidelines, comparison, conclusions, and feedback. Audit in palliative care does more than provide a mechanism for monitoring and review. Training in audit methods can provide an opportunity for training staff in palliative care and for improving their assessment of patients, in the same way that the present state examination (PSE) is used as a method for for patient evaluation and student training in history taking in psychiatry.[22] Using audit measures systematically can help ensure that the staff performs a broader assessment of the patient and family. We suggest that staff training in audit should take place in two stages:

1. A basic introduction to audit—objectives, benefits, tools.
2. A focus on advanced skills—motivation, data analysis and interpretation, feedback.

Table 5.3. Questionnaire on staff experience with audit

Please complete the following questionnaire about the audit. The purpose of the questionnaire is to find out about your experience with audit. It should only take a few minutes to complete and will help to plan the training and implementation of audit.

Please check the box or comment as appropriate. Thank you.

1. What is your reaction to the introduction of audit in your unit? *(please check all that apply)*

   - a good idea   ☐
   - might be useful   ☐
   - unsure   ☐
   - more work   ☐
   - more paperwork   ☐
   - more change   ☐
   - of no use   ☐
   - other comments _____

2. What do you think may be the main advantage of audit? _____

3. What do you think might be the main disadvantage of audit? _____

4. Have you ever had any training in audit, e.g., seminars, workshops, formal courses? Yes/No
   If Yes:
   > How long was the course/session? _____
   > What did you cover? _____

5. Have you been involved in any audit previously? Yes/No
   If Yes:
   > Please give further details: _____
   > Was it helpful? Yes/No

6. What do you think is needed to start audit or keep it going? _____

7. What do you think you might be gained by taking part in audit?
   (please consider both yourself and the whole unit) _____

What do staff think and know about audit?

Before training in audit can begin, it is essential to understand how much those involved already know about audit and what their attitudes are. In this way training can be focused, and staff members with prior audit experience can be enlisted to assist with the training sessions. Moreover, the introduction of an audit may be seen as less threatening if comprehensive, targeted training is provided and the teams involved are given the opportunity to discuss their concerns. McKee[23] reported the value of "selling" audit to staff and allowing ample time for discussion and agreement on methods. It this is done, the audit will not be viewed by staff as an imposition by managers—a factor often given as a reason for the difficulties that arise during the audit process.[24]

This applies to staff at all levels of the organization. Training needs to be targeted to needs, and this can be achieved only if the trainer is aware of current attitudes toward and knowledge of audit. Staff attitudes and knowledge can be determined during the initial stages of audit implementation, either through group discussion or by using a simple questionnaire. A group discussion is probably the quickest and easiest way to get an idea of what is known, but those with less experience or bad experiences may be less likely to volunteer this information. A questionnaire could ask what the staff thinks the advantages and disadvantages of audit might be, whether they have received any previous training or been involved in any audit, whether they have found audit useful, and what changes they may have seen as a result of any audit. An example of a questionnaire we have used for this purpose is given in Table 5.3.

The process for the first stage of training can be outlined using the mnemonic *ASTRA*:

- *Assess* current knowledge and attitudes.
- *Sell* the reasons for the audit.
- *Target* training to areas of need.
- *Review* concerns and likely problems.
- *Agree* on an audit to be introduced and any further training required.

How can the right people be involved?

It is essential that the audit is implemented using both a bottom-up and a top-down approach; audit meetings can be used to facilitate this. While it would be counterproductive to enforce attendance at audit meetings, participation should be made explicit in staff contracts and the reason for this discussed. Managers and staff need to agree on the time allocated to participation in audit and find ways to incorporate this into the review of staff progress.

The responsibility for audit should be shared by the entire staff, throughout all grades and across all professions. Staff at both ends of the managerial spectrum need to appreciate the concerns of others, and should be given the opportunity to question the purpose of a proposed audit in a nonjudgmental atmosphere. Each member of a team will approach a topic from a different perspective, and the opinions of all should be given equal value, irrespective of who is taking the lead at any stage. Specific time needs to be allocated to audit within the usual working hours, and sufficient coverage provided during this time to reassure the staff that patient care is being maintained. In this way, audit can become part of routine practice, whether once a day, once a week, one every two weeks, or once a month. Those unable to attend audit meetings should be updated by a named colleague, or audit "buddy," whom they have agreed to liaise with in order to keep informed.

How should we go about starting audit?

The initial stages of audit are very important and often determine whether the audit is a success. The mnemonic *SPREE* can be used for guidance when starting audit:

- *Small:* When audit is introduced it should be inexpensive and simple, and cause minimum disruption of routine care. It is better to begin small and expand as audit becomes established.
- *Plan:* There should be a clear audit plan and a commitment to it by all staff. This requires leadership from senior staff and participation of all staff, plus a clear view of how the audit will evolve. There should be discussion among all staff about the audit plan at an early stage.
- *Regular:* Audit meetings, data collection, and the review of results must occur regularly; otherwise, these may become lost in other aspects of care.
- *Exchange:* It is helpful to exchange ideas within the audit group and with other groups locally to learn of each other's successes and mistakes.
- *Enjoy:* This is perhaps the most important aspect of audit. The intention of audit must be educational and relevant to clinical care. It is important that staff do not see audit as a threat, but instead feel that they own it. This attitude can be promoted if participation is voluntary and if the staff feel that they have had a hand in developing or choosing the methods.

For audit to be successful it is important to be able to measure successfully what we intend to audit. Some of the key issues to keep in mind are included in the mnemonic *BRAVE*:

- *Borrow* standards, methods, and measures from others to save time and resources, if possible, and adapt these to local circumstances as necessary. Developing new measures and standards can be very time-consuming. It may lead to "reinventing the wheel" and developing a standard or measure similar to one already published.
- *Reliable:* Reliable measures or criteria are needed if more than one person will assess the standards; otherwise, time will be wasted and the results can be meaningless. *Reliability* is the stability and consistency of information provided by the measure, also sometimes referred to as the *precision* of the instrument. A measure is reliable to the extent that repeated measures under constant conditions will give the same result. Reliability can be enhanced by using the measure under controlled conditions, by ensuring that the assessors are adequately trained, by using unambiguous items, and by providing clear rating instructions.[25]
- *Appropriate:* Appropriate standards and measures are needed so that the staff feel that the work in their setting is being assessed accurately.
- *Valid:* Measures and criteria that accurately assess what the investigator sets out to measure are important if the audit is to be effective and to achieve the goal of improving the care of the patient and family. Validity has a number of components,[26] and measures shown to be valid must also have some demonstrable reliability. Note: a measure may be totally reliable but not valid at all!
- *Easy:* The methods must be simple enough to be understood and applied

in routine practice. Ideally, information for an audit should be collected in monthly, weekly, or daily practice.

Tools for Clinical Audit in Palliative Care

A systematic literature review of outcome measures in palliative care for advanced cancer patients identified 12 potential clinical audit tools.[27] Information on these tools came from a comprehensive search of published literature, with the assistance of a multiprofessional steering group, through personal communications with other professionals working in palliative care, and from an investigation of the grey (unpublished) literature. Measures were considered suitable if they met the following criteria:

1. The target population included cancer patients, or patients with advanced disease receiving palliative care, or was considered by the authors to be appropriate for this patient group.
2. The measure contained more than one domain.
3. The measure could be used with patients who had all types of cancer.

To summarize the 12 measures: 3 are completed by a professional,[28–30] 7 by the patient alone,[31–37] and 2 contain both patient and professional completion elements[38,39]; 8 assess items relating only to the patient,[28,31–35,37,39] and 4 may also consider the family/carer unit[29,30,36,38]; 7 have been validated in just one setting, 5 contain 30 or more items, and 2 were designed for the assessment of clinical trial interventions. These measures are described in more detail below; their validity and reliability are summarized in Table 5.4.

Initial Assessment of Suffering[32]

This measure was developed on the basis of interviews of 259 advanced cancer patients in acute hospitals. A 5-point Likert scale with scores ranging from 5 ("good") to 1 ("bad") was used to record the answers to 43 questions either by the patient or by a trained nurse interviewer. The questions have been refined to give a shorter 20-item questionnaire suitable for use during the initial assessment by any member of the hospice/palliative care team.

Edmonton Symptom Assessment Schedule (ESAS)[34]

The ESAS was developed for quick assessment of outcomes in routine practice. It consists of nine Visual Analogue Scales (VASs). Patients draw a mark along a 100-mm line corresponding to how they feel, with the left end of the line corresponding to the mildest degree of symptoms, and the far right to the most intense symptoms. The ESAS is completed on admission to the hospital and twice daily thereafter, either by the patient alone or with the assistance of a nurse.

Table 5.4. Measures for assessing the outcome of palliative care patients are people with advanced cancer

Name of measure	Number of items and domains covered	Validity	Reliability	Responsiveness to change	Setting	Appropriateness of format	
						Time	Administration
Initial Assessment of Suffering[32]	43 (patient); mood, symptoms, fears and family worries, knowledge and involvement, support	Correlates with Spitzer Quality of Life Index of physical health	Internal consistency	Stable over time	Inpatient	Not known	Patient completion or by professional interview
Edmonton Symptom Assessment Schedule (ESAS)[34]	9 (patient); pain activity, nausea, depression, anxiety, drowsiness, appetite, well-being, shortness of breath	Correlates with STAS (except for activity)	Interrater consistency (0.5–0.9)	Improvement demonstrated in palliative care	Inpatient	A few minutes	Patient completion or with nurse assistance
European Organisation for Research on Treatment of Cancer (EORTC QLQ-C30)[35]	30 (patient); 9 multi-item scales including 5 functional scales, 3 symptom scales, and a global quality of life scale	Interscale correlation; correlates with clinical status	Internal consistency (0.54–0.86)	Palliative care module being evaluated in Europe	Outpatient	11–12 min	Patient completion
Hebrew Rehabilitation Center for Aged Quality of Life Index (-HRCA-QL)[28] (Morris et al, 1986)	5 (patient); mobility, daily living, health, attitude, support	Correlates with single and Multi scale version and with the Karnofsky Performance Index	Internal consistency (0.77) and interrater (0.6–0.81)	Scores correlate with survival	Community inpatient	1–2 min	Professional completion
McGill Quality of Life Questionnaire (MQOL)[37]	17 (patient); physical symptoms, psychological symptoms, outlook on life and meaningful existence	Correlates with Spitzer Quality of Life and Symptom Impact Scale (SIS)	Internal consistency (0.89)	Distinguishes between patients	Inpatient, outpatient	Not known	Patient completion

Instrument	Validity	Reliability	Responsiveness	Setting	Time	Completion
McMaster Quality of Life Scale (MQLS)[39]	32 (patient); physical symptoms, functional status, social functioning, emotional status, cognition, sleep and rest, energy and vitality, general life satisfaction, meaning of life	Correlates with Spitzer Quality of Life Index	Internal consistency (0.62–0.79) interrater consistency (0.83–0.95)	Changes in scores were related to whether patients felt they had changed	community, inpatient, outpatient	Patients, 3–30 min; staff, <3 min; family, ~3 min	Patient, family, or staff completion
Palliative Care Assessment (PACA)[30]	12 (patient and relatives); symptom control, insight, and future placement	Symptom scores correlate with the McCorkle Symptom Distress Scale	Interrater consistency (0.44–1)	Improvement demonstrated in palliative care	Inpatient	A few minutes	Professional completion
Palliative Care Core Standards - PCCS (Hunt, 1993)	6 core standards and 56 process and outcome items (patient and carer); symptom control, information, support, bereavement care and emotional support, specialist education for staff	currently being tested	Currently being tested	Not evaluated	Inpatient	Expected to take ~10 min	Professional, patient, carer, and the bereaved complete separate questionnaires
Rotterdam Symptom Checklist (RSCL)[33]	34 (patient); physical and psychosocial symptoms	Interscale correlation for psychological dimension, less for physical distress items	Internal consistency (0.82–0.88)	Not evaluated	Outpatient	8 min	Patient completion

(continued)

Table 5.4. Measures for assessing the outcome of palliative care patients are people with advanced cancer—Continued

Name of measure	Number of items and domains covered	Validity	Reliability	Responsiveness to change	Appropriateness of format Setting	Time	Administration
Support Team Assessment Schedule (STAS)[29]	17 (patient and carer); pain and symptom control insight, psychosocial, family needs, planning affairs, home services communication, and support of other professionals	Correlates with patients' and families' ratings and with HRCA-QL	Interrater consistency (0.65–0.94) Internal consistency (0.68–0.89) Test-retest consistency (0.36–0.76)	Improvement demonstrated in palliative care	Community, hospice	2 min	Professional completion
Symptom Distress Scale (SDS)[31]	13 (patient); nausea, mood, loss of appetite, insomnia, pain, mobility, fatigue, appearance, bowel pattern, concentration	Correlates with global quality of life measures	Internal consistency (0.78–0.89)	Sensitive to changes in treatment over time	Inpatient	Not known	Patient completion in presence of an interviewer
The Schedule for the Evaluation of Individual Quality of Life (SEIQoL)[36]	5 domains chosen by the individuals; 30 hypothetical scenarios rated based on these domains, and weights are derived for each domain	Correlates with McMaster health index questionnaire subscales for health status and physical function	Internal consistency (0.48–0.74) Internal validity (0.62–0.79)	Does not distinguish between patients and controls before treatment)	Community; inpatient	Not known	Patient completion as part of a structured interview

Patients who are unable to respond due to cognitive failure are assessed by their nurse or a specially trained family member. The score for each item is recorded on a bar graph, allowing the staff to visualize patterns of symptom control over time. Further testing of the validity and reliability of the ESAS are required, particularly with reference to the potential bias introduced by a change in the person recording the answers on the VASs as care continues.

European Organization for Research on Cancer Treatment (EORTC QLQ-C30)[35]

Developed with lung cancer patients to evaluate the quality of life of those patients participating in international clinical trials, this self-report questionnaire is both a reliable and a valid measure of the quality of life of cancer patients in research settings. Questions cover the past week, and responses are mainly in the format of a straightforward 4-point Likert Scale ranging from 1 ("not at all") to 4 ("very much"). The questionnaire contains a generic core with cancer-specific modules, and work is being done to extend it for use with patients with more advanced cancer. At present, some questions are thought to be inappropriate for this patient group and have caused distress in patients with advanced disease in a French community setting (LaGabrielle D, personal communication).

Hebrew Rehabilitation Centre for Aged Quality of Life (HRCA-QL)[28]

This instrument was adapted from the Spitzer Quality of Life Index (a scale developed for doctors to measure the quality of life of their cancer patients), with the item activity being replaced by mobility for the older target patient group. It has not been re-validated and has been criticized for lack of responsiveness in patients with advanced disease. Ratings for each item are scored from 0 to 2 to give a total score ranging 0 to 10 (higher scores indicate a better quality of life). It has been used to evaluate treatments and support services.

McGill Quality of Life Questionnaire (MQOL)[37]

Developed for advanced cancer patients treated at home or in an inpatient unit, the MQOL was designed to measure overall quality of life in patients with a life-threatening illness and to indicate the areas in which the patient is doing well or poorly. The patient circles a number on a 10-point categorical scale, with the least desirable and most desirable extremes at either end. The MQOL includes an existential domain that the authors propose plays a greater role in determining quality of life in patients with local or metastatic disease than in patients with no evidence of disease.

McMaster Quality of Life Scale (MQLS)[39]

This scale was developed on 83 patients to measure the quality of life in a palliative patient population, including cancer patients. Items are rated on a 7-point numerical scale, with the direction of positive and negative descriptors varied. The MQLS is currently being refined, and patients are now asked which 10 items of the scale are most important to their quality of life. Patients who begin to experience difficulty filling in answers are then asked to rate only these 10 most important items.

Palliative Care Assessment (PACA)[30]

The PACA was developed on 125 patients to assess the outcome of interventions made within 2 weeks of referral to a hospital palliative care team. The form comprises three rating scales. Symptoms are scored on a 4-point scale from 0 ("absent") to 3 ("daily life dominated by the symptom") assessing the severity of each symptom from the patient's perspective using a semistructured interview. Insight is assessed by an observer on a 5-point scale, and questions about plans for future care are asked of the patient and recorded on a 4-point scale. Facilitation of appropriate placement for hospital patients is a fundamental element of this measure.

Palliative Care Core Standards (PCCS)[38]

Originally a set of standards for inpatient hospice care and community teams, this tool has been refined and is currently being piloted in inpatient units as separate questionnaires for all those involved with the patient's well-being, including professionals, the patient, and the carer. Structure, process, education, and training are also covered, resulting in a comprehensive but lengthy tool.

Rotterdam Symptom Checklist (RSCL)[33]

Developed primarily as a tool to measure the symptoms reported by cancer patients participating in clinical research, this questionnaire uses a 4-point Likert scale to record responses on the trouble caused by various symptoms over the past 3 days or 1 week. Categories range from "not at all" to "very much." The authors suggest that it may be useful in the evaluation of supportive care, but it may be inappropriate for patients to complete as disease advances.[40]

Support Team Assessment Schedule (STAS)[29]

Developed for use with multidisciplinary cancer support teams, STAS is a validated measure of the effectiveness of palliative care. Items were developed by cancer support teams to reflect the goals of palliative care. The effect of the items on the daily life of the patient over the last week is scored by a professional on a 5-point Likert scale ranging from 0 ("none"—no effect) to 4 ("overwhelming effect"). STAS is widely used in community settings, and has been adapted for use in inpatient settings and to assess individual symptoms.

Symptom Distress Scale (SDS)[31]

This scale was developed for patients with a life-threatening disease, either cancer or heart disease, and can be used for all types of cancer. The scale is self-administered (usually in the presence of an interviewer), with responses rated on a 5-point Likert scale ranging from 1 ("no distress") to 5 ("extreme distress"). It concentrates mainly on the patient's symptoms and mood in relation to quality of life.

Schedule for the Evaluation of Individual Quality of Life (SEIQoL)[36]

This measure was developed from the technique of *judgement analysis* to measure patients' level of functioning. It allows respondents to name the five areas of life that are most important to them, rate their level of functioning or satisfaction with each, and indicate the relative importance of each area to their total quality of life. The SEIQoL has been tested with a variety of patient populations and healthy individuals and has recently been reported for clinical use with patients who have human immunodeficiency virus or acquired immune deficiency virus and are managed in general practice.

Measures under development

The purpose of measuring quality of life and the outcomes of patient care are reiterated in Table 5.5. Each of the measures described fulfills the objectives to varying degrees, but none of them does so completely. It is questionable whether any such tool can be developed that will meet all the requirements for patient assessment.

After carrying out the systematic literature review, we used the information obtained on the 12 measures to develop a new outcome measure for clinical audit

Table 5.5. Purposes for measuring the patient's quality of life and the outcomes of patient care

1. To obtain more detailed information about the patient for clinical monitoring in order to aid and improve patient care

2. To audit the care provided by determining whether standards are being met and to identify potential areas for improvement

3. To compare services, or to compare care before and after the introduction of a service, which can be of value in assessing the efficacy and cost effectiveness of a service

4. To analyze data generated using outcome measures and use the data to inform purchasing bodies, thereby securing resources for future services.

in palliative care, the Palliative Care Outcome Scale. Evidence on the validity and reliability of the tool is currently in press. We will use this core audit measure for palliative care as an example of a model for training staff in assessment, monitoring, and review. Other measures described above could also be used for training in the same way.

Training Staff Using the Palliative Care Outcome Scale (POS)

The measure

A variety of clinical audit tools and systems for palliative care have been developed, as described above. Many do not consider quality of life, and many are not applicable across the range of palliative care settings. We have developed a core clinical audit system to measure the outcome of care for patients with advanced cancer and their families and have tested its validity in a variety of settings. The POS was developed from other outcome measures that have been used or proposed for use in the palliative care of patients with advanced cancer.[27] This work was carried out in collaboration with a multidisciplinary steering group. The steering group consisted of representatives of the main palliative care organizations in the United Kingdom covering the range of professionals involved in providing palliative care, plus a patient representative and local researchers involved in similar projects. The original questionnaire was pilot tested on 25 patients from five of the centers. The questionnaire was revised accordingly to yield the final version, and then was validated using data from 450 patients receiving care from eight palliative care units in England and Scotland.

The POS consists of a core of 10 items covering the physical, psychological, and spiritual domains of life within the remit of palliative care, along with room to write down main problems (Table 5.6). A box is checked in reply to each item, and answers are scored on a 5-point Likert scale ranging from 0 for no problem to 4 representing an overwhelming problem. There is a staff-completed version of the questionnaire and a patient-completed version for use by those patients who are able to contribute. Data can therefore be gathered on all patients by the staff throughout the course of a patient's care, avoiding the problem of incomplete data if only a patient-completed outcome measure is used. However, patients can provide additional input to the measurement of their outcomes if they are able to do so.

Stage 1. Basic training in audit

The objectives and benefits of the audit should be described, as outlined earlier in this chapter and summarized in Table 5.7. The barriers to audit should be explained, along with suggestions on how to overcome them. Trainees should be presented with an overview of the tools available to carry out audit, as described earlier in this chapter. The relevance of these tools to the individual organization

Table 5.6. POS Staff Questionnaire

Patient	Care setting
Assessment No.	Date

Please answer the following questions by checking the box next to the answer that you think most accurately describes how the patients have been feeling. Thank you.

1. Over the past 3 days, has the patient been affected by pain?

   Not at all, no effect ☐ 0

   Slightly—but not bothered to be rid of it ☐ 1

   Moderately—pain limits some activity ☐ 2

   Severely—activities or concentration markedly affected ☐ 3

   Overwhelming—unable to think of anything else ☐ 4

2. Over the past 3 days, have other symptoms (e.g., nausea, coughing, or constipation) seemed to be affecting how they feel?

   No, not at all ☐ 0

   Slightly ☐ 1

   Moderately ☐ 2

   Severely ☐ 3

   Overwhelmingly ☐ 4

3. Over the past 3 days, have they been feeling anxious or worried about their illness or treatment?

   No, not at all ☐ 0

   Occasionally ☐ 1

   Sometimes—affects their concentration now and then ☐ 2

   Most of the time—often affects their concentration ☐ 3

   Patient does not seem to think of anything else—completely preoccupied by worry and anxiety ☐ 4

4. Over the past 3 days, have any of their family or friends been anxious or worried about the patient?

   No, not at all ☐ 0

   Occasionally ☐ 1

   Sometimes—it seems to affect their concentration ☐ 2

   Most of the time ☐ 3

   Yes, they always seem preoccupied with worry ☐ 4

5. Over the past 3 days, how much information has been given to the patients and their families or friends?

   Full information—patient feels free to ask ☐ 0

   Information given but not always understood by patient ☐ 1

   Information given to patient on request—patient would have liked more ☐ 2

   Very little given, and some questions have been avoided ☐ 3

   None at all ☐ 4

(continued)

Table 5.6. POS Staff Questionnaire—Continued

6. Over the past 3 days, have patients been able to share how they are feeling with family or friends?

Yes, as much as they wanted to	☐ 0
Most of the time	☐ 1
Sometimes	☐ 2
Occasionally	☐ 3
No, not at all with anyone	☐ 4

7. Over the past 3 days, do you think they have felt that life was worth living?

Yes, all the time	☐ 0
Most of the time	☐ 1
Sometimes	☐ 2
Occasionally	☐ 3
No, not at all	☐ 4

8. Over the past 3 days, do you think they have felt good about themselves?

Yes, all the time	☐ 0
Most of the time	☐ 1
Sometimes	☐ 2
Occasionally	☐ 3
No, not at all	☐ 4

9. Over the past 3 days, how much time do you feel has been wasted on appointments relating to the health care of this patient (e.g., waiting for transport or repeating tests)?

None at all	☐ 0
Up to half a day wasted	☐ 1
More than half a day wasted	☐ 2

10. Over the past 3 days, have any practical matters resulting from patients illness, either financial or personal, been addressed?

Practical problems have been addressed, and their affairs are as up-to-date as they would wish	☐ 0
Practical problems are in the process of being addressed	☐ 1
Practical problems exist that were not addressed	☐ 2
The patient has had no practical problem	☐ 8

11. If any, what have been the patient's main problems in the last 3 days?

    a. _____

    b. _____

12. What is the patient's ECOG scale performance status?

    (0-fully active; 1-restricted; 2-ambulatory; 3-limited self-care; 4-completely disabled)   ☐

Table 5.7. Objectives, benefits, and difficulties in auditing palliative care

Objectives

1. Need to review a relatively new specialty that is expanding rapidly
2. Personal goal of improving care
3. External pressures to improve
4. Practice varies throughout the country

Benefits

1. The problems of patients and their families are considered in more detail.
2. Staff members are able to monitor the quality of their work and seek ways of improving it.
3. Audit provides a systematic way of thinking about the objectives and outcomes of care.
4. Audit identifies areas where care is effective and ineffective.

Difficulties in implementing change as a result of audit

1. There is inadequate communication of information from those present at the audit meeting to others.
2. It is difficult to ensure that those with hands-on patient contact feel ownership of changes.
3. Difficulties exist if the main communicator is resistant to change.

should be assessed. Boyle and Torrance[41] outlined the following seven points as key criteria in maximizing the usefulness of a measure:

1. Is it easy to apply?
2. Is it acceptable to its responders?
3. Is it brief and inexpensive to administer?
4. Does it use precoded response categories?
5. Does it use an explicit time period of assessment (e.g., today, the last week or month)?
6. Does it use unambiguous instructions for respondents?
7. Does it require prior access to or use of clinical or laboratory services?

The commitment of all organizational or team members to the audit must be obtained before going any further. Both the staff dealing with patients on a day-to-day basis, who will probably be responsible for collecting data and implementing changes in patient care, and those with less patient contact but with the power to implement major changes need to show that they will support the objectives of audit. Well-planned audit meetings can help facilitate this process.

Stage 2. Advanced training in audit using the POS

The individual needs of patients with advanced cancer in day-to-day clinical practice may vary greatly as a result of the diverse nature of the disease.[42] Patients with advanced cancer experience deterioration of physical health over time, as well as a variety of acute complications. Hence, patients with the same primary tumor may have different symptomatology, and patients with different primary tumors may have a common clinical pathway in advanced disease.[6] For this reason, it is important not to rely solely on the control of specific symptoms as a measure of improved outcome. Quality of life therefore also needs to be considered. Quality of life is a multidimensional construct including not only the physical aspects of life, but also the psychological and social domains.[27]

Systematized audit measures can be used to help ensure that the staff performs a broad assessment of patients and their families. The POS can assist in training staff to take a holistic approach to patients and their families. If each item of an audit measure is considered in turn, the key components of palliative care provision can be discussed. The proposed solutions to a problem can be debated, and practice among the staff and across professions can be reviewed. New staff may bring new experience or may need to be introduced to methods they have not previously used. The mechanisms for communication within an organization, and access both to services within the organization and to local agencies, can also be discussed.

The first question on the staff-rated version of the POS questionnaire will now be used to explore in depth the mechanisms to train staff by using an audit tool.

Question 1. Over the past 3 days, has the patient been affected by pain?

Total pain
Using the first question in the questionnaire on the effect of pain provides an opportunity to discuss the concept of *total pain*. Total pain encompasses not only the physical problem, but also the mental attitude, the social circumstances, and the spiritual or existential approach of patients to their perception of pain. The perception of pain is therefore modulated by the patient's mood, the patient's morale, and the meaning of pain for the patient.[43]

The wider picture
Further information can be given at this stage, putting the questionnaire item into the broader context. This may enhance training. For example, information on the epidemiology of pain can illustrate the extent of the problem. Data from 19 studies on the prevalence of pain in advanced or terminal cancer populations reported a combined mean pain prevalence of 72% (range, 53–100%).[44] This problem is not confined to those countries in the developing world where access to pharmacological therapies may be limited. In evaluation studies using the STATS as the outcome measure, of the 695 patients with advanced cancer referred to 11 multidisciplinary teams in the United Kingdom, 70% reported pain to be a problem at the time of referral to the service.[45] These patients had advanced disease and were already receiving medical and nursing care.

Why is pain unrelieved?
Pain and cancer are not synonymous.[43] Evaluation of pain in advanced cancer is primarily clinical and is based on pattern recognition. Attention to detail is necessary to prevent inappropriate treatment.[46] Those evaluating pain in a patient should always believe the patient's report of pain.[47]

Doctors and nurses need to be able to directly assess and treat pain or to know when to refer a patient to other professionals. Fears about morphine or lack of attention to detail in management, coupled with failure to monitor effects and side effects, all contribute to unrelieved pain for the patient with cancer. By discussing the questionnaire item on pain within the context of the audit tool, the staff can be reminded of the mechanisms available to treat a symptom such as pain using both pharmacological and nonpharmacological methods.

Should we implement a standard?
Using an audit tool and training in this way can provide an opportunity to introduce mutually agreed-on standards into practice. The following standards could be set:

1. There must be a full assessment of all patients by the second or third time they are seen by the service unless the patient is unconscious; carry out multiprofessional review if information is incomplete.
2. Any patient with two consecutive ratings of "severe" for any item should undergo a multiprofessional review of management; this can be made more specific for each individual item by outlining suggested action plans.
3. Specific standards can be developed for outcomes to be achieved for specific patient groups (e.g., patients in primary care).

What does severe pain mean?
The concept of pain *severity* also needs to be discussed at this stage. Staff need to be consistent in their rating of an item on an audit tool, not only to ensure that meaningful audit data are collected, but also to facilitate communication between staffing shifts and across professions. Case studies or fictional patients can be used to train the staff to rate patients in the same way. This training should be done in a positive way as a means of improving communication by staff caring for the same patient, not as competition with other staff to get the "right" answer.

"I don't know enough" is not good enough
On beginning an audit, staff members often remark that they are unable to assess an item because they "do not know enough." If this is the case, the audit tool should be used as part of routine note-taking at referral or entry to the service. The above answer would not be satisfactory from any health care professional treating any patient. Staff should recognize that some questions may need input both from patients and from the person who has referred them to the palliative

care service. Standards can be developed, as suggested above, to help ensure that complete information is recorded.

What if a patient is confused?
In cases of patient confusion, it is important to establish whether the confusion is iatrogenic and if the condition reversible. Data cannot easily be collected on severely confused patients, and a the palliative care team must decide how to incorporate such patients into any audit they carry out.

Conclusions

Audit approaches and methods are now well advanced in palliative care, especially in clinical audit. We have a variety of new and proven methods and measures that we can adapt for our own needs, rather than having to undertake much of the development ourselves. Apart from completing the audit cycle, we can use clinical audit for educating and training the staff to work effectively and consistently. Audit can be used to develop clinical protocols for treatment or algorithms to predict patient problems and the need for specialized care.

Audit is perceived by most health professionals as beneficial to a service, but finding the time for an audit can be difficult. Thomson and Barton[48] suggest that this problem can be solved by incorporating the audit into the daily routine. With increasing knowledge and experience, this would become possible as people identify the best and simplest ways to perform particular audits.

Audit is here to stay and is now widely accepted, but it requires resources. Hence it must be sure to benefit patients and families, kept as simple and efficient as possible, and have a strong educational component. Further work is needed to evaluate the impact of different audit approaches and methods on improving care so that we know which approach is most cost-effective. If palliative approaches extend backward to include patients earlier in care, rather than just those close to death, the audit could become a means for clinical dialogue and education among specialties. Palliative medicine staff could take the lead in encouraging this movement, promoting methods among their medical and surgical colleagues and presenting their own results.

References

1. Parkes CM. Terminal care: evaluation of in-patient service at St Christopher's Hospice. Part I. Views of surviving spouse on effects of the service on the patient. *Postgrad Med J* 1979; 55:517–522.
2. Parkes CM. Terminal care: home, hospital, or hospice? *Lancet* 1985; 1:155–157.
3. Hinton J. A comparison of places and policies for terminal care. *Lancet* 1979; 1:29–32.

4. Higginson I. Palliative care: a review of past changes and future trends. *J Public Health Med* 1993; 15(1):3–8.

5. Hodgson CS, Hearn J, Higginson IJ. The role of palliative care in cancer. *Oncol Today* 1997; 16:7–10.

6. Rinck GC, van den Bos GAM, Kleijnen J, et al. Methodologic issues in palliative cancer care: a systematic review. *J Clin Oncol* 1997; 15:1697–1707.

7. Higginson I. Clinical and organisational audit in palliative care. In: Doyle D, Hanks GWC, MacDonald N, eds. *Oxford Textbook of Palliative Medicine,* 2nd ed. Oxford: Oxford University Press, 1998:67–81.

8. Shaw CD. Aspect of audit. 1. The background. *Br Med J* 1980; 280:1256–1258.

9. Shaw CD. *Medical Audit. A Hospital Handbook.* London: King's Fund Centre, 1989.

10. Department of Health. Working for Patients. *Medical Audit: Working Paper 6.* London: HMSO, 1989.

11. Department of Health. *Medical Audit in the Hospital and Community Health Services.* HC(91)2. London: Department of Health, 1991.

12. Donabedian A. *Explorations in Quality Assessment and Monitoring. Volume 1: The Definition of Quality Approaches to Its Assessment.* Michigan: Health Administration Press, 1980.

13. Shaw CD. Introduction to audit in palliative care. In: Higginson I, ed. *Clinical Audit in Palliative Care.* Oxford: Radcliffe Medical Press, 1993:

14. Ford G. Constructive audit. *Palliat Med* 1990; 4:1–2.

15. Shaw CD. Quality assurance in the United kingdom. *Qual Assur Health Care* 1993; 5(2):107–118.

16. Higginson I, Webb D. What do palliative staff think about audit? *J Palliat Care* 1995; 11(3):17–19.

17. Higginson IJ, Hearn J, Webb D. Audit in palliative care: does practice change? *Eur J Cancer Care* 1996; 5:233–236.

18. Clark D, Neale B, Heather P. Contacting for palliative care. *Soc Sci Med* 1995; 40(9):1193–1202.

19. Haines A, Jones R. Implementing findings of research. *Br Med J* 1994; 308:1488–1492.

20. Higginson I. *Quality, Standards, Clinical and Organisational Audit for Palliative Care.* London: National Council for Hospice and Specialist Palliative Care Services, 1992.

21. Higginson I. Clinical audit: getting started, keeping going. In: Higginson I, ed. *Clinical Audit in Palliative Care.* Oxford: Radcliffe Medical Press, 1993:

22. Wing JK. Use and misuse of the PSE. *Br J Psychiatry* 1983; 143:111–117.

23. McKee E. Audit experience: a nurse manager in home care. In: Higginson I, ed. *Clinical Audit in Palliative Care.* Oxford: Radcliffe Medical Press, 1993:128–137.

24. Hunt J. Audit methods: palliative care core standards. In: Higginson I, ed. *Clinical Audit in Palliative Care.* Oxford: Radcliffe Medical Press, 1993:78–87.

25. Moser CA, Kalton G. *Survey Methods in Social Investigation,* 2nd ed. London: Heinemann, 1971.

26. Bowling A. *Research Methods in Health.* Buckingham: Open University Press, 1997.

27. Hearn J, Higginson IJ. Outcome measures in palliative care for advanced cancer patients: a review. *J Pub Health Med* 1997; 19(2):193–199.

28. Morris J, Suissa S, Sherwood S, et al. Last days: a study of the quality of life of terminally ill cancer patients. *J Chronic Dis* 1986; 39:47–62.

29. Higginson I. A community schedule. In: Higginson I, ed. *Clinical Audit in Palliative Care*. Oxford: Radcliffe Medical Press, 1993:34–37.
30. Ellershaw JE, Peat SJ, Boys LC. Assessing the effectiveness of a hospital palliative care team. *Palliat Med* 1995; 9:145–152.
31. McCorkle R, Young K. Development of a symptom distress scale. *Cancer Nurs* 1978; 101:373–378.
32. MacAdam DB, Smith M. An initial assessment of suffering in terminal illness. *Palliat Med* 1987; 1:37–47.
33. de Haes JCJM, van Knippenberg FCE; Neijt JP. Measuring psychological and physical distress in cancer patients: structure and application of the Rotterdam Symptom Checklist. *Br J Cancer* 1990; 62:1034–1038.
34. Bruera E, Kuehn N, Miller MJ, et al. The Edmonton Symptom Assessment System (ESAS): a simple method for the assessment of palliative care patients. *J Palliat Care* 1991; 7(2):6–9.
35. Aaronson NK, Ahmedzai S, Bergman B, et al. The European Organisation for Research and Treatment of Cancer QLQ-C30: a quality-of-life instrument for use in international clinical trials in oncology. *J Natl Cancer Inst* 1993; 85:365–376.
36. O'Boyle CA, McGee H, Joyce CRB. Quality of life: assessing the individual. *Adv Med Soc* 1994; 5:159–180.
37. Cohen SR, Mount BM, Strobel MG, et al. The McGill Quality of Life Questionnaire: a measure of quality of life appropriate for people with advanced disease. A preliminary study of validity and acceptability. *Palliat Med* 1995; 9(3):207–219.
38. Trent Hospice Audit Group. Palliative Core Core Standards; a multi-disciplinary approach. Trent Hospice Audit 1992, c/o Nightingale Macmillan Continuing Care Unit, Trinity Street, Derby, UK.
39. Sterkenburg CA, Woodward CA. A reliability and validity study of the McMaster Quality of Life Scale (MQLS) for a palliative population. *J Palliat Care* 1996; 12(1):18–25.
40. Rathbone GV, Horsley S, Goacher J. A self-evaluated assessment suitable for seriously ill hospice patients. *Palliat Med* 1994; 8(1):29–34.
41. Boyle MH, Torrance GW. Developing multiattribute health indexes. *Med Care* 1971; 22(11):1045–1057.
42. Porzsolt F. Goals of cancer therapy: scope of the problem. *Cancer Treat Rev* 1993; 19(suppl A):3–14.
43. Twycross R. Cancer pain classification. *Acta Anaesth Scand* 1997; 41:141–145.
44. Hearn J, Higginson IJ. Pain associated with cancer. The *Epidemiology of Chronic Pain*. Internal report.
45. Higginson IJ, Hearn J. A multicenter evaluation of cancer pain control by palliative care teams. *J Pain Symptom Manage* 1997; 14:29–35.
46. Twycross R. Attention to detail. *Progr Palliat Care* 1994; 2:222–227.
47. World Health Organisation (WHO). *Cancer Pain Relief: With a Guide to Opioid Availability*, 2nd ed. Geneva: WHO, 1996.
48. Thomson R, Barton AG. Is audit running out of steam? *Quality Health Care* 1994; 3:225–229.

6

Cancer Pain as a Model for the Training of Physicians in Palliative Care

DAVID E. WEISSMAN

From the standpoint of medical education, cancer pain has received far greater attention over the past 10 years than all other topics in palliative care. This is undoubtedly due to the widespread acceptance of a standardized assessment approach and well-accepted treatment algorithms, combined with the tremendous attention that cancer pain has received on a national and international basis.[1,2] During this time, consensus statements, curriculum guides, and cancer pain teaching materials have been developed and published.[1–7]

Much of the recent focus on cancer pain education was stimulated by a 1990 article by Dr. Mitchell Max, "Improving Outcomes in Analgesic Treatment: Is Education Enough?"[8] This review of the problems in cancer pain education was a wake-up call to medical educators, highlighting the fallacy that conventional medical education (e.g., lectures, books, journal articles) could significantly impact physicians' *practice behavior*, which is rooted in a medical tradition replete with inappropriate attitudes about pain, pain treatment, and the role of the physician in treating pain. Dr. Max challenged educators to develop a new paradigm for cancer pain education—one that would focus on changing the system which physicians operate through patient education, development of systems of accountability, and work with state drug control authorities to encourage appropriate opioid use.

In the realm of palliative care, the effective assessment and management of pain is the first duty of a physician caring for a dying patient. Pain must be controlled before physicians can assist patients with the myriad of physical, psychological, and spiritual problems encountered at the end of life. Many of the challenges of physician pain education are mirrored in other areas of end-of-life care—management of nonpain symptoms, communication skills, and application of basic bioethical concepts to end-of-life care. Thus, understanding the particular problems and opportunities in physician pain education can provide insights into the design of education programs for other topics in end-of-life care. This chapter will review the current state of cancer pain education and discuss implications for related topics in palliative care.

Why Is Physician Education About Pain So Hard?

The primary reason conventional pain education formats fail to translate into a change in clinical practice is that physicians harbor a host of attitudes about pain and pain management that inhibit the appropriate application of knowledge and skills. These attitudes have been well studied and can be divided into two broad categories. First are the physician attitudes about pain that merely reflect societal views about the meaning of pain and pain treatment.[9] We live in a society that struggles between two polar views of pain. On the one hand, physicians are professionally encultured to relieve pain; pain treatment is viewed as a basic duty and obligation of physicians. The modern model of medical practice would like to view pain as something that can be defined and measured, to the point where, if pain cannot be measured, it is often assumed by physicians to be "false pain."[10,11] On the other hand, since the dawn of Western civilization, society has viewed pain as having special value to the individual sufferer, something that can lead to "meaningful social status and the promise for redemption," best exemplified by the expression "no pain, no gain."[10] Thus, there exists a modern tension between pain as something to be valued and pain that physicians are professionally challenged to investigate and alleviate. In the words of Dr. Thomas Johnson, "with the view of pain as an experience that has been taken away from the patient, physicians now find themselves in the thankless, impossible position of judging which pains are authentic, which have a physical and which have a psychic base, which are simulated and which are real. Faced with feelings of impotence, clinicians may fall back on the vestiges of Judeo-Christian construction of pain in which suffering is not only laudable but even essential."[10]

A second category of physician attitudes that inhibit pain education consists of the many fears and myths about opioid analgesics. Chief among these are fears of addiction, respiratory depression, and regulatory scrutiny, along with the secondary consequences of these fears—malpractice claims, professional sanctions, loss of practice privileges, and personal guilt about potential culpability for causing death. These attitudes, often referred to as *opiophobia,* directly reinforce societal attitudes about pain and pain treatment, especially as they apply to the notion that the need to use drugs to control pain represents personal weakness.[11–13]

Beyond such attitudes are the many deficits in basic cancer pain knowledge and skills, subjects never taught in medical school or graduate training programs. These subjects include how to conduct a pain assessment; clinical pharmacology involving opioid and nonopioid analgesics: use of nondrug analgesic treatments including antineoplastic, anesthetic, and behavioral treatments and skills in patient education and counseling regarding pain and pain treatment.

What Education Techniques Are Used to Improve Cancer Pain Education and Do They Work?

As discussed by Dr. Max, the conventional methods of medical education have failed to change clinical practice.[8] Since the publication his article, a number of new cancer pain educational programs have been developed, largely reflecting the general trend in medical education toward application of adult-learning theory.

Techniques used to address attitudes toward cancer pain

Attitudes cannot be *taught;* thus, the idea of changing deeply held societal and professional attitudes about cancer pain is an enormous task. In particular, lectures or written educational material, when used alone, are ineffective in overcoming deeply held attitudes. To address attitudes, some type of small-group, mentoring, or preceptorship experience is needed. Guidelines to keep in mind when considering how to *teach* attitudes are listed in Table 6.1.

There is only a single literature report documenting an educational effort specifically designed to change physician attitudes about pain.[14] Wilson, using a pre/post test design, reported that an educational intervention among first-year medical students led to a favorable change in attitudes, measured 5 months later. Unfortunately, there have been no further studies on attitude changes among medical students, especially into the clinical years. In fact, there are virtually no

Table 6.1. Guidelines for the teaching of attitudes°

---

1. Exhortation, information, and rational argument have a limited role in the learning or changing of attitudes.

2. Effective teaching capitalizes on "teachable moments" when the learner is emotionally or intellectually aroused by a question, contradiction, or problem.

3. Attitudinal development is fostered in situations in which the learner can be active and can engage with others in addressing problems.

4. Attitudes are best learned/changed when (a) the learner is able to examine personal feelings/attitudes in an open and nonthreatening dialogue with peers; (b) concrete knowledge and skills are taught that relate to the desired attitudes; (c) the learner has an opportunity to practice the new behavior, thus making a commitment; and (d) the learner has an opportunity to reflect on the meaning, difficulties, and rewards of attitude change.

5. Role playing and role reversal encourage the learner to take an alternative perspective and may foster an empathic awareness of the other's experience.

6. Role models and mentors are crucial to the process of learning attitudes, especially when the learner is making a transition.

7. Feedback about the learner's progress toward explicitly desired attitudinal objectives can help promote self-reflection and self-learning.

°Provided by Susan Block, M.D., with assistance from Luann Wilkerson, Ed.D.

descriptions of education programming for physicians-in-training that directly address the issue of attitudes, even though it is well accepted that attitudes play a central role in the problem of cancer pain management.

The Cancer Pain Role Model Program of the Wisconsin Cancer Pain Initiative uses small-group, case-based workshops to address attitude concerns of physicians in practice, along with their clinical partners (teams of physicians, nurses, and pharmacists).[15,16] As in many cancer pain education programs, physicians attending the Role Model Program already had "appropriate" attitudes, as measured by an attitude pretest.[15] However, the Role Model Program uses case studies that are designed not only to explore personal attitudes, but also to help participants develop strategies to use when approaching colleagues with attitude barriers. Although this program has demonstrated the ability to help physicians teach others the facts about pain management and to change the institutional culture of pain, there are no data documenting whether this educational approach has any direct impact on physicians' practice.

Techniques to improve knowledge and skills

Key physician knowledge of and skills in cancer pain management have been outlined in several publications.[1-5] One's knowledge of cancer pain management facts (e.g., differential diagnosis of back pain) can be improved using many formats, including lectures, audio- or videotapes, clinical consultations, question/answer sessions, small-group workshops, mentoring, and self-study guides. By using a pre/post test format, one can easily document improvement in knowledge directly following an educational intervention. This has now been demonstrated in a variety of cancer pain educational programs.[14-18] Long-term retention of facts can also be assessed through simple testing procedures and has been documented for at least one cancer pain education program.[19] The more difficult task is to document that new knowledge has been applied to clinical practice (see "Techniques to Change Practice Behavior" below).

Teaching new skills in pain management requires a combination of providing knowledge and the opportunity to practice the desired skill. An example is teaching others how to perform a cancer pain assessment. A body of facts need to be provided (e.g., what questions need to be asked), followed by an experiential opportunity to practice the skill. The latter can be done in a role-playing format or through practice with actual patients under observation. An excellent example of this technique is the recent report by Sloan et al., in which an objective, structured, performance-based testing method was used first to assess family practitioners skill in performing a pain assessment and then to provide immediate feedback and instruction.[20] This type of performance-based assessment is crucial to document appropriate acquisition of new skills. However, data describing continued improvement and application of new pain management skills over time as a result of an educational intervention are lacking.

Techniques to change practice behavior

The subject of changing practice behavior is quite complex and has been thoroughly reviewed by Greco and Eisenberg.[21] They noted that there is no single optimal method for changing practice behavior. Instead, it is best to consider a combination of methods that are most suitable for the particular circumstances to be addressed.

While there are no research data demonstrating that a cancer pain educational program has a direct impact on the cancer pain practice of individual physicians, there are data on the effects of changing practice behavior within communities of physicians. In a nonrandomized, uncontrolled pharmacy practice survey, Strobusch and Ott documented a shift in community physician (New London, Wisconsin) opioid analgesic prescribing—less meperidine use and greater morphine use—following participation in the Wisconsin Cancer Pain Initiative's Role Model Program.[22]

Elliot et al. reported the results of a randomized community pain education project, involving intensive education of community physicians, nurses, pharmacists, social workers, and leading clergy, to effect practice change.[23] Education formats included lectures, small-group discussions, case studies, and practicums, followed by the formation of community education task forces to disseminate cancer pain information. The results of this trial, obtained 15 months after the initial intervention, were small, nonstatistically significant improvements in all measures of pain and practitioner pain attitudes.[23] This study, by far the most comprehensive and well-designed cancer pain education trial to date, demonstrated that the use of community opinion leaders can lead to modest improvements in community practice but that, among other causes, "secular trends towards improved cancer pain management may have diminished the chances of any intervention having a significant effect."[23]

The latter issue, the gradual improvement in cancer pain management unrelated to a specific educational intervention, is certain to confound any future attempts to measure changes in clinical practice. Although this issue is difficult to measure, there has probably been a gradual improvement in cancer pain practice due to greater public and health professional recognition of the cancer pain problem, widespread dissemination of national cancer pain treatment guidelines, and greater availability of cancer pain treatment options.

Perhaps the most exciting advance in cancer pain education has been recent evaluation of the ability of educational programming to change the institutional culture and practice of pain management. Clearly, physician practice behavior is more likely to change if it is supported by an institutional culture that promotes such change.[24-26] Examples of institutional pain management practices that support better physician practice include pain education for nurses and allied health professionals, regular use of standardized pain assessment procedures, good pain assessment and treatment documentation, and a system of quality assurance for pain management. Gordon et al. have studied the mechanics of institutional pain practice and have developed a workbook to guide practitioners through the change process.[27]

Several large pain education projects have been published that have attempted to use institutional change as one vehicle for practice change.[15,16,26,28] All these projects have demonstrated success in helping participants begin the process of making institutional changes. In particular, Bookbinder et al., in the first report of a single hospital making sweeping institutional changes, documented improvement in patient satisfaction and in nurse knowledge and attitude scores.[28] However, to date, there have been no direct measures of physician practice change as a result of any of these institutional change projects. One universal finding is that these projects are time-consuming and require a major and continuing commitment, both by participants and by their health care institutions.

Lessons for Palliative Care Education

The past 10 years have seen a variety of new educational projects developed to improve physician pain education: small-group teaching to address attitude concerns, use of performance-based techniques to evaluate cancer pain skills, and projects to help change practice behavior through institutional change. Part of this effort is merely a reflection of the greater use of all of these techniques throughout medical education, as it is recognized that the conventional lecture format (turn off the lights, turn on the slides, turn off the students) is not appropriate for the affective and skill components of medical practice.

It is clear that the concept and practice of physician pain education, once thought of as involving no more than a simple lecture or new journal article, must be broadened to include discussion of attitudes and knowledge, practice of defined skills, education of other health care professionals, and changes in institutional culture/practice. This same idea can be applied to all other topics of palliative care. However, before discussing educational techniques suitable for palliative care, it is important to review some of the barriers to palliative care education.

What Are the Barriers to Physician Education on Palliative Care?

There is little formal teaching about end-of-life care during medical school or postgraduate training. There is, however, much negative so-called informal teaching about end-of-life care: for example, death represents a medical failure, physicians should not express personal emotions about their patients, and dying patients should not be disturbed.[29,30] Part of this problem is related to the lack of faculty role models for good end-of-life care. Supervising physicians often have no training experience in caring for a dying patient and are generally unaware of what they do not know about good end-of-life care. They often lack essential communication and symptom control skills and are poorly prepared to manage the clinical application of basic bioethical principles.

Little or no emphasis is placed on clinical care using an interdisciplinary model of care, even though it is widely accepted that all health disciplines are needed to care effectively for the dying. In addition, little importance is placed on the recognition, validation, and discussion of the patient's and family's reactions to either the hospital environment (e.g., the personal losses engendered by being ill) or the fatal illness. This is equally true of the reactions of physicians and other health care workers. Finally, in the increasingly fast-paced world of inpatient and outpatient medicine, faculty have little time to explore any but the most superficial aspects of end-of-life care.

What Are the Domains of Palliative Care Education?

Symptom control

Besides pain, other common end-of-life symptoms include nausea and vomiting, anorexia, constipation, delirium, depression, fatigue, skin and mouth problems, and dyspnea. Educational objectives should include an understanding of symptom epidemiology, pathophysiology, and differential diagnoses, along with a demonstration of symptom assessment skills and application of knowledge related to drug and non-drug treatments. In general, these symptoms do not involve the same degree of attitude barriers that exist with pain. One notable exception are the negative attitudes and fears surrounding use of opioids to control terminal dyspnea.

Communication skills/ethics

End-of-life communication skills, and the closely related ethical principles that provide a framework for decision making, include discussing the diagnosis and prognosis; conducting a family conference; performing a spiritual assessment; and discussing treatment withdrawal, do-not-resuscitate orders, and hospice referrals. Of particular educational importance is the observation that discussing end-of-life issues with patients and families will stir a host of personal feelings within the physician, issues that need to be discussed in a safe and comfortable learning environment.[31] Therefore, any communication skills training program must also include an opportunity to share feelings and discuss attitudes.

Use of technology in end-of-life care

The common interventions in this domain include use of oxygen, mechanical ventilation, artificial hydration, nonoral feeding, blood products, intravenous an-

tibiotics, pulse oximetry, laboratory/radiological testing, radiotherapy, chemotherapy, and kidney dialysis. The key challenge for this educational domain is to
demonstrate that physicians learn the indications and contraindications for these
interventions and that any educational program leads to improved practice behavior (e.g., not ordering blood tests for a dying patient).

Needs of the patient and family

Understanding the needs and value systems of dying patients and their families
is perhaps at the core of palliative care education. Trainees need to learn how to
recognize the various physical, psychological, and spiritual needs that are part of
the dying experience and how these differ among cultures.

Alternative care settings

The major alternatives for end-of-life care include the acute-care hospital, home
care with specialized nursing services, home or free-standing inpatient hospice
care, and hospice care within a hospital or long-term care setting. Education
concerning this domain is largely related to knowledge (e.g., eligibility criteria for
the Medicare Hospice Benefit) but also includes understanding personal attitudes
toward end-of-life care (e.g., difficulty in referring to home hospice care).

What Education Formats Are Most Desirable for Palliative Care Education?

As with pain education, education formats to address attitudes and values (e.g.,
the meaning to the doctor of treatment withdrawal) are best addressed in a
small-group or one-on-one setting (e.g., mentorship). Topics that involve specific
facts (e.g., use of antiemetics) can be taught in a lecture format or via self-study
guides reinforced by case discussion. Teaching end-of-life skills (e.g., conducting
a spiritual assessment) is best done by role modeling, followed by a chance to
practice via role playing and/or by actual performance under direct observation
with immediate feedback. Experiential opportunities for training (e.g., visits to
home hospice patients) are an invaluable educational tool to reinforce appropriate attitudes, knowledge, and skills.

As with pain control, there are many aspects of end-of-life care that can be
institutionalized to support improved physician performance. These can be divided into five key areas: commitment, assessment, responsibility, education, and
standards (CARES)[32]:

- Facility commitment: Administrators are clearly commited to the concept
  that end-of-life care is a priority and that resources (staff, time, money) will
  be directed to improving clinical care.

- Assessment: An institutional program of symptom assessment and documentation is established.
- Responsibility: A system is established to ensure that poorly managed end-of-life care is identified in a timely manner and that the underlying causes for such problems are corrected.
- Education: Programs for new and existing staff are in place to provide education about end-of-life care, and educational resources are made available to staff, patients, and families.
- Standards: Explicit standards of care are established that outline staff responsibilities and expected patient outcomes.

Conclusion

Physician education in the realm of pain and palliative care is immensely challenging. Unlike many areas of physician education, in which knowledge of facts and their application to clinical practice is paramount, end-of-life care is filled with attitudes, values, and myths, both personal and societal. Addressing these issues in conjunction with the myriad facts and skills necessary to provide excellent end-of-life care is perhaps the most daunting task currently facing medical educators at the millennium. The recent trend in medical education to better understand and apply the principles of adult learning, practice change, and interdisciplinary education holds great promise for improving physician palliative care education.

Acknowledgment

Dr. Weissman is a recipient of the Open Society Institute's Project on Death in America Faculty Scholar Program.

References

1. Jacox A, Carr DB, Payne R, et al. *Management of Cancer Pain.* Clinical Practice Guideline No. 9. AHCPR Publication No. 94-0592. Rockville, Md.: Agency for Health Care Policy and Research, U.S. Department of Health and Human Services, Public Health Service, March 1994.
2. World Health Organization. *Cancer Pain Relief and Palliative Care.* Geneva: World Health Organization, 1990.
3. Fields HL, ed. *Core Curriculum for Professional Education in Pain.* Seattle: IASP Publications, 1991.
4. Ad-Hoc Committee on Cancer Pain. The American Society of Clinical Oncology. Cancer pain assessment and treatment guidelines. *J Clin Oncol* 1992; 10:1976–1982.
5. Palliative Oncology Education Section of the American Association for Cancer Edu-

cation. Cancer pain education: objectives for medical students and residents in primary care specialties. *J Cancer Education* 1996; 11:7–10.

6. Max M, Donovan M, Misakowski C, et al. American Pain Society Quality Improvement Guidelines for the treatment of acute and chronic pain. *JAMA* 1995; 274: 1874–1880.

7. Weissman D, Dahl J. *Cancer Pain: Diagnosis and Treatment, 5th ed.* Madison, Wisc.: Wisconsin Cancer Pain Initiative, 1996.

8. Max MB. Improving outcomes in analgesic treatment: is education enough? *Ann Intern Med* 1990; 13:885–889.

9. Weissman DE, Dahl JL. Attitudes about cancer pain: a survey of Wisconsin's first year medical students. *J Pain Symptom Manage* 1990; 5:345–349.

10. Johnson TM. Contradictions in the cultural construction of pain in America. In: Hill CS, Fields WS, eds. *Advances in Pain Research and Therapy, Vol. 11.* New York: Raven Press, 1989:27–30.

11. Von Roenn JH, Cleeland CS, Gonin R, et al. Physician attitudes and practice in cancer pain management: a survey from the Eastern Cooperative Oncology Group. *Ann Intern Med* 1993; 119:121–126.

12. Cleeland CS. Pain control: Public and physician attitudes. In: Hill CS, Fields WS, eds. *Advances in Pain Research and Therapy, Vol. 11.* New York: Raven Press, 1989: 81–89.

13. Morgan JP. American opioiphobia: customary under-utilization of opioid analgesics. In: *Controversies in Alcoholism and Substance Abuse.* Binghampton, NY: Haworth Press, 1986:163–172.

14. Wilson JF, Brockopp GW, Kryst S, et al. Medical students attitudes toward pain before and after a brief course on pain. *Pain* 1992; 50:251–256.

15. Weissman DE, Dahl JL, Bealsey JW. The cancer pain role model program of the Wisconsin Cancer Pain Initiative. *J Pain Symptom Manage* 1993; 8:29–35.

16. Weissman DE, Dahl JL. Update on the cancer pain role model education program. *J Pain Symptom Manage* 1995; 10:292–297.

17. Weissman DE, Griffie J, Gordon DB, et al. A role model program to promote institutional changes for management of acute and cancer pain. *J Pain Symptom Manage* 1997; 14:274–279.

18. Von Gunten CF, Von Roenn FH, Weitzman S. House staff training in cancer pain education. *J Cancer Education* 1994; 9:230–234.

19. Janjan NA, Martin CG, Payne R, et al. Durability of education in cancer pain management principles with the role model program. *Cancer* 1996; 77:996–1021.

20. Sloan PA, Donnelly MB, Vanderveer B, et al. Cancer pain education among family physicians. *J Pain Symptom Manage* 1997; 14:74–81.

21. Greco PJ, Eisenberg JM. Changing physicians' practices. *N Engl J Med* 1993; 329: 1271–1274.

22. Strobusch AD, Ott N. Impact of physician/nurse role models on cancer pain management in clinical practice. *Wisconsin Family Physician* 1992; June:24–25.

23. Elliot TE, Murray DM, Oken MM, et al. Improving cancer pain management in communities: main results from a randomized controlled trial. *J Pain Symptom Manage* 1997; 13:191–203.

24. McMenamin E, McMorkle, Barg F, et al. Implementing a multidisciplinary cancer pain education program. *Cancer Pract* 1995; 3:303–309.

25. Foley KM. Pain relief into practice: rhetoric without reform. *J Clin Oncol* 1995; 13:2149–2151.

26. Ferrell BR, Dean GE, Grant M, et al. An institutional commitment to pain management. *J Clin Oncol* 1995; 13:2158–2165.

27. Gordon DB, Dahl JL, Stevenson KK. *Building an Institutional Commitment to Pain Management.* Madison, Wisc.: Wisconsin Cancer Pain Initiative, 1996.

28. Bookbinder M, Coyle N, Kiss M, et al. Implementing national standards for cancer pain management: program model and evaluation. *J Pain Symptom Manage* 1996; 12:334–347.

29. Billings JA, Block S. Palliative care in undergraduate medical education. *JAMA* 1997; 278:733–743.

30. Hafferty FW, Franks R. The hidden curriculum, ethics teaching and the structure of medical education. *Academic Med* 1994; 11:862–871.

31. Novack DH, Suchman AL, Clark W, et al. Calibrating the physician: personal awareness and effective patient care. *JAMA* 1997; 278:502–509.

32. Weissman DE. Educating home health professionals in cancer pain management. *Home Health Care Consultant* 1995; 2:10–18.

7

The Palliative Care Unit as a Focus for Professional Education

J. CAMERON MUIR AND CHARLES F. VON GUNTEN

Deficiencies in the provision of palliative care have been widely documented. The 1992 U.S. Census confirmed that the vast majority of Americans (63%) die in a hospital. An additional 17% die in other institutional settings such as nursing homes. Only 15% of Americans die while cared for in a hospice program in which palliative care is provided predominantly at home.[1] Furthermore, the SUPPORT study,[2] one of the largest studies of hospitalized critically ill patients, demonstrated that death in the hospital is still often associated with prolonged, painful suffering. Among the deaths reported in SUPPORT, the median number of days spent in the intensive care unit (ICU) comatose or on mechanical ventilation was 8, with more than 30% of patients spending at least 10 days in the ICU. In addition, the study found that nearly one-quarter of patients were in moderate to severe pain more than half of the time, and their families indicated that 50% of all conscious patients who died in the hospital had moderate to severe pain at least half of the time during their last 3 days of life. Paris et al. claim that "these data call into question how well physicians take seriously and attempt to honor patient preferences on treatment choices. They also force us to ask what, if anything, will reduce or eliminate what the investigators label 'undesirable days' for dying patients."[3] Clearly, these data point to the need for improved palliative care in hospitals.

These deficiencies have come to the attention of the public. Countless newspaper articles, magazine articles, and books on these subjects have been published within the last 5 years.[4-7] Television shows have also been covering these issues. The average person cannot help but be exposed to such topics as prolonged painful suffering, "mercy" killing, and Dr. Kevorkian. In addition to the public, the medical and legal professions have been heatedly and publicly debating the merits of physician-assisted suicide, withdrawal of life-sustaining therapy, and euthanasia.

This broad concern about suffering and death is justified. Prior to the twentieth century, physicians had little to offer patients with advanced progressive illness except to visit them at home and offer comfort as the disease took its natural course to either recovery or death. In contrast, the vitalistic medicine of the late twentieth century has seen the development of medical science and technologies that allow for significant prolongation of life. The development of therapeutics such as antibiotics, hemodialysis, mechanical ventilation, and anesthesia has brought the focus of medical care for patients from the home to "the institution" for these interventions. These discoveries have dramatically altered the outcomes of medical care, at least for some patients.

This shift toward scientific medicine has had unintended consequences. The majority of patients now die of chronic diseases. Further, in the overweening focus on the treatment of the underlying disease, patients and their families may suffer longstanding, poorly palliated, or even unaddressed, debilitating symptoms such as intractable nausea, dyspnea, delirium, or severe pain. As described in the SUPPORT study, their finances are often exhausted, and their need for information and self-determination is neglected.

The public outcry for mercy killing and physician-assisted suicide may be interpreted as a call for better care rather than as a societal wish to die. Attention must be paid to pain and symptom management, spiritual and psychosocial suffering, as well as to the scientific treatment of disease. Further, when life-prolonging care is either not desired or impossible, medical care should appropriately focus on providing comfort without either shortening or unnecessarily prolonging dying. When it is possible, an attempt to return patients to their homes for their last days, weeks, or months should be made.

The medical care that specializes in the care of patients with advanced progressive disease, for whom the prognosis is limited and the focus is the relief of suffering, has been termed *hospice care* or, more aptly, *palliative medicine.* Unfortunately, palliative medicine is not a significant part of medical education or postgraduate training for those in clinical practice.

In its decisions regarding the lack of a constitutionally based right to die, the U.S. Supreme Court found that Americans have the right to expect palliative care.[8] The report issued in 1997 by the Institute of Medicine[9] also indicated that palliative medicine should be incorporated into the training and clinical practice of physicians. This implies that a formal educational program that establishes a firm knowledge base in these important issues early in the medical educational process and reinforces them throughout medical school, postgraduate training, and clinical practice is needed. Only an integrated and coordinated program of education in hospice and palliative medicine will shape the knowledge, attitudes, skills, and practice of physicians.

The purpose of this chapter is to describe elements of such an academic program in Hospice and Palliative Medicine at Northwestern University Medical

School (NUMS) and Northwestern Memorial Hospital (NMH), an independent private hospital that is the principal teaching affiliate of the medical school. Because the majority of physician education continues to occur in hospitals, we will emphasize the role of the inpatient palliative care unit in achieving the educational goals of the program. We believe the structure of this program may serve as an example of an effective system of physician education in this important area. In this chapter, we will first describe the background for the field. Then we will describe the specific elements of the clinical program on which the educational program is based. Next, we will discuss our palliative care educational curriculum, with emphasis on the inpatient unit. Finally, we will review data evaluating some of the educational outcomes of the program.

Background

The modern hospice movement began with the work of Dr. Cicely Saunders in England. Based on her observations of the care of terminally ill cancer patients in both acute care hospitals and hospices run by religious communities, she formulated the concepts that led her to establish the first modern hospice. St. Christopher's Hospice was founded in 1967 in south suburban London as an inpatient facility dedicated to the care of patients with poorly controlled symptoms due to either cancer or motor neuron disease. The principles of palliative care that Dr. Saunders articulated have become synonymous with hospice care: the unit of care is both the patient and the family; the relief of suffering or "total pain" requires consideration not only of the physical element of suffering, but also 1 of the psychological, social, and spiritual components; and interdisciplinary team is best equipped to meet these needs. Furthermore, St. Christopher's founding mission was not only to look after patients using a biopsychosocial model of care, but also to pursue solid research into the best care of patients with advanced terminal illness and to train others to do similar hospice work. As a result of the success and achievements of St. Christopher's Hospice, hospice and palliative care programs proliferated in a variety of health care settings throughout Great Britain and the rest of the world. Because the three missions of patient care, research, and education are inextricably linked in the day-to-day affairs of St. Christopher's Hospice, it can also be regarded as the first modern academic hospice.

By 1987, the multidisciplinary field of palliative medicine was recognized as a medical specialty by the Royal College of Physicians in Great Britain. This recognition came only after it had been demonstrated that there was an established body of medical knowledge that pertained uniquely to a distinct patient population. Further, there was recognition of a 4-year training program to follow general medical training for those physicians who wished to be recognized as specialists in the field.

Other countries have instituted similar programs for training physicians in hospice and palliative medicine at various levels. In Australia, the University of Adelaide established a degree-granting academic program in hospice and palliative medicine for practicing physicians. In Canada, the Canadian Committee on Palliative Care Education developed a Palliative Care Curriculum for implementation in 16 Canadian medical schools.

The United States has followed a somewhat different course. The first hospice program in the United States was established in 1974. In the next 15 years, more than 1700 active programs developed. However, the primary impetus for their initiation was different. In the United States, hospice programs were introduced largely by nurses and volunteers as a reaction against the perceived inadequacies of the medical establishment in caring for terminally ill patients.[10] Consequently, there developed a polarity that prevented hospice medicine from becoming incorporated into the academic mainstream.

If physicians in general are to incorporate good palliative care into their practice patterns and use hospice programs appropriately, and if, as a recent article by Quill et al. suggest, "palliative care is the standard of care for dying patients,"[11] then good palliative care must be taught as part of physicians' medical education. It seems essential, then, that education about the principles of palliative medicine and hospice care should be integrated throughout the system of medical education, from student to attending physician, in order to have the broadest impact within the academic medical centers where doctors train and where the principles and practice of medicine are established. At NUMS, we have been pursuing this objective for many years.

Clinical Program in Palliative Care

The clinical program at Northwestern is ostensibly a trinity: a 12-bed acute inpatient hospice/palliative care unit,[12] a hospice/palliative medicine consultation service,[13] and a Medicare-certified home hospice program. One of the key features of this clinical program is that movement of patients among the three elements is relatively seamless. A physician and a patient can access the program at any point. Inpatients may be seen by the consultation service and/or transferred to the inpatient unit. Outpatients can be seen in the office, directly admitted to the inpatient unit, or seen at home. This integrated system is designed to ensure smooth, easy access to palliative care expertise in the home or hospital without having to call 911 or go through the emergency room and/or admitting office—care systems not designed to meet the needs of patients with advanced progressive illness and their families.

Consultation service

In the hospital, a request for consultation is transmitted to the service through the hospital computer or by directly paging a member of the service. The consultation service, consisting of an attending physician, a nurse, and any fellows, residents, and medical students rotating on the service, reviews the patient's medical chart, takes a history, and examines the patient. The elements of the palliative medicine consultation have recently been described by Weissman.[14] Medical issues are clarified, and the goals of care are discussed with the patient, the family, and the primary medical team. The full consultation may take several days. Often, the consultation marks the beginning of an elegant process of "transition" for the patient and family. Daily visits to the bedside are made during rounds. Patients may make a transition from a narrow focus on eradicating disease and prolonging life to a broader consideration of maximizing function, achieving important goals, and optimizing the quality of life. They may focus explicitly on minimizing pain and suffering. Specific recommendations regarding pain and symptom management are made. Issues surrounding care planning are raised with both the family and the primary medical service. Recommendations to include or direct ancillary services such as social work, chaplaincy, physical therapy, and occupational therapy are made.

The range of issues presented to the consultation service is broad (13): recommendations for the management of pain and other distressing symptoms; facilitating communication about disease status and prognosis; end-of-life planning; clarifying resuscitation wishes; convening family meetings; facilitating nurse, social work, physical therapy, occupational therapy, or chaplaincy interventions; or providing information about home and/or inpatient hospice care programs. The consultation team facilitates appropriate discharge planning to home hospice, home health, or other care settings. If the patient requires continued hospitalization due to ongoing medical treatments, symptoms that are difficult to manage, or a very limited prognosis whereby death is anticipated in a short period of time, or if there are acute psychosocial issues for the patient and/or family, then the consultation team may recommend a transfer to the inpatient unit. Not all patients seen by the service have imminent life-threatening disease. Where appropriate, members of the consultation service may also provide recommendations for management of pain and other symptoms in patients whose disease is not end-stage.

As with other consultation services in teaching hospitals, an important purpose of the daily rounds is to teach. Rounds often begin in the office of the medical director, where topics pertinent to hospice/palliative medicine are discussed in a didactic/Socratic format. These topics are drawn from both the formal syllabus (see "Palliative Care Curriculum") and as from issues raised by specific patient encounters. Next, the team proceeds to bedside rounds, where communication skills are first role modeled and then practiced and assessed. The team approach at the bedside allows a trainee to lead a discussion with a patient and family while other, more experienced members of the interdisciplinary team are present. This discussion often includes the topics of death, dying, advance directives, and the hospice approach to terminal illness. Using the patients and families interviewed and the experience of the individual interviewing them, general points can be illustrated about effective and ineffective interviewing techniques; institutional, cultural, ethnic, language, and spiritual components of a patient's illness; and their effect on decision making. In addition, considerations about the members of the hospice team that may be beneficial or components of the hospice program that may be most helpful can be discussed. Suggested changes to and/or additions of medications for the treatment of specific symptoms can also be reviewed.

Outpatients may be seen in an ambulatory outpatient clinic staffed by one of the attending physicians on the service.

Inpatient unit

There are only two general requirements for admission to the unit: the focus of care should be palliative, and the patient must carry a do-not-resuscitate (DNR) status. There are no stipulations about what modalities may or may not be used to achieve the goals set by patients, their families, and their physicians. Patients must be sick enough to be admitted to the hospital. This 12-bed unit is a ward of the general hospital and is not separately licensed as a dedicated hospice unit. For patients who are admitted after having accessed their Medicare Hospice Benefit, the hospital agrees to accept that reimbursement for inpatient care. The vast majority of patients (>80%), however, have not accessed special hospice benefits at the time of admission. Because patients are covered under acute care reimbursement, the medical team has maximum flexibility in determining appropriate care for patients and their families. The characteristics of the inpatient unit and the rationale for its establishment have been described in detail elsewhere.[12] Suffice it to say that a specialty unit for palliative care serves patients in an analogous way to other specialty units in the hospital where patients and families are better served by an organized team of individuals with special training and expertise. Examples of patients who are admitted include those who require acute care for management of their illness and symptoms, those who are acutely dying and cannot be moved to another setting, and those for whom acute psychosocial support and discharged planning are needed.

The daily routine begins with the medical team (nurse practioner, medical student, resident, fellow) conferring with the night nurses working on the unit to get information about what happened overnight. Next, they make work rounds to visit their inpatients and write a daily progress note. After work rounds, the team gathers for formal bedside teaching rounds later in the morning, where the rationale for medication adjustments and their resulting effects can be ascertained and discussed, and challenges in home arrangements and/or family dynamics can be clarified. Many of the same issues seen in the consultation setting are reinforced as the transition process continues, while the acute management of symptoms and psychosocial issues takes on increased importance. Trainees participate in scheduled patient care meetings and family meetings as they are arranged.

Patients continue to have their attending physician of record while in the inpatient unit. The medical team writes orders for the patient with the consent and advice of the attending physician. The hospice/palliative medicine attending physician and fellow serve as consultants. However, when requested, they assume primary responsibility for patient care.

The entire inpatient hospice/palliative care team, which includes the nurses, physicians (and physician trainees), social workers, bereavement coordinator, chaplain, pharmacist, nutritionist, and volunteers, assesses symptoms and psychosocial issues and helps to coordinate a comprehensive treatment plan. Trainees note that this means spending more time with families and communicating about terminal illness issues than would characterize a general medical unit. This allows an individual trainee to experience the vast array of issues that are characteristic of caring for patients and their families within an interdisciplinary palliative care framework. Many trainees remark that it is the first time they have experienced real teamwork. They learn the benefit of working directly with allied health care providers in the care of patients and families by helping to care for patients hospitalized on the unit. The attending physicians working on the unit model this teamwork by working as team members rather than as team leaders. As Twycross recently wrote "The concept of specialist palliative-care units still elicits a mixture of responses. For most people, however, actually visiting one leads to the strange discovery of life and joy in the midst of death and distress."[15] Our experience supports this finding. Trainees witness "human compassion in action" during one of the most challenging and potentially rewarding times of a patient's life. Trainees are encouraged to spend time at the bedside of a patient to understand the issues more intimately and personally, rather than remaining at a distance, as would likely occur on general medical units.

Home program

There is a hospital-based, Medicare-certified home hospice program that serves patients and families living within the Chicago city limits. Patients may be admitted while in their homes or on leaving the hospital. Trainees see patients in the home as team physicians, initially accompanied by a hospice team member such as a nurse, social worker, chaplain, or hospice physician. As these individuals gain experience, they are encouraged to make a home visit alone to patients with whom they are familiar. In the home setting, adjustments in medication may be made; further discussions about the nature of the disease, the prognosis, and the effects on the patient and family may be discussed; and valuable insight is gained by team members as they see patients on the patients' terms in their own environment. This often provides insights that can uniquely be gained in the home and are invaluable to understanding the situation and modifying the care plan.

Palliative Care Curriculum

In 1987, Von Roenn et al. reviewed many of the studies verifying "that palliative care skills and principles receive minimal attention in medical schools and medicine training programs," leaving physicians with "marked deficiencies in medical knowledge relevant to terminal care."[16] Additionally, there is evidence that inadequate preparation in the area of palliative care of patients with advanced terminal illness is the single most important qualitative factor leading to oncologist "burnout."[17] As a result, the team at NUMS/NMH worked to define a set of goals for medical students, residents and fellows in palliative medicine:

1. Learn the principles of palliation:
    - The adoption of a caring, as opposed to curing, role for health care providers
    - The psychological stages of the dying process, grief reactions, and the pathophysiology of death and dying
    - Concepts and structure of hospice programs; reimbursement for home care and hospice care
    - Ethical and legal issues in the care of the terminally ill
2. Learn specific skills required in providing palliative care:
    - Accurate prognostication and communication of the prognosis
    - Communication of other issues to the patient and family, including management of emotional and psychological issues
    - Effective methods of symptom control, including relief of pain, fever, nausea, dyspnea, pruritus, and other gastrointestinal, respiratory, urinary, cutaneous, central nervous system, musculoskeletal, and systemic symptoms
3. Gain an understanding of the patient and family in the context of the home environment, and acquire experience in conducting home visits
4. Learn to provide care as a member of a coordinated, multidisciplinary team of physicians, nurses, social workers, physical and occupational therapists, and clergy

To achieve these goals, a formal curriculum was designed in the early 1990s. It was important that the curriculum have three major components: (1) supervised clinical experience; (2) a formal lecture series and a bibliography on pain and symptom management; and (3) seminars focusing on physicians' attitudes toward death and dying and physicians' coping skills.

In the first component, the supervised clinical experience, residents and fourth-year medical students have an opportunity take a 1-month clinical elective in hospice and palliative medicine. Fellows specializing in hematology/oncology are required to take the course. The curriculum as it is outlined is designed to be covered didactically during the first 30 min of the afternoon consultation rounds three times per week. Over the course of a 4-week rotation, all topics are covered. In general, the needed skills for the rotation are covered earlier in the month, while philosophical, ethical, and legal issues are covered later, using the experiences with specific patients as a basis for discussion. The core content of the clinical elective is given in the following outline:

1. Hospice/Palliative Medicine (Week 1/Day 1)
   A. History of the hospice
   B. Palliative medicine
   C. Medical model versus the biopsychosocial model of illness
   D. The hospice interdisciplinary team approach to palliative care
2. Breaking Bad News (Week 1/Day 3)
   A. Guidelines for the interview
   B. Important factors that influence patient/family decision making
      (1) Cultural
      (2) Ethnic
      (3) Language
      (4) Institutional
      (5) Spiritual
3. Cancer Pain Management
   A. Assessment/pathophysiology (Week 1/Day 5)
   B. Opioid pharmacology and use (Week 2/Day 1)
   C. Adjuvant analgesics (Week 2/Day 3)
   D. Barriers to cancer pain management (Week 2/Day 5)
4. Nausea and Vomiting (Week 3/Day 1)
5. Symptoms of Advanced Illness (Week 3/Day 3)
6. Advance Directives (Week 3/Day 5)
7. Diagnostic and Therapeutic Procedures (Week 4/Day 1)
8. Terminal Illness and the Process of Dying (Week 4/Day 3)
   A. Physiologic responses
   B. Family responses
   C. Spiritual issues
9. Managing Personal Stress (Week 4/Day 5)

The area of communication skills is of particular importance to medical educators in general and is critical to hospice and palliative medicine. NUMS has the good fortune to have an excellent Center of Clinical Education and Evaluation (CCEE), which uses patient instructors as part of a comprehensive course in communication skills for medical students and house staff. All of the Clinical Education and Evaluation activities rely heavily on standardized patients in role playing for teaching and assessment. The educational content is enhanced by videotaping the interaction and then reviewing it with the student, resident, or fellow. For the hospice/palliative medicine rotation, we have drawn on this resource and incorporated a specific module for each trainee. The standardized patient is described below:

Mr(s) P has Dukes Stage D colon cancer with liver metastases diagnosed 2 years ago. The primary lesion was resected and the patient referred to a medical oncologist. The patient was treated with a course of fluorouracil and leukovorin on a bolus schedule for 6 months. CT [Computed tomography] scan of the abdomen revealed progressive disease. The patient declined investigational therapy but pursued a course of continuous infusion fluorouracil as an outpatient. The overall course has been relatively uncomplicated. The patient has completed 6 months of this therapy. A CT scan was recently performed on an outpatient basis. The patient has made an appointment because of progressive fatigue. The patient does not know the results of the CT scan. At today's interview, she describes progressive fatigue and some right upper quadrant discomfort. The examination shows increased abdominal girth and a palpable nodular liver. Percussion for shifting dullness is equivocal. The CT scan is reported to show progressive liver disease. The videotaped interview begins when the student/physician invites the patient into the consultation room.

Goals for physician: to discuss results of exam and CT scan
                        to discuss DNR status
                        to clarify future patient goals
                        and introduce hospice concept

The standardized patient encounter has proven to be a very valuable and illuminating tool for educating physicians in various aspects of communication while providing an additional forum for experience and feedback in a clinical palliative care setting. Communication skills are essential in hospice and palliative care and are applicable to the entire physician–patient encounter. Von Roenn et al. note that "hospice programs are designed to provide a humanistic, holistic approach to the care of terminally ill patients and their families. A comprehensive clinical and didactic experience within a hospice thus creates an opportunity to teach much more than the skills of palliation. As medical educators become more concerned with the nurturing of humanistic qualities, they are finding few effective ways to integrate such teaching into the ongoing clinical activities of medical students, residents and fellows. The hospice environment, as described here, with students and housestaff actively involved in the comprehensive, continuing care of terminally ill patients, is an ideal setting for the teaching of health care as a humanistic endeavor."[16] Thus, the goal of our educational program in palliative medicine is to teach skills and encourage development of attitudes by students and physicians that are not only useful in the care of the terminally ill, but are applicable to all the patients for whom they care.

Central Role of the Palliative Care Unit

Besides serving the useful clinical needs described earlier, an inpatient palliative care unit located within the principal teaching hospital serves the same educational purposes that specialist inpatient care in general serves. In this respect, it is useful to reflect on the pronounced emphasis on training physicians in inpatient settings that has developed since the publication of the Flexner Report. It is widely acknowledged that medical students and residents need to be exposed to real patients in the setting where they are receiving real care by real medical professionals in order to achieve an adequate medical education. A similar case has been made for the training of nurses and other health care givers. Although multiple forces have driven the development of inpatient medical centers, the efficiency with which a team of physicians and other health care givers can deliver care to an inpatient population is paramount. Such hospital care lends itself well to the important task of supervising trainees at various levels of training and incorporating them into the medical care plan for patients.

The palliative care unit is a potent educational resource beyond the conventional clinical rotations described earlier. As mentioned, the overall curriculum calls for seminars focusing on physicians' attitudes toward palliative care. We have found that such seminars, whether for medical students, residents, or other physicians, are much more productive when they are patient based and located in the setting where care is given. Seminars and course meetings may occur on the unit in the conference room or the office of the medical director at the request of various course directors in the medical school and hospital. Didactic material can be presented and then taken to the bedside of a patient on the unit (with their permission, of course). Because the unit is always active, such seminars can occur flexibly, sometimes with little advance notice. In our experience, patients and their families are eager to participate in this educational enterprise.

In addition to providing a convenient location for patient-centered education, the palliative care unit serves an additional educational function that is difficult to measure but that we believe is quite important. The mere presence of a palliative care unit in a large teaching hospital is a potent statement of the importance of this kind of care. This can be imputed from the data shown in Figure 7.1. The home

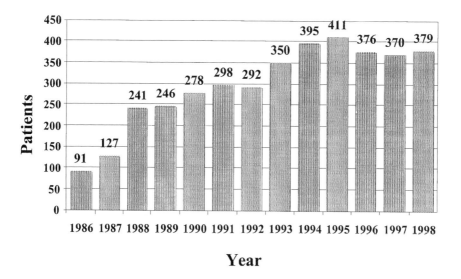

Figure 7.1. Total number of patients dying in the Hospice/Palliative Care Program of Northwestern Memorial Hospital as a function of calendar year.

hospice program began in 1982, and the inpatient unit opened in early 1987. One can clearly see the increase in overall patient volume that came as a result of opening the unit. The consultation service was begun in 1993. One can also see the contribution that this made to the patient volume. In a medical culture where dedicated inpatient space correlates with power and prestige, the presence of a palliative care unit within the hospital itself serves to reinforce the importance of palliative care as part of the total program of care delivered to patients and families. When the hospital staff were surveyed, more than 90% of respondents though that the program was an important hospital resource.[18]

While quantitation is difficult, it is our conviction that the unit, and the program administered from it, have affected the culture of care throughout the hospital. For example, 24-hr visitation is now permitted in the ICUs. Families commonly stay overnight with patients throughout the hospital. In fact, in the replacement hospital facility currently under construction (at a cost of $300 per square foot), all rooms will be private, with sleeping capacity for family members. Of course, there will be a new palliative care unit in the new facility.

Educational Outcomes

We have attempted to measure some of the educational outcomes of the program in palliative care education that involves medical students, medical residents, and fellows in the comprehensive care of hospice patients in the home as well as in the hospital.

Medical students

Beginning in the fall of 1993, NUMS restructured the medical student curriculum. For first-year medical students, the class of 175 students was divided into four "colleges," each with approximately 44 students and a theme. One college chose cancer as its theme and, as part of a pilot integration scheme, was offered the opportunity to spend on afternoon with a hospice nurse making home visits and one afternoon making rounds with the consultation service. Half of the students in this college participated. To assess this experience, the students were given a questionnaire. Fourteen of them turned in evaluations of their experience: 11/14 (79%) rated their satisfaction as "excellent" and 3/14 (21%) as "good." None reported a "fair" or "poor" reaction. In addition 13/14 (93%) rated this experience as "definitely" important for a medical student, and 12/14 (86%) thought medical students should definitely know more about this area. This response led to incorporation of death and dying issues into the teaching curriculum of another college whose theme was acquired immune deficiency syndrome. (The experience was again rated enthusiastically and is now part of the core college curriculum.) After gaining an academic stronghold in the curriculum, further reinforcement of hospice/palliative care and of death and dying issues has been facilitated by incorporation of these themes into ongoing seminars run by the Ethics and Human Values program at the medical school that focus on providing direct student–patient encounters on the inpatient unit and at home.

Residents

At the resident level, there are three major efforts at education in palliative medicine. The first is the month-long elective on the hospice/palliative care service doing inpatient rounds, consultations, and home visits described earlier. The second is a curriculum in pain education for house staff rotating on the inpatient oncology unit. Each month, house staff receive a questionnaire on basic knowledge about cancer pain at the beginning of the 4-week rotation. They then receive a series of lectures on cancer pain management. As part of the series, a quiz on analgesic dosing was administered before and after the pertinent lecture. The questionnaire and quiz were then repeated at the end of the rotation. On the questionnaire, the house staff scored an average 58% correct at the beginning of the rotation. This improved to 83% correct at the conclusion of the rotation ($p <$ .0001). The initial score did not correlate with the month of the academic year or with the year of training. On the analgesic dosing quiz, house staff answered an average 38% correct before the lecture. This improved to 83% correct after the lecture ($p = $ .001). However, by the conclusion of the rotation, the percent correct dropped to 57%. We have subsequently instituted an analgesic dosing service that incorporates this pain education curriculum to improve cancer pain education for medicine house staff.

The second effort at palliative medicine education for house staff is an extension of the curriculum in palliative care—an ambulatory clinical elective in hospice and palliative medicine for second- and third-year residents. Nineteen residents (predominantly on the primary care track) have participated in this elective, in which they spend one-half day per week over the 2-month elective with a general internist who makes home visits for patients in the hospice program. Nineteen residents have participated in this rotation. Eighteen of them (95%) were on the primary care track, and the majority (95%) were in their third year of training. They were asked to complete an evaluation of their experience. Sixteen evaluations were received. In this group, 8/16 (50%) reported their skills in managing pain and symptoms to be "much improved," 8/16 (50%) "improved," and none reported "no change." In addition, 9/16 (56%) reported their comfort and skill in discussing death/dying/advance directives with patients/families to be "much improved," 5/16 (31%) were "improved" and 2/16 reported "no change." Further, 11/16 (69%) reported their understanding of hospice/palliative care as a program and philosophy to be "much improved," 5/16 (31%) were "improved," and none reported "no change." Finally, 16/16 (100%) would recommend the rotation to others.

Fellows

Fellows enrolled in a 3-year hematology/oncology training program are required to spend 1 to 2 months on the hospice/palliative care service at NMH. During this period, the fellows are expected to see all new patient referrals to the hospice/palliative medicine consultation service, supervise the care of inpatients on the 12-bed Hospice/Palliative Care Unit, participate in care of patients in the home hospice program including making home visits, and participate in teaching medical students and residents who may be on the service. At the conclusion of each month, the fellows were asked to complete a brief assessment of their experience. After a pilot period of 9 months, nine evaluations were received; 7/9 (78%) were from second- year fellows (PGY-5), and 2/9 were from third-year fellows (PGY-6). Regarding in skills acquired in managing pain and symptoms, 4/9 (44%) reported them to be "much improved," 5/9 (56%) reported them to be "improved," and none reported "no change." In comfort and skill with discussing death/dying/advance directives with patients/families, 6/9 (67%) reported that they were "much improved," 2/9 (22%) were "improved," and 1/9 (11%) reported "no change." In understanding hospice/palliative care as a program and a philosophy, 5/9 (56%) were "much improved," 2/9 (22%) were "improved," and 2/9 (22%) reported "no change." Finally, 9/9 (100%) would recommend this rotation to others. As a result, the month on the hospice/palliative care service has become a required rotation in the oncology fellowship.

Attending Physicians

After formal training ends, much of the knowledge is disseminated through a physician's experience with a patient referred to the program or by word of mouth from a colleague. In order to assess the attitudes and practices of attending physician faculty at NMH, we initially surveyed the entire faculty about their opinion of hospice care. Of the respondents, 75% had referred patients or knew of colleagues who had referred patients to a hospice program. Of those who had referred patients to a hospice program, 94% were satisfied with their care. Ninety-four percent would refer patients in the future, and 96% thought that the hospice program was a valuable resource to the medical center. A second survey assessed all attending physicians who had referred patients to the hospice through the hospice/palliative care consultation service over a 12-month period. Of the responders, nearly 100% thought that the handling of the referral was "excellent" or "good," that communication with hospice staff was "excellent" or "good," that symptom control was "excellent" or "good," that their patients and families had received "excellent" or "good" psychosocial support, and that their patients and families were satisfied with the hospice care they received. When asked if they would refer another patient to the hospice program, 95% responded "definitely" and 5% responded "possibly." Thus, the integration of a hospice program within an academic hospital leads to broad acceptance of hospice care by physician faculty.

Visiting Scholars

There are many physicians and other health care providers who would like additional training after they begin to practice. While there is a broadly accepted literature describing elements of good palliative care, there are few places in the United States where professionals can go for practical training in this area. As a result, we have developed a program funded by an unrestricted grant from Roxane Laboratories, Inc., to provide a practical educational experience in hospice/palliative medicine for health care professionals from other institutions that is tailored to the self-identified needs of the "visiting scholar." After a 1- to 2-week visit, the scholar is asked to complete a survey to evaluate the experience both at the end of the visit and 6 months later. After 2 years of the visiting scholars program, there have been 190 requests for applications from 22 states and abroad, with 35 health care professionals completing the visit—17 nurses, 16 physicians, 1 psychologist, and 1 chaplain.

The evaluation (from 1-strongly disagree to 5-strongly agree) found that, at the conclusion of the program, scholars achieved their specific goal (4.6), the experience was worthwhile (4.9), and the scholars would recommend it (4.9). After 6 months, the ratings were unchanged.

Summary and Conclusions

The palliative care unit serves as the fundamental anchor of a program of palliative care education in a teaching hospital. It is the base of operation for a clinical program of palliative care that extends to inpatient and office consultation as well as to home hospice care. Moreover, its presence in the academic hospital serves the broad educational mission of improving the palliative care of patients throughout the course of their disease by testifying to the importance of palliative care. During the past 3 years, more than 300 physicians at various stages of training have been exposed to the care on the unit and the principles of palliative care. We hope this model will be extended to other teaching hospitals.

References

1. National Center for Health Statistics. *Vital Statistics of the United States: Mortality.* 1993.
2. The SUPPORT Principle Investigators. A controlled trial to improve care for seriously

ill hospitalized patients: the study to understand prognosis and preferences for outcomes and risks of treatment (SUPPORT). *JAMA* 1995; 274:1591–1598.

3. Paris JJ, Muir JC, Reardon FE. Ethical and legal issues in intensive care. *J Intensive Care Med* 12; 6:298–309.

4. Nuland SB. *How We Die*. New York: Random House, 1993.

5. Byock I. *Dying Well: The Prospect for Growth at the End of Life*. New York: River-Head Books, 1977.

6. Goopman J. *The Measure of Our Days*. New York: Penguin Putnam, 1997.

7. Vaux K, Vaux S. *Dying Well*. Nashville, Tenn.: Abingdon Press, 1996.

8. Burt RA. The Supreme Court speaks: not assisted suicide but a constitutional right to palliative care. *N Engl J Med* 1997; 337(17):1234–1236.

9. Institute of Medicine, Committee on Care at the End of Life. *Approaching death: improving care at the end of life*. Washington, D.C.: National Academy Press, 1997.

10. Stoddard S. Hospice in the United States: an overview. *J Palliat Care* 1989; 5:10–19.

11. Quill TE, Lo B, Brock DW. Palliative options of last resort: a comparison of voluntarily stopping eating, drinking, terminal sedation, physician-assisted suicide, and voluntary active euthanasia. *JAMA* 1997; 278(23):2099–2104.

12. Kellar N, Martinez J, Finis N, et al. Characterization of an acute inpatient hospice palliative care unit in a U.S. teaching hospital. *J Nursing Admin* 1996; 26;16–20.

13. von Gunten CF, Camden B, Neely KJ, et al. Prospective evaluation of referrals to a hospice/palliative medicine consultation service. *J Palliat Med* 1998; 1(1):45–53.

14. Weissman D. Consultation in palliative medicine. *Arch Intern Med* 1997; 157:733–737.

15. Twycross R. The joy of death. *Lancet* 1997; 350(Suppl 3):20.

16. Von Roenn JH, Neely KJ, Curry RH, et al. A curriculum in palliative care for internal medicine housestaff: a pilot project. *J Cancer Ed* 1988; 3:259–263.

17. von Gunten CF, Von Roenn JH, Gradishar W, et al. Palliative medicine rotation for hematology/oncology fellows. *J Cancer Ed* 1994; 9(Suppl 3):23.

18. von Gunten CF, Von Roenn JH, Johnson-Neely K, et al. Hospice and palliative care: attitudes and practices of the physician faculty of an academic hospital. *Am J Hospice Palliat Care* 1995; 12(4):38–42.

8

The Palliative Care Consultation Team as a Model for Palliative Care Education

JANET L. ABRAHM

In the best circumstances, dying can be a peaceful time during which important memories are shared. In Fred Chappell's novel *Farewell, I'm Bound to Leave You,*[1] a beloved grandmother is dying, and for her family, "The wind had got into the clocks and blown the hours awry." The grandson asks his father, "' . . . what are we going to do?' 'We will watch the clocks at their strange antics', my father said. 'We will listen to the wind whisper and weep and tell again those stories of women that your mother and grandmother needed for you to hear.'" When the telling is done the father explains, "Not long from now there will come an icy cold into this room. There will be a darkness like we were trapped inside a vein of coal. I want you to be brave and show me what you are made of, and I will try to be brave, too. Then it will pass off like a slow and painful eclipse of the sun and moon and stars. It will be terrible. But we must overmaster it. So hang on tight, Jess. It is coming soon."

It is our duty as physicians to enable the telling of these stories and to help the survivors withstand that darkness. We must manage the physical symptoms of our dying patients expertly, be attuned to sources of psychological and spiritual distress, and, if we cannot deal with them ourselves, obtain the help of those who can. And we must help our patients achieve their goals.

But the literature has amply documented our failure in these areas. Care is often fragmented, especially for the 65% of the population who have the misfortune to die in a hospital.[2] As Morrison et al. state in their recent poignant case discussion, "Most physicians in the United States receive no formal training in palliative care, lack exposure to those who practice palliative medicine, and do not know how to refer their patients to hospice programs."[3] Physician education in pain management is inadequate,[4–12] and as a consequence, pain remains undertreated in an astonishingly high proportion of patients—85% of those with acquired immune deficiency syndrome[8] and 40–50% of those with cancer.[9,10] A similar lack of physician education exists in end-of-life issues,[13] and nurses have had to take it on themselves to relieve what they felt was intolerable suffering.[14] Physicians are reluctant to discuss advance directives with patients,[6,15] and we do not heed them even when they are made known to us.[10] Even patients who trust their physicians to fulfill their wishes may fear that we will not be able to help them die with dignity when the time comes, and rather than confront us with their lack of faith in our abilities, they ask us to kill them.[16]

Unfortunately, we not only fail to fulfill our contracts with our dying patients, but we often abandon their families as well. The courage demanded of the bereaved is eloquently captured by Fred Chappell in another of his novels, *I Am One of You Forever,*[17] in the chapter entitled "The Telegram." It is a story full of magic and truth in which the telegram that announces a tragic death cannot be discarded or destroyed. We hear from the son in the family: "Then one evening I pulled a chair to the table and sat down to stare at the telegram. *Let it do to me what it can,* I thought. It was just at dusk and the telegram was the brightest object in the room. I don't know how long I sat looking. The room darkened and stars appeared in the upper windowpanes. At last the telegram began to change shape. Slowly wrinkling and furling inward, it took the form of a yellow rose, hand-sized, with a layer of glowing yellow petals. It seemed to hover an inch or so above the tablecloth. It uttered a mournful little whimper then, a sound I had once heard a blind puppy make when it could not find its mother's warm flank. And with that sound it disappeared from my sight forever, tumbled spiraling down a hole in the darkness. I watched it go away and my heart lightened then and I was able to rise, shaken and confused, and walk from the room without shame, not looking back, finding my way confidently in the dark."

"I think that my grandmother and mother and father each had to undergo this ritual, and I think that we each saw the telegram take a different transformation before it disappeared, but we never spoke of that either."

We need to support these family members as they find the strength to face their grief. There are many effective techniques for helping the bereaved and for identifying those at high risk for an especially painful experience so that they can receive assistance even before the patient dies.[18] But outside of hospice programs, it is unclear how much clinicians know about the needs of the bereaved.

Barriers to Delivery of Palliative Care

Definitional diversity[19]

What physicians, nurses, social workers, and others who work with the dying and their families need is expertise in palliative care, which is defined by the World Health Organization as "The active total care of patients whose disease is not responsive to curative treatment. Control of pain, of other symptoms, and of psychological, social and spiritual problems, is paramount. The goal of palliative care is achievement of the best quality of life for patients and their families. Many aspects of palliative care are also applicable earlier in the course of the illness in conjunction with anticancer treatment."[20] Dr. Russell Portenoy adds that "palliative care may be distinguished from traditional hospice approaches by its concern with the comfort and functioning of patients and their families at all stages of disease, strong physician input on an ongoing basis, willingness to use aggressive 'tertiary' interventions (such as primary anticancer therapies and invasive treatments of symptom control) for appropriate patients, and acceptance of research for quality improvement and scientific advancement. . . . Oncologists must endorse the importance of good quality of life during the period of active treatment and must reject the unfortunate, and untrue, position that the lack of an antineoplastic treatment means that "nothing can be done."[21]

In this broader definition, which I support, palliative care should begin at the time of diagnosis, complementing disease-oriented treatment. As the disease advances, disease-oriented treatment should support palliative goals (Figure 8.1).

This "definitional diversity"[19] can lead to confusion concerning the appropriate timing of consultation. Physicians may delay consulting palliative care experts until patients are clearly terminal, neglecting the symptom-management support they could offer patients during periods of intensive care.[19] In addition, rather than considering palliative care as just another consultative service, such as surgery or radiation oncology, physicians may mistakenly believe that when they bring in the palliative care consultation team, they must relinquish care of the patient to them. Their consequent reluctance to initiate a consultation is understandable. Definitional diversity also affects patients and their families: if palliative care is considered to be appropriate only for patients for whom no disease-directed therapies remain, patients and their families may be reluctant to consult palliative care experts.

Attitudes

Physicians may resist developing their own expertise in palliative care of terminal patients because they are not accustomed to placing the values of patients and

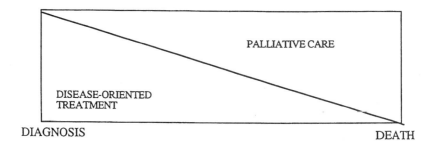

Figure 8.1. The complementary relationship between disease-oriented treatment and palliative care.

their families at the center of the decision-making process. As von Gunten et al, stated: "To provide palliative care, practitioners must shift their focus to the patient's point of view. The patient becomes the expert on suffering, and the physician becomes the consultant. Often, health-care professionals find this to be a striking contrast to providing therapy with curative or remissive intent: in that paradigm, practitioners' knowledge of the science of medicine and the management of disease is paramount."[22] Other attitudinal barriers include "confusion about decisions to forego life-sustaining treatment and euthanasia, fear and denial of death among medical professionals,"[23] and the public, and a belief that prolongation of life is the predominant goal of medicine.[2] Physicians are therefore reluctant to discuss death, to help patients complete advance directives,[3,4,15,24–27] and to advise them to appoint durable powers of attorney for health care. Families report that they feel isolated, misinformed, and unprepared, especially about the expected course of the patient and his or her death.[19]

Insufficient training

Until recently, physicians in training[7] and in practice,[6] nurses, and social workers had very little formal education in palliative care and therefore lacked expertise.[6,28] In U.S. medical and nursing schools, curricula were lacking,[6,11,29–34] and there were few role models in teaching institutions, even for palliative care of the dying, because any expertise that existed was found in hospices.[3] This situation offers little help to those who die in hospitals.[2]

Solutions

Improved delivery of palliative care to patients and their families will require profound changes in the attitudes of health care providers, along with increased knowledge and development of the skills that will enable them to alleviate physical, social, psychological, and spiritual distress. Training in all these dimensions of palliative care can be provided in a number of ways. Textbooks[35,36] pain guidelines,[37,38] and course work using the newly available curricula on cancer pain[39–44] and palliative care[38,45–47] can remedy the knowledge deficit for those motivated to do so. Dr. Neil MacDonald, for example, has edited a case-based learning text that can be integrated into seminar series, ward rounds, clinical conferences, grand rounds, nursing inservices, or social work case conferences.[48]

Additional methods are needed to reach clinicians with the attitudinal barriers described above who are unlikely to seek out available information or participate voluntarily in formal educational programs. Even for those who are motivated, experience with solving the problems of patients and their families in inpatient and outpatient settings and in the home will be required to help them develop the necessary skills. Working with an inpatient or outpatient hospice team would be very useful,[49–51] but it is not a practical solution for graduate physicians or nurses, and hospice teams would be unlikely to provide optimal experience in solving the problems of nonterminal patients. Palliative care units are an excellent educational venue as well (as discussed elsewhere in this volume), but they can train only a small minority of interested clinicians.

Educational opportunities for palliative care consultation teams

Palliative care consultation teams, on the other hand, can be developed at any clinical site. They can overcome the barriers posed by definitional diversity by performing consultations for patients at all stages of disease and by demonstrating to hospital staff how to implement the hospice philosophy, when indicated, for hospitalized patients.[52] Palliative care consultation teams can produce attitudinal changes in physicians and nurses by demonstrating the enormous impact of expert symptom control on quality of life at any point along the disease trajectory. The teams can also help those with insufficient training by serving as a source of palliative care education for patients, their families, and their friends, as well as for an unlimited number of clinicians who wish to improve their expertise.

In the common academic model, however, individual clinical experts are the educators—knowledgeable people whose opinion is respected, who are good teachers, and who serve as role models for the staff. In intensive care units, for example, house staff learn from cardiologists how to administer very dangerous medications to reverse life-threatening arrhythmias. Similarly, a physician who is a pain expert could instruct house staff at the bedside of a patient in excruciating pain in how to increase the morphine dose safely in order to resolve a different, but equally serious, patient problem. An analgesic dosing service has, in fact, been effective in improving pain management in inpatients.[53] But educating clinicians in how to manage the medical, psychosocial, and spiritual concerns of the dying requires a team of experts such as the physician, nurse coordinator, social worker, and chaplain usually available in palliative care consultation teams or services.[6,54–59] As dictated by the clinical site, this team may be staffed only by nurse specialists with physician backup.[60]

In their paper describing the status of undergraduate education in palliative care and presenting recommendations for improvement, Billings and Block outline a number of key content areas for palliative care education for undergraduate medical students.[7] These same content areas need to be mastered by any clinician caring for patients who need palliative care. By working with a palliative care consultation team, students from a variety of disciplines at any level of training would acquire knowledge and skills in several of these content areas, such as "skillfully managing pain and other distressing symptoms commonly occurring in end-stage disease; working with an interdisciplinary team to provide comprehensive, coordinated care; acknowledging and responding to the personal stresses of professionals working with dying persons; and developing an awareness of one's own attitudes, feelings, and expectations regarding death and loss."

In addition, Billings and Block suggest a number of educational principles, many of which the team would embody: "respect for patients' personal values and an appreciation of cultural and spiritual diversity in approaching death and dying"; "a comprehensive integrated understanding of and approach to death, dying and bereavement is enhanced when students are exposed to the perspectives of multiple disciplines working together"; and "faculty should be taught how to teach about end-of-life care, including how to be mentors and to model ideal behaviors and skills." Sheldon and Smith echo these principles: "Balancing risk and safety, and promoting growth while yet ensuring maintenance of a basic level of functioning are then the tasks of educators in palliative care in relation to students, just as they are for the multiprofessional team surrounding the person who is dying and [his or her] carers. Students are exposed to the uncertainties of joining and belonging to a new group, with handling disagreements and conflicts and with the challenge of whether to welcome learning or to retreat into former comfortable certainties."[47]

Palliative care consultation teams also serve as excellent models of truly collaborative practice with a biopsychosocial focus. As Sheldon and Smith stated, "It is a process that is *with* and *for* people rather than *on* people."[47] Since suffering has physical, emotional, psychological, spiritual, and social components, a multidisciplinary team is required to address it; the consultation team can teach all types of health professionals how they can contribute. Physicians in particular may profit from exposure to the benefits of working with a team in solving such complex problems. Oncology fellows, for example, have responded very favorably.[61]

Clinical effectiveness of a palliative care consultation team

To be role models and mentors and to change attitudes, the consultation team first has to prove that it can make a clinical contribution. When we started our team at the Philadelphia Veterans Affairs Medical Center (VAMC), the local administration raised concerns about duplication of services. They noted that there were already several active oncology clinics and an oncology consultation service that included medical oncologists, nurses with master's degrees in oncology nursing, and an oncology social worker, and that the chaplain was available to us on request. They questioned how assembling a palliative care team (which we called a *hospice consultation team*) would deliver services more efficiently to veterans and the families who helped care for them.

We therefore conducted a prospective study of all consultations received during the first year of the team's operation to determine whether the team approach would simply duplicate already available services or would provide improved care.[59] All members of the hospice consultation team saw the patients initially and prospectively completed data collection forms, which included demographic and medical information, as well as an assessment of the medical, nursing, psychosocial, and spiritual needs of the patients and their families. Team meetings were held weekly or more often if clinically indicated.

Data collection

Demographic information included age, sex, race, religion, discharge and read-mission dates, the date and location of death (hospital, home, nursing home), whether a do-not-resuscitate (DNR) status had been established, and whether the patient was currently followed in one of our four medical oncology clinics.

Medical information included the type of cancer, metastatic sites, other medical illnesses, smoking, and any alcohol and drug abuse history. An extensive list of possible symptoms, derived from an early version of the Memorial Symptom Assessment Scale,[62] was reviewed with the patient to ascertain the number of symptoms currently being experienced. We also documented physical findings, performance status, and weight loss of more or less than 10%. We recorded the type and source of the patient's nutrition, all medications and their side effects (especially sedation, delirium, constipation, and diarrhea), skin or oral care regimens, and equipment required to maintain mobility.

Psychosocial information included the presence or absence of psychological disorders (anxiety, depression, anger), lack of understanding of the patient's medical condition, type of insurance and other financial resources, names of caregivers and their relationship to the patient, and current living situation. Spiritual assessment included the importance of religion or faith to the patients, their need for prayer, and their fear of death. Patients were seen daily, and their progress was documented. During the data collection period, problems discovered by the hospice consultation team were distinguished from those noted by the physicians, nurses, and social workers who consulted us.

The medical data recorded during our subsequent follow-up visits to the patients included changes in the medical or nursing regimen; changes in DNR status; relief of previously incompletely treated pain; changes in the opioid drug, dose, or route of administration; addition of adjuvant pain-relieving agents; changes in the agent or dose of laxative or sleep medication; appearance and resolution of mental status changes (sedation, delirium), nausea, or diarrhea; changes in skin or oral care regimens, or in the nursing management plan, or in nutrition; and identification and provision of equipment to maintain mobility or meet physical or occupational therapy needs.

Psychosocial and spiritual data recorded during follow-ups included referral to home care services or placement in a nursing home; identification of financial resources, insurance, or caregivers; identification and resolution of knowledge deficits by clinicians, caregivers, or the patient; identification of the need for patient or family counseling; identification of patient psychological disorders (anger, anxiety, depression); success in finding family members; identification and resolution of spiritual concerns; need for delivery of the sacraments or of prayer; and fear of death.

Records of problem resolution included the inpatient team's responses to our suggestions, as well as the patients' assessments of whether their symptoms were adequately relieved.

Results

Patient characteristics

The hospice consultation team received 80 consultations in its first year of operation; complete data were available on 75 (95%). Sixty percent of the patients were African-American, 37% were white, and 3% were Hispanic. Ninety-eight percent were male and 2% were female. Forty percent were Catholic, 59% were Protestant, and 1% were Jewish. Only 50% of the patients has a caregiver in the home.

Patients were generally very debilitated: 72% had an Eastern Cooperative Oncology Group (ECOG) performance status of 3. Half of the patients had experienced a loss of more than 10% of their usual body weight. Forty percent of patients had lung cancer, 22% prostate cancer, 21% gastrointestinal cancers, and 17% other cancer types. Bone metastases (often accompanied by spinal cord compression) were found in 37% of the patients, epidural metastases in 17%, brain metastases in 16%, liver metastases in 14%, and other metastatic sites in 16%.

Problems identified by the hospice consultation team

The hospice consultation team identified a large number of medical, psychosocial, and spiritual problems not previously identified or inadequately treated by the hospital team. In all, we identified 164 medical problems in the 75 patients. The majority of these (123) centered on managing the patients' pain. There were problems with the opioid being used: a change in agent, dose, route, or frequency of administration was required. Side effects of the opioid, such as constipation, change in mental status, or nausea, were also common, and many patients required addition of an adjuvant agent. Other medical and nursing problems included inadequate skin care, oral care, or nutrition, or nonopioid-related problems with laxatives, mental status, nausea, or diarrhea. Of interest, 15 patients who had been referred to us for hospice care had not had their wishes regarding resuscitation recorded.

The hospice consultation team identified 152 psychosocial problems in the 75 patients, including a need for family counseling and unappreciated anxiety, depression, and/or anger. Despite the presence of a social worker on each of the inpatient units, the hospice consultation team noted the lack of information about insurance or an agency to deliver home care or placement in a nursing home. Overall, only 54% of our patients were found to have medical insurance. Fifty percent of our patients had either general spiritual needs or requested prayer or sacraments.

Of special interest were the hospice consultation team referrals already being followed in one of our medical oncology clinics. Of these 22 patients, 21 had one or more problems identified by the hospice consultation team. Most of these were financial, social, or spiritual, but 11 patients reported inadequate pain relief and 4 had other medical problems identified.

Problems resolved

Of the 164 new medical/nursing problems, we were able to resolve 85%. Ninety percent of the patients who initially suffered from unacceptable pain achieved acceptable pain relief from changes in the route, dose, or type of opioid or adjuvant medication. Opioid side effects were resolved in 25 of 27 patients (96%). Of 22 patients followed in oncology clinics, new problems were identified and resolved in 21. Unfortunately, of the 152 new psychosocial and spiritual problems, only 40% and 61%, respectively, were resolved. It may be that psychosocial problems are resistant to resolution in these patients, but we felt that our failure was more likely due to the absence of a psychologist or psychiatrist on the team. We subsequently arranged an affiliation with a graduate school of psychology. Both first- and third-year clinical psychology students are now available to the team and the patients several days a week, and their hospital-based preceptor is available at all times. We conclude that the expertise of the hospice consultation team members, along with the team process provided, improved care to these patients.

As our population was largely African-American and male, the results of our study are not directly generalizable to all populations. However, while the frequency of the problems we identified may be different, it is likely that the types of medical and psychosocial problems we identified and resolved are similar to those in any institution lacking professionals who are experts in palliative care.

Clinical and educational role of palliative care consultation teams in a disease management program for patients at the end of life

In view of our positive results, we plan to establish more palliative care consultation teams as part of a disease management program for care of patients at the end of life in the University of Pennsylvania Health System (UPHS). These teams will assist in the critical implementation phase of our symptom management program, which requires support from local opinion leaders, as well as a combination of intense physician and patient education and compliance programs.

The literature supports the educational efficacy both of local opinion leaders[63–67] and of palliative care services.[68,69] Local opinion leaders (physicians, nurses, social workers) have been found to be as good as or better than audit and feedback techniques in inducing practitioners to implement practice guidelines.[66,67] Ferrell and colleagues, for example, have developed the *PRN* nursing model (*Pain Resource Nurse*),[63] which trains nurses to be institutional pain management resources; these nurses provide expertise and education and act as role models. Weissman and Dahl have developed a *role model* program in which clinician pairs (nurses or social workers plus a physician) undergo intensive training in pain management, at the end of which they contract to complete a project in their home institution.[64]

Similarly, community palliative care teams, using guidelines, have been effective in improving pain management.[68,69] We are in the process of creating a network of teams in selected inpatient, outpatient, and long-term care facilities to enable clinicians throughout the UPHS to benefit from their expertise. Clinicians (nurses and doctors) and social workers who care for patients with cancer, human immunodeficiency virus, or pulmonary diseases, or for the elderly, will form the core teams and will have help from psychiatry, pharmacy, chaplain, and nutrition services.

Our palliative care consultation teams will be taught how to assess and manage a wide range of problems faced by dying patients and their families and will learn about bereavement care.[70,71] They will then serve as the local program leaders and play a key role in educating clinicians about the care of dying patients using clinical practice guidelines, algorithms, and protocols,[4,46,72–74] which they will help develop and implement. The symptom management guidelines will be supplied to primary care and specialty physicians in their offices, as well as to clinicians based in community or academic hospitals or long-term care facilities. The palliative care consultation team members will be involved in helping other clinicians to use the guidelines and educational materials provided, and will serve as mentors and role models as well as clinical consultants. Teams will also help specialists, primary care physicians, and nurse practitioners coordinate patient care with community agencies and hospices.

Summary

Palliative care consultation teams can play a number of important roles in the education of health professionals, patients, and their families. They can educate their colleagues both in the specifics of managing many of the severe physical, psychological, social, and spiritual problems of patients and in how to recognize other disorders that require referral to specialists. They demonstrate that symptoms should be minimized whenever possible and that even for patients whose disease cannot be reversed, much can still be done to maximize their quality of life and enable them to accomplish their final goals. Teams teach patients and their families how they can participate in the process, a process that, after all, is centered on them and their values. As clinicians begin to care for dying patients with the support of team members, the clinicians will learn how satisfying caring for patients at the end can often be—how discharging our duty not to abandon the patient can bring us the closure we need and enable us to be secure in the knowledge that we really did everything we could for our patients and their families.

References

1. Chappell F. *Farewell, I'm Bound to Leave You.* New York: Picador, 1996:3–5.
2. Meier DE, Morrison RS, Cassel CK. Improving palliative care. *Ann Intern Med* 1997; 127:225–230.
3. Morrison SR, Meier DE, Cassel CK. When too much is too little. *N Engl J Med* 1996; 335:1755–1760.

4. Hill CS. When will adequate pain treatment be the norm? *JAMA* 1995; 274:1881–1882.

5. Council on Scientific Affairs, American Medical Association. Good care of the dying patient. *JAMA* 1996; 275:474–478.

6. Committee on Care at the End of Life. Educating clinicians and other professionals. In: Field MJ, Cassel CK, eds. *Approaching Death: Improving Care at the End of Life.* Washington, D.C.: National Academy Press, 1997:207–234.

7. Billings JA, Block S. Palliative care in undergraduate medical education: status report and future directions. *JAMA* 1997; 278:733–738.

8. Breitbart W, Rosenfeld BD, Passik SD, et al. The undertreatment of pain in ambulatory AIDS patients. *Pain* 1996; 65:243–249.

9. Cleeland CS, Gonin R, Hatfield NK, et al. Pain and its treatment in outpatients with metastatic cancer. *N Engl J Med* 1994; 330:592–596.

10. The SUPPORT Principal Investigators. A controlled trial to improve care for seriously-ill hospitalized patients. *JAMA* 1995; 274:1591–1598.

11. Von Roenn JH, Cleeland CS, Gonin R, et al. Physician attitudes and practice in cancer pain management. A survey from the Eastern Cooperative Oncology Group. *Ann Intern Med* 1993; 119:121–126.

12. Cherny NI, Catane R. Professional negligence in the management of cancer pain. A case for urgent reforms. *Cancer* 1995; 7:2181–2185.

13. Ogle KS, Mavis B, Rohrer J. Graduating medical students' competencies and educational experiences in palliative care. *J Pain Symptom Manage* 1997; 14:280–285.

14. Asch DA. The role of critical care nurses in euthanasia and assisted suicide. *N Engl J Med* 1996; 334:1374–1379.

15. Morrison RS, Morrison EW, Glickman DF. Physician reluctance to discuss advance directives. *Arch Intern Med* 1994; 154:2311–2318.

16. Block SD, Billings JA. Patient requests to hasten death: evaluation and management in terminal care. *Arch Intern Med* 1994; 154:2039–2047.

17. Chappell F. *I Am One of You Forever.* Baton Rouge: LSU Press, 1985:93–96.

18. Rando TA. *Treatment of Complicated Mourning.* Champaigne, IL: Research Press, 1993.

19. Zuckerman C. Project Director, Hospital Palliative Care Initiative, United Hospital Fund. Presentation: "Dying in New York City Hospitals," delivered June 17, 1997, at "Care for Dying Patients: Building Palliative Care Programs," sponsored by the United Hospital Fund, New York.

20. Doyle D, Hanks G, MacDonald N. Introduction. In: Doyle D, Hanks G, MacDonald N, eds. *Oxford Textbook of Palliative Medicine.* New York, Oxford University Press, 1998:3–8.

21. Portenoy RP. The von Gunten et al. article reviewed. *Oncology* 1996; 10:1074–1079.

22. von Gunten CF, Neely KJ, Martinez J. Hospice and palliative care: program needs and academic issues. *Oncology* 1996; 10:1070–1074.

23. Seravalli E. The dying patient, the physician, and the fear of death. *N Engl J Med* 1988; 319:1728–1730.

24. Lo B. Improving care near the end of life: why is it so hard? *JAMA* 1995; 274:1634–1636.

25. Gilligan T, Raffin TA. Whose death is it anyway? *Ann Intern Med* 1996; 125:137–141.

26. Teno JM, Hakim RB, Knaus WA, et al. Preferences for cardiopulmonary resuscitation:

physician-patient agreement and hospital resource use. *J Gen Intern Med* 1995; 10:179–186.

27. Tulsky JA, Chesney MA, Lo B. See one, do one, teach one? House staff experience discussing do-not-resuscitate orders. *J Gen Intern Med* 1996; 156:1285–1290.

28. Mortimer JE, Bartlett NL. Assessment of knowledge about cancer pain management by physicians in training. *J Pain Symptom Manage* 1997; 14:21–28.

29. Tolle SW, Elliot DL, Hickam DH. Physician attitudes and practices at the time of patient death. *Arch Intern Med* 1984; 144:2389–2391.

30. Dickinson GE. Changes in death education in U.S. medical schools during 1975–1985. *J Med Educ* 1985; 60:942–943.

31. Mermann AC, Gunn DB, Dickinson GE. Learning to care for the dying: a survey of medical schools and a model course. *Acad Med* 1991; 66:35–38.

32. Plumb JD, Segraves M. Terminal care in primary postgraduate medical education programs: a national survey. *Am J Hosp Palliat Care* 1992; 9:32–35.

33. Martini CJ, Grenholm G. Institutional responsibility in graduate medical education and highlights of historical data *JAMA* 1993; 270:1053–1060.

34. Rappaport W, Witzke D. Education about death and dying during the clinical years of medical school. *Surgery* 1993; 113:163–165.

35. Doyle D, Hanks GWC, MacDonald N, eds. *Oxford Textbook of Palliative Medicine, 2nd ed.* New York: Oxford University Press, 1998.

36. Berger AM, Portenoy RK, Weissman DE, eds. *Principles and Practice of Supportive Oncology.* Philadelphia: Lippincott-Raven, 1998.

37. American Pain Society Quality of Care Committee. Quality improvement guidelines for the treatment of acute pain and cancer pain. *JAMA* 1995; 274:1875–1880.

38. Jacox A, Carr DB, Payne R, et al. *Management of Cancer Pain: Clinical Practice Guideline No 9. Agency for Health Care Policy and Research* Washington, D.C.: U.S. Public Health Service, 1994.

39. Weissman DE. Cancer pain education: objectives for medical students and residents in primary care specialties — Palliative Oncology Committee of the AACE. *J Cancer Educ* 1995; 11:7–10.

40. Ad Hoc Committee on Cancer Pain of the American Society of Clinical Oncology. Cancer pain assessment and treatment curriculum guidelines. *J Clin Oncol* 1992; 10:1830–1832.

41. Fields HL, ed. *Core Curriculum for Professional Education in Pain, 2nd ed.* Seattle: IASP Press 1995.

42. Weissman DE, Dahl JL. Update on the cancer pain role model education program. *J Pain Symptom Manage* 1995; 10:292–297.

43. World Health Organization Expert Committee Report. *Cancer Pain Relief and Palliative Care.* Technical Report Series 804. Geneva: World Health Organization, 1990.

44. American Pain Society Quality of Care Committee. Quality improvement guidelines for the treatment of acute pain and cancer pain. *JAMA* 1995; 274:1874–1880.

45. American Board of Internal Medicine. *Caring for the Dying: Identification and Promotion of Physician Competency.* Educational Resource Document. Philadelphia: American Board of Internal Medicine, 1996.

46. MacDonald N, Mount B, Boston W, et al. The Canadian palliative care undergraduate curriculum. *J Cancer Educ* 1993; 8:197–201.

47. Sheldon F, Smith P. The life so short, the craft so hard to learn: a model for post-basic education in palliative care. *J Palliat Care* 1996; 10:99–104.
48. MacDonald N, ed. *Palliative Medicine: A Case-Based Manual.* New York: Oxford University Press, 1997.
49. Ross DD, O'Mara A., Pickens N. et al Hospice and palliative care education in medical school: a module on the role of the physician in end-of-life care. *J Cancer Educ* 1997; 12:(3)152–6.
50. Seligman P, Massey E, Fink R, et al. Practicing physicians' assessment of the impact of their medical school clinical hospice experience. *J Cancer Educ* 1997; 12(suppl): 29. (abstract)
51. Neely KJ, von Gunten C. First year medical students' narrative accounts of hospice home visits. *J Cancer Educ* 1996; 11(suppl):27. (Abstract)
52. Esper P, Redman BG. Supportive care pain management and quality of life in advanced prostate cancer. *Urd Clin NA* 1999; 26:375–89.
53. von Gunten CF, Lothian ST, Fotis MA, et al. Cancer pain management through a pharmacist-based analgesic dosing service. *Am J Health-System Pharmacy* 1999; 56:1119–25.
54. Goldstein P, Walsh D, Horvitz LU. The Cleveland Clinic Foundation Harry R. Horvitz Palliative Care Center. *Support Care Cancer* 1996; 4:329–333.
55. Jarvis H, Burge FI, Scott CA. Evaluating a palliative care program: methodology and limitations. *J Palliat Care* 1996; 12:23–33.
56. Vohr F, Wacker M. Palliative care service, a nurse-driven consulting service. *J Palliat Care* 1995; 11:69.
57. Camden B, Franz G, Twaddle M, et al. Prospective study of referrals to a hospice/palliative medicine consultation team. *J Palliat Care* 1995; 11:63.
58. Yeomans W, Spring B, Porterfield P. Consultation services within the continuum of palliative care. *J Palliat Care* 1995; 11:69.
59. Abrahm JL, Callahan J, Rossetti K, et al. The impact of a hospice consultation team on the care of veterans with advanced cancer. *J Pain Symptom Manage* 1996; 12:23–31.
60. Committee on Care at the End of Life. The health care system and the dying patient. In: Field MJ, Cassel CK, eds. *Approaching Death: Improving Care at the End of Life.* Washington, DC: National Academy Press, 1997:87–121.
61. von Gunten CF, Von Roenn JH, Gradishar W, et al. Hospice/palliative medicine rotation for fellows training in hematology-oncology. *J Cancer Educ* 1995; 10:200–202.
62. Portenoy RK, Thaler HT, Kornblith AB, et al. The Memorial Symptom Assessment Scale: an instrument for the evaluation of symptom prevalence, characteristics and distress. *Eur J Cancer* 1994; 30A:1326–1336.
63. Ferrell BR, Grant M, Ritchey KJ, et al. The pain resource nurse training program: a unique approach to pain management. *J Pain Symptom Manage* 1993; 8:549–556.
64. Weissman DE, Dahl JL. Update on the cancer pain role model education program. *J Pain Symptom Manage* 1995; 10:292–297.
65. Weissman DE. Cancer pain education for physicians in practice: establishing a new paradigm. *J Pain Symptom Manage* 1996; 12:364–371.
66. Lomas J, Enkin M, Anderson GM, et al. Opinion leaders vs. audit and feedback to implement practice guidelines. *JAMA* 1991; 265:2202–2207.

67. Karuza J, Calkins E, Feather J, et al. Enhancing physician adoption of practice guidelines. *Arch Intern Med* 1995; 155:625–632.
68. McQuillan R, Finlay I, Branch C, et al. Improving analgesic prescribing in a general teaching hospital. *J Pain Symptom Manage* 1996; 11:172–180.
69. Higginson IJ, Hearn J. A multicenter evaluation of cancer pain control by palliative care teams. *J Pain Symptom Manage* 1997; 14:29–35.
70. Bromberg MH, Higginson I. Bereavement follow-up: what do palliative support teams actually do? *J Palliat Care* 1996; 12:12–17.
71. Abrahm JL, Cooley ME, Ricacho L. Efficacy of an educational bereavement program for families of veterans with cancer. *J Cancer Educ* 1995; 10:207–212.
72. Robinson L, Stacy R. Palliative care in the community setting: practice guidelines for primary care teams. *Br J Gen Pract* 1994; 44:461–464.
73. National Hospice Organization Standards and Accreditation Committee 1995–1996. *A Pathway for Patients and Families Facing Terminal Illness.* National Hospice Organization, 1997.
74. Weissman DE, Griffie J, Gordon DB, et al. A role model program to promote institutional changes for management of acute and cancer pain. *J Pain Symptom Manage* 1997; 14:274–279.

III

PROCOAGULANT AND ANTICOAGULANT THERAPY IN PALLIATIVE CARE

9

The Management of Bleeding in
Advanced Cancer Patients

JOSE PEREIRA, ISABELLE MANCINI,
AND EDUARDO BRUERA

Bleeding is a common presenting problem at the time of the original diagnosis of several different types of cancers. Ninety percent of patients with endometrial cancer report vaginal bleeding at the time of their diagnosis, 10–20% of patients with colorectal cancer report rectal bleeding, and 25–50% of patients with lung cancer describe hemoptysis at the time of the initial diagnosis.[1] Just over one-half of patients with a renal malignancy first present with hematuria. However, hemorrhaging in the palliative care setting occurs less frequently and has been estimated to affect approximately 6–10% of patients.[2,3] However, although they are less frequent, these bleeding events can be frightening experiences for patients, their families, and health care professionals alike, especially if the hemorrhaging is considerable.[4] Moreover, a massive bleed, whether external or occult, is said to be the immediate cause of death in 6% of cancer patients.

The chapter will focus on external hemorrhages. Although occult intra-abdominal, intrathoracic, or intracranial hemorrhages following the rupture of a large blood vessel by a malignant process do occur, and are often fatal, they do not necessarily give rise to the severe distress that massive external hemorrhages do. Moreover, because they are not always as apparent as external hemorrhages are, little is known about their frequency and their course.

Clinical Approach

In the palliative setting, management of bleeding must consider many factors. Not only does the clinician have to consider the underlying cause and the clinical presentation, including the severity and nature of such an event, but he or she also needs to take into account other salient factors such as the setting of care, availability of various resources, overall disease burden, predicted life expectancy, the patient's overall quality of life, and the wishes of the patient and family. This chapter will discuss and review the various treatment modalities that are available to manage bleeding events in the palliative setting. These modalities vary from local, topical treatments to therapies that require systemic administration. Some treatments are noninvasive, and others require invasive interventions such as endoscopy or surgery. Some are widely available to palliative care practitioners and others, such as interventional radiology, require specialist resources.

The decision to use one or another treatment modality must balance the risk of overaggressive management, with increased treatment-related toxicity, on the one hand, with the failure to use treatments that have potential symptomatic benefits on the other.[5] Although many of the simple treatment modalities can be initiated by oncology or palliative care staff, definitive management may require an interdisciplinary approach and the expertise of various other specialists.

As an example of the need to balance priorities, it is evident that interventional radiology or surgical ligation of a pelvic vessel would be less likely considered in a homebound, cachectic patient who has expressed the desire to remain at home, particularly if the patient has an estimated life expectancy ranging from a few days to perhaps a few weeks. On the other hand, had the same patient presented with significant hemorrhaging soon after the diagnosis was made, it would have been reasonable to at least consider these treatment modalities as options, particularly if specialists with the required skills and equipment were available. Similarly, administering fresh–frozen plasma or other blood components to a patient who is bleeding secondary to disseminated intravascular coagulopathy brought on by extensive metastatic adenocarcinoma is unlikely to significantly improve the long-term quality of life of that patient. Conversely, a patient with advanced cancer who is experiencing frequent episodes of epistaxis secondary to thrombocytopenia may have an improved quality of life, at least temporarily, by a transfusion of platelets. In the latter case, the disadvantages of continued, ongoing transfusions of platelets would probably at some point outweigh the benefits, and the patient and family, in collaboration with the attending clinicians, would need to make a decision regarding termination of the transfusions. It goes without saying that patients and families faced with such a profound decision would require extensive psychological support, as would any other patient and family faced with the prospect, or the reality, of a massive bleeding episode.

Clinical Presentation and Underlying Causes of Hemorrhaging in Palliative Patients

The nature and severity of the hemorrhage will impact on management and is often determined by the underlying malignancy and its clinical course. A large, ulcerating head and neck tumor, for example, can erode a large blood vessel in the neck and result in massive external hemorrhaging. The erosion of a large vessel in the groin by a malignancy in the genitalia can give rise to similar consequences, as can a large anal tumor or a tumor in the chest wall from metastatic breast cancer.[6] The source of a massive hemorrhage could also be an internal organ. Malignancies involving the upper and lower gastrointestinal tracts, lungs, kidneys, bladder, and female genital tract can produce massive bleeds that present as hematemesis, hematochezia, melena, hemoptysis, hematuria, and vaginal bleeding, respectively.

These hemorrhages can result in catastrophic events that may cause hypovolemic shock and are immediately life-threatening. They can also give rise to chronic, low-volume bleeding or episodic hemorrhages of low to medium intensity. An ulcerating exophytic neck mass, for example, can result in distressing episodic hemorrhages. Chronic hematuria or melena from genitourinary or gastrointestinal malignancies can result in anemia that, in turn, can aggravate other symptoms such as shortness of breath or fatigue.

Mechanisms other than the local erosion of small or large blood vessels are sometimes responsible for hemorrhaging in patients with advanced cancer. Systemic processes such as coagulation and platelet abnormalities may be responsible.[6,7] Clotting and fibrinolysis abnormalities are relatively common—detectable in up to 50% of palliative care patients. These occur most often in the presence of metastatic spread and result in bleeding or thrombosis in only approximately 15% of cases.[8] Disseminated intravascular coagulation (DIC), which is characterized pathophysiologically by excessive thrombin activation, extensive consumption and depletion of circulating clotting factors, and deposition of fibrin-platelet thrombi in the microvasculature, results from malignancy-associated procoagulants and activators of fibrinolysis released by some acute leukemias and adenocarcinomas of the prostate, pancreas, stomach, colon, gallbladder, lung, ovary, and breast. Abnormalities of coagulation times, clotting factors, platelets, fibrinogen, and D-dimers may ensue. Liver failure following extensive involvement by the malignancy or following multiorgan failure may be the cause of deficiencies in vitamin K–related coagulation factors. Other cancer-related causes of vitamin K deficiency, such as malabsorption and malnutrition, may aggravate the situation. Thrombocytopenia or abnormal platelet function may be the underlying cause of the bleeding and may be secondary to bone marrow suppression following chemotherapy or radiation therapy, marrow infiltration by malignancies such as prostate cancer and leukemia, sepsis, and DIC. Occasionally, immune-based mechanisms are responsible. These may be related to lymphoproliferative disorders; certain drugs such as anticonvulsants, heparin, and nonsteroidal anti-inflammatory drugs; and, on occasion, solid tumors. Thrombocytopenia or abnormal platelet function, when it does occur, is not necessarily caused by the malignancy or its treatment. Pre-existing conditions such idiopathic thrombocytopenia may be responsible. These abnormalities may manifest clinically as purpura, petechiae, epistaxis, melena, hematuria, vaginal bleeding, and excessive bleeding after procedures such as venipuncture or the insertion of a subcutaneous needle.

General Measures

The first step in approaching the problem of hemorrhaging in patients with advanced cancer is to identify those patients who are at increased risk of hemorrhaging, particularly those at risk of massive external hemorrhages. Factors that place the patient at risk include large, fungating head and neck or lung tumors that are anatomically close to large blood vessels; recurrent episodes of mild hemoptysis, hematemesis, or hematuria; and large intra-abdominal tumors. Patients with liver failure, bone marrow suppression, or hematological diseases may also be at increased risk. Patients with an increased risk of hidden internal bleeds that could have catastrophic results also need to be identified. In patients with thrombocytopenia, for example, the risk of spontaneous bleeding increases as the platelet count drops below 20,000/μl.

In patients who present with bleeding, a review of current medications is required. In particular, the concurrent use of drugs such as a nonsteroidal anti-inflammatory drug, acetylsalicylic acid, and anticoagulants needs to be identified. This was recently highlighted in an audit of hospice patients taking warfarin for indications such as venous thromboembolism, dysrhythmias, and heart valve abnormalities.[9,10] The audit revealed a high incidence of hemorrhaging and problems in maintaining therapeutic warfarin levels, as measured by the international normalized ratio (INR). The audit resulted in the increased use of low molecular weight heparins for hospice-based patients requiring anticoagulation because these medications are associated with for less risk of bleeding than is warfarin. In addition, their pharmacokinetics are more predictable, their interactions with other drugs are fewer, they are not affected by liver dysfunction, and they require much less monitoring.[11] A survey of 174 palliative care physicians based in the United Kingdom revealed that one in four of them have abandoned warfarin in favor of low molecular weight heparins.[12]

The next step in the management of patients at increased risk of significant bleeding is to inform their families, particularly those members who are caring for them. Other professional caregivers also need to be informed. This allows them to be prepared for such an event and to feel empowered to respond as best they can. However, it must be recognized that even the best coaching and preparation may sometimes not be enough to prepare families or other caregivers for the trauma of a major bleeding event, and support both before and after such an event is critical. If an occult bleeding source, such as intracranial hemorrhage, is predicted, the need to inform caregivers is less acute. However, families may need to be aware of this so as to prepare themselves for the possibility of a sudden deterioration in their loved one's condition. This may also be important for some patients, especially those who indicate that they wish to know so as to prepare themselves, make the necessary financial and legal preparations, and bid their farewells in a timely manner. Given the potentially distressing nature of the topic, great sensitivity is required when discussing it with the patient and relatives. It can be argued that patients at a high risk of large external bleeds do not necessarily need to know and should be spared the details, which may increase their distress. This may certainly be true in many cases. Dark towels and dark-colored bassinets need to be at hand to make the blood loss less evident than it would be with white or light-colored utensils and bed sheets. The family may need to be instructed on how to apply pressure to a site that is bleeding. In the case of massive hemoptysis or hematemesis, the family and caregivers should be taught to place the patient in the left lateral position to avoid suffocation. The appropriate support mechanisms need to be discussed and put in place. The authors of this chapter are aware of incidents in which families, who, despite extensive coaching and preparation beforehand, panicked at the time of the event and summoned emergency paramedic and ambulance services, which are generally trained to respond by implementing full resuscitative measures when confronted with massive hemorrhaging. This not only underscores the psychological impact of such an event on families and caregivers, but also reminds health care professionals of the importance of discussing and documenting issues related to resuscitation versus nonresuscitation in these patients.

A massive hemorrhage can obviously be extremely distressing to the patient as well. Although it can be massive and rapidly result in death, it can also be more prolonged. In those bleeds that are significant but more prolonged, sedation of the patient may be required to spare the patient great distress. This is different from the management of patients who are experiencing a small blood loss, which usually does not result in the level of distress caused by more pronounced bleeding and, therefore, does not require sedation. The availability of a sedating drug that can be administered rapidly and acts quickly may be useful under these circumstances. If given promptly, it can relieve the patient and give the family and caregivers a means of providing comfort. Midazolam is a benzodiazepine with properties that allow it to be used in such a role.[13] If an intravenous line is available, which is seldom the case in palliative care, the drug can be given intravenously. Alternatively, it can be given via the subcutaneous or intramuscular route at a dose of 2.5–5 mg.[4] It can be argued that the subcutaneous route is not pharmacodynamically ideal in cases of hypovolemia since systemic absorption may be compromised. However, families are seldom comfortable administering drugs by intramuscular injection or, for that matter, subcutaneously. A subcutaneous butterfly needle may therefore need to be inserted prophylactically to allow families to administer the drug in patients at a very high risk of a major bleed. Midazolam is effective within a few minutes.[14] Unlike some of the other benzodiazepines such as lorazepam, which require refrigeration, prefilled syringes of midazolam can be stored at room temperature in a dark area or in a dark envelope for periods of up to 30 days.

Local Interventions

Local measures include local packing, wound dressings, reduction of the frequency of dressing if possible, the use of nonadherent dressings, and, in some cases, local radiation therapy. Occasionally, in selected patients and if the expertise is available, more invasive measures such as endoscopy and interventional radiology may be used. The decision to use one or more of these modalities, particularly the most invasive ones, must consider their potential benefits and risks for the particular patient.

Local packing, hemostatic agents, and dressings

Packing can be used with or without pressure to achieve hemostasis, particularly in the case of bleeding from organs such as the rectum,[15] nose,[16] or vagina.[17] Depending on the area involved, packing can be achieved with small or large surgical swabs. In some cases, these swabs can be coated with various chemicals to facilitate hemostasis. Examples include the use of acetone in vaginal packing[17] and cocaine in nasal packing. Pressure to stem local blood flow can also be applied by using catheters and other similar devices. Catheters, including Foley catheters, have been used to stem severe hemorrhaging from the posterior nasal cavity by maneuvering the catheters into position and then inflating their balloons in the area of the bleed.

Local pressure by surgical dressings and swabs can also be applied on areas of surface bleeding. More specialized products and dressings to improve hemostasis are available (Table 9.1). They are useful mainly in managing oozing blood from capillaries and small venules that are accessible. Some of these hemostatic dressings and products are used more often in the surgical setting to stop oozing from small sites that are not amenable to vessel ligation, but some of them may be useful in the palliative setting. Purified gelatin solution is available in either powder or a compressed pack form (Gelfoam).[18] As a pad, this hemostatic, absorbable agent is available in an assortment of sizes that can be cut to cover areas of bleeding. When it is placed on an area of capillary bleeding, fibrin is deposited in the interstices of the foam, resulting in swelling of the sponge and the formation of a large, synthetic clot. In some cases, Gelfoam is soaked with local vasoconstrictors such as epinephrine or cocaine 1% solutions. The foam is absorbable and therefore may need to be replaced.

Another approach is to apply dressings or mesh impregnated with topical thromboplastin (Thrombostat).[19] This topical hemostatic agent is a natural blood-clotting agent that is obtained from bovine plasma as a sterile, water-soluble powder and standardized in National Insitutes of Health units. Thrombin clots the fibrinogen of the blood directly, and the speed of clotting is dependent on its concentration. For example, the contents of a 5000 NIH unit vial dissolved in 5 ml of saline diluent is capable of clotting 5 ml of blood in less than 1 sec.[19] In the surgical

Table 9.1. Local interventions and products for the control of bleeding in palliative care

- Reduction of fequency of dressings

Local dressings and pressure

Use of nonadherent dressings

  Algisate

  Allevyn

  Mepitel

Hemostatic agents and dressings

  Gelatin solution (Gelfoam)

  Thrombin (Thrombostat)

  Collagen (Colagen)

  Cellulose compounds (Oxycel, Nu-kit)

  Fibrinogen + Clotting Factors

  Tissue Glue (Tissel-sealant)

  Kaltostat

Vasoconstricting and cauterizing drugs

  Formalin 2% or 4%

  Solutions of 1% alum

  Prostaglandins E_2 and F_2

  Silver nitrate

  Epinephrine

  Cocaine

Interventional radiology

Surgical ligation

Endoscopy

Radiation

setting, the intended use of the solution determines its strength. Where bleeding is profuse, such as from cut surfaces of the liver and spleen, concentrations as high as 1000 to 2000 units/ml may be required. For this, the 5000 unit vial is dissolved in 5 or 2.5 ml, respectively. Readers need to be aware of the solution and powder strengths that are available in their own countries. Thrombin can also be used in dry form and sprinkled as a powder over the site of oozing. This may be the preferred approach in large, fungating lesions that are seen in the palliative care setting. It must be stressed that this product cannot be injected systemically or allowed to enter large vessels since this will result in extensive intravascular clotting.

Another substance that is used to impregnate mesh to promote hemostasis is bovine-derived collagen (Colagen).[20] When it is placed in contact with a bleeding surface, hemostasis is achieved by aggregation of platelets and fibrin deposition.

More recently, cellulose compounds (Oxycel, Nu-Kit) have become available as dressings.[20] These products may be sutured to, wrapped around, or held firmly against a bleeding site until hemostasis is obtained. When oxidized cellulose comes into contact with whole blood, clots form rapidly. As it reacts with blood, it increases in size to form a gel.

Aluminium astringents such as 1% alum solution or sucralfate can be useful in controlling cutaneous oozing or gastrointestinal bleeding from cancer. Sucralfate paste can be prepared by dispersing 1 g tablet of sucralfate in 5 ml of water-soluble gel (e.g., KY jelly), and this solution can be applied to the bleeding site once or twice daily.[21]

Fibrinogen is available in highly concentrated fibrinogen solutions.[22] One such product (Tissel Kit V) contains clotting factor XIII and a solution of thrombin and calcium chloride. When applied to the wound area, the mixture coagulates. The presence of factor XIII causes the fibrin to cross-link, which gives the coagulum additional resilience. It is also available as a tissue glue (Tissel-sealant) with sealing, hemostatic, and gluing properties, which may enhance wound healing. Other hemostatic agents containing calcium, such as calcium alginate (Kaltostat), have been reported to promote local hemostasis.[22]

Vasoconstricting or cauterizing agents provide an alternative means of managing local areas of capillary oozing. The use of formalin, alum solutions, prostaglandins, and silver nitrate to control bleeding, including bleeding from more concealed sites such as the bladder, has been described.[23] Formalin 2% or 4% acts as a chemical cautery that can occasionally control bleeding from mucosal and submucosal vessels. Formalin, administered intrarectally, has been applied to treat hemorrhagic radiation proctitis, with up to 80% effectiveness.[24,25] It has also been described in the control of hemorrhaging from the bladder when irrigation and fulguration were unsuccessful.[23] Solutions of 1% alum can be delivered by continuous bladder irrigation.[23] During instillation bladder spasms may occur, but they are usually well controlled by antispasmodic medications. An advantage of this modality is that it can be delivered at the bedside, without the need for anesthesia, using a three-way indwelling catheter. A drawback that may limit its application is that, on occasion, it may take as long as 7 days to control bleeding effectively.

Some authors have recommended the initial use of alum for hematuria, with formalin as a second-line therapy. Prostaglandins E_2 and F_2 have been reported to be effective in controlling intractable hemorrhagic cystitis.[23] The mechanism of action is not well known, but it may involve protection of the microvasculature and epithelium and inhibition of the development of tissue edema. Severe bladder spasms may limit its overall utility. Silver nitrate, an inorganic silver salt, has been used locally to control epistaxis and, by instillation, to treat hematuria arising from the bladder.[20,26] Its mechanism of action is essentially chemically induced cauterization. Subsequent scarring and healing induced by the cauterization may help prevent recurrent endothelial breakdown and thereby diminish the chance of recurrent bleeding. The compound's concentration and contact time determine its clinical effect.

Vasoconstrictors such as epinephrine are available mainly in combination with local anesthetic agents.[20] Liberal use is not advised because of the potential for overdoses from either the epinephrine or the local anesthetic. The maximum dose of lidocaine appears to be 3 mg/kg when no epinephrine is used and 7 mg/kg when a vasoconstrictor is added.

The role of all these local hemostatic agents is limited to small areas of capillary bleeding. They are not effective in larger hemorrhages. Unfortunately, there are no randomized controlled trials comparing these various agents with one another, particularly in the setting of cancer. Therefore, the decision to use one or another agent must be based on factors such as the location of the bleeding, the amount of bleeding, the response to more conservative and less costly measures such as local pressure and the use of nonadherent dressings, clinical experience of the treating clinician with the various products, cost, and local availability.

Radiotherapy

The palliative role of radiotherapy in controlling bleeding, particularly lung, vaginal, bladder, and rectal bleeding, has been well documented and should always be considered fairly early.[27–30] In lung cancer, small fractionation strategies are as effective as multiple fractions in controlling hemoptysis, with control occurring in about 85% of patients.[27,28,30] The optimal dose and fractionation remain controversial. A single fraction of 10 GY has been shown to be as effective as multiple fractions in patients with hemoptysis due to lung cancer.[30] A retrospective study conducted by Srinivasan et al. suggested that reduced fractionation may be the palliative treatment of choice for advanced bladder cancer, with control of hematuria occurring in approximately 60% of patients.[29] Radiotherapy has also been found to be of value in controlling uterine and vaginal bleeding, either by external beam or by intracavity irradiation.[30,31] When previous radical radiation has been administered to the pelvis, a further small dose may be tolerated well and may be sufficient to achieve hemostasis. There are few data on the success of radiotherapy in controlling tumor-induced bleeding from the upper gastrointestinal tract.[30] In the lower gastrointestinal tract, an overall response rate of 85% and a complete control rate of 63% have been reported after palliative irradiation of bleeding rectal carcinoma.[30] This success was achieved with radiation doses of 30 to 35 GY delivered in 10 fractions over 2 weeks. In the case of skin or superficial lesions, radiotherapy may reduce the size of the tumor and have a hemostatic effect.[32] However, head and neck malignancies have often already been treated with extensive radiation therapy by the time the patient enters the palliative care setting, and repeat radiation therapy may not always be feasible.[33]

Endoscopy

Treatment with endoscopy may be considered in selected cases, particularly where surgical resection is not an option.[34] Endoscopy may be considered in upper gastrointestinal and bladder-related bleeding and, to a lesser extent, in bleeding from the lower gastrointestinal tract and the lungs. Recently, new endoscopic techniques have been introduced, including the injection of substances such as pure ethanol,[35,36] hyperosmotic saline epinephrine,[34] gelatin solutions,[37] and sodium tetradecyl sulfate.[34] Severe active bleeding may, however, pose a technical problem by limiting visibility. If a bleeding vessel is identified, it is cauterized by heater probe coagulation,[38,40] polar coagulation,[36,38] or laser.[39,40] These methods of cauterization have been compared in the treatment of malignant and nonmalignant gastrointestinal ulcers. In upper gastrointestinal tract bleeds, these methods all appear to be comparable in safety and efficacy, with effective hemostasis being achieved in about 70%[34] to 100%[38] of cases. Complications occur in 5–15% of cases, including worsening of the bleeding, perforation of the bowel, and cardiac arrest. Unfortunately, endoscopic-mediated therapy does not seem to offer long-lasting benefits in patients with advanced gastroduodenal tumors, and 30–80% of these lesions either bleed persistently or the bleeding recurs.[38]

Malignant ulcers and erosions are not the only sources of bleeding from the upper gastrointestinal tract in patients with advanced cancer. Occasionally, esophageal, gastric, and duodenal varices are involved as a result of portal hypertension brought on by liver or pancreatic involvement. If pharmacologic therapy with systemic agents such as vasopressin or somatostatin analogues fails to control bleeding, various endoscopic procedures may be considered. Endoscopic treatment has been shown to be superior to balloon tamponade in cancer-related bleeding.[41] Endoscopic-mediated procedures involve either injection of sclerosing agents into the varices or ligation of the vessels. Sclerotherapy of varices and variceal ligation in the setting of chronic liver disease have rebleeding rates of approximately 35% and 25%, respectively.[42] Their complication rates, 20%, are similar. When these modalities are combined, rebleeding rates do not change significantly. Endoscopic variceal ligation may be preferred to sclerotherapy, especially when varices are large and there is no active bleeding.[43]

Although surgery is often the best approach to manage hemorrhaging from the lower gastrointestinal tract, endoscopic measures may be considered in symptomatic patients who are unsuitable for surgery or present with a recurrent neoplasm.[44,45] Colonoscopic methods vary widely and include bipolar electrocoagulation (Bicap Prob), heater probe, and argon[46] or Nd:Yag lasers.[45]

Cystoscope-assisted cautery by either heat or laser probes has been used in the treatment of hematuria in patients with bladder cancer.[47] It is used mainly in patients in whom continuous bladder irrigation and lavage have been tried and failed. Under direct vision, the urologist can inspect the bladder, identify the source of bleeding, and fulgurate any bleeding vessel or tumor. Diffuse bleeding for any reason that persists despite clot evacuation and fulguration is an indication for intravesical instillation of a hemostatic agent, radiotherapy, or surgery.[23,30,47]

The use of bronchoscopy has been described in the management of malignant hemoptysis.[48,49] This procedure requires lavage of the bronchial tree with an iced saline solution.[50] Other bronchoscopy-mediated modalities include balloon tamponade,[50,51] laser phototherapy,[50] and the use of topical agents such as thrombin or fibrinogen.[50] As a last resort in selected patients with severe hemoptysis, options other than bronchoscopy, such as surgery[49] or embolization, may be considered.[50] Once again, the invasiveness and discomfort of such procedures may limit their use in patients with advanced cancer.

Interventional radiology

Transcatheter arterial embolization is a well-recognized radiological technique that has been used for many years. Hemostatic material, usually in the form of coils, is inserted into a blood vessel supplying the hemorrhaging area. The procedure is performed under local anesthesia via a femoral or axillary approach.[52] The procedure is generally very well tolerated and requires only mild sedation. Limiting factors include the availability of radiologists with the appropriate expertise and skills and the presence of a bleeding disorder. Embolization has been well described in the management of hemorrhaging due to head and neck tumors,[53] pelvic malignancies,[49,50,54–57] and lung cancers[54]—especially if the source of hemorrhage cannot be localized endoscopically. Embolization is obviously restricted to areas where the catheter can be easily guided into a blood vessel and where embolization of the blood vessel does not result in devastating adverse consequences.

Surgery

Surgical intervention in critically ill patients is often not feasible and should be considered only if conservative measures have failed and if a useful symptomatic benefit is expected. Surgery usually consists of ligation of a bleeding vessels or removal of bleeding tissue.[58]

Systemic Interventions

Systemic measures include the use of vitamin K, vasopressin, somatostatin analogues, antifibrinolytic agents, and the transfusion of blood products (Table 9.2). These modalities may be considered in specific situations and can be used alone or in combination with local measures.

Vitamin K

Vitamin K is necessary for the hepatic production of a number of clotting factors, including factors II, VII, IX, and X. The primary source of vitamin K, a fat-soluble vitamin, is bacterial synthesis in the intestine, and it requires a functional biliary system for absorption. Therefore, liver disease, decreased intake of leafy green

Table 9.2. Systemic interventions and products for
the control of bleeding in palliative care

Vitamin K

Vasopressin

Somatostatin analogues

Antifibrinolytic agents

   Tranexamic acid

   Aminocaproic acid

Blood component transfusions

   Platelets

   Fresh–frozen plasma

   Coagulation factors

vegetables (a source of vitamin K), decreased bowel production because of small bowel disease or decreased absorption because of small bowel resection or disease, and intrahepatic and extrahepatic biliary obstruction can all lead to deficiencies in the above-mentioned clotting factors. Often other signs of liver involvement, such as jaundice or encephalopathy, are present. Coagulation screening studies will reveal a prolonged prothrombin time (PT) and partial thromboplastin time (PTT), with a normal thrombin time (TT), fibrinogin, and serum fibrin-fibrinogen degradation products (FDP). Parenteral administration (intravascular or subcutaneous) of 5–10 mg of vitamin K once or twice a week could potentially prevent some hemorrhagic complications.

Vasopressin

Vasopressin is a posterior pituitary hormone that causes splanchnic arteriolar constriction and reduction of portal pressure when injected intravenously or intra-arterially.[43] In a controlled trial, vasopressin therapy stopped bleeding in about one-half of patients with active upper malignancy–related gastrointestinal bleeding.[59] The optimal intravenous dosage appears to be 0.3 unit/min; complications increase with dosages of 0.4 to 0.6 unit/min. The vasoconstrictor effects on the myocardial, mesenteric, and cerebral circulations are the most important side effects, but these can be partially offset by the concomitant use of nitroglycerin.

Somatostatin analogues

Octreotide, an analogue of somatostatin, is more commonly used in the palliative setting for management of malignant bowel obstruction.[60] It is also can play a role in the systemic management of upper gastrointestinal bleeds.[61] However, most of the data related to its use in bleeding problems are from noncancer patients, so one can only speculate on its possible role in palliative care. Recent studies show equal effectiveness of systemic octreotide therapy and emergency sclerotherapy in the acute control of variceal bleeding.[62,63] In the treatment of bleeding peptic ulcers, the literature includes contradictory reports of its effectiveness.[64–67]

The benefit of somatostatin probably derives from its effect on mesenteric blood flow and pressure, and possibly its concomitant cytoprotective effects and suppression of gastric acid secretion. The reduction in splanchnic flow and pressure is presumably due to venous dilatation, which decompresses the esophogeal varices. Octreotide significantly decreases portal pressure, portal venous flow, and hepatic artery flow. These effects are mediated by an increase in splanchnic vascular resistance without influencing portal venous resistance, suggesting an action on prehepatic splanchnic vascular resistance. Generally, a starting dose of 50–100 µg twice daily seems appropriate.[68] The dose should be increased according to the clinical response but seldom needs to exceed 600 µg/day An alternative regimen consists of a bolus of 50 µg given intravenously or subcutaneously, followed by a continuous subcutaneous or intravenous infusion of 50 µg/hr for 48 hr.[69] At low doses very few side effects are reported, but at doses above 100 µg/hr, brief episodes of nausea immediately following the injection or delayed abdominal discomfort and diarrhea have been described. Its high cost limits general use.

Antifibrinolytic agents

Tranexamic acid (TA) and aminocaproic acid (EACA) are synthetic antifibrinolytic agents that act by blocking the lysine binding sites of plasminogen, thereby inhibiting the conversion of plasminogen into plasmin by tissue plasminogen activator.[70] The end result is decreased lysis of fibrin clots. These agents, in theory at least, should therefore be most effective when bleeding is secondary to hyperfibrinolysis. TA in vitro is approximately 10 times more potent than EACA.[71,72] Fibrinolytic inhibitors have been used successfully in a variety of nononcology settings, including the control of bleeding following dental extractions,[73] subarachnoid hemorrhages,[74] and gastrointestinal bleeds.[75] Several case reports and a few studies have been published suggesting a role for these agents in the oncology and palliative care settings.[70,76–81]

Dean and Tuffin recently reported on a prospective open pilot study that enrolled 16 palliative care patients over a period of 2 years.[70] The patients presented with various types of malignancies. Bleeding occurred from fungating lesions and from the bladder, lung, and gastrointestinal tract. All of these patients had normal coagulation profiles. Ten patients received A and 6 EACA. Patients who were started on TA received an initial dose of 1.5 g orally, followed by 1 g three times daily, and those started on EACA acid were given an initial dose of 5 g orally followed by 1 g four times a day. The investigators comment that there are few data to guide practitioners on the optimum duration of treatment for cancer-associated bleeding. Therefore, in this study, they decided to continue administering the drugs until the bleeding resolved. Thereafter, patients were advised to continue treatment for at least another 7 days. Fifteen of the 16 patients noted a reduction in bleeding, and 14 had complete cessation. The average time until significant reduction of bleeding was just 2 days, and the average time for complete cessation was 4 days. The treatment period ranged from 1 to 54 days. Only three patients experienced rebleeding cessation of treatment.

These antifibrinolytic agents have been used in a number of ways and for bleeding in a variety of cancers. Two patients who did not desire oral therapy in the study by Dean and Tuffin were given topical TA, one as a solution applied to a skin would and the other as a bladder instillation.[70] TA has also been administered by intrapleural instillation for hemorrhagic pleural infusion complicating malignant mesothelioma[77]; a marked decrease in transfusion requirements was noted in two patients. TA has also been used in rectal installition for colonic bleeding.[82] EACA has been used for the treatment of a diffuse intravascular coagulopathy and excessive fibrinolysis in a patient with metastatic carcinoma.[78] It has also been used to control bleeding in severely thrombocytopenic patients.[83]

The effectiveness of antifibrinolytics in preventing or controlling hemorrhage in severely thrombocytopenic patients seems to require the presence of enhanced fibrinolysis.[83,84] TA has been suggested for bleeding in acute promyelocytic leukemia[80] and for bleeding in patients undergoing active treatment of acute leukemia, chronic lymphocytic leukemia, and dysmyelopoietic syndrome.[79] Several case reports and studies, including one randomized, placebo-controlled, double-blind study,[80] have suggested that TA may be a prophylactic option to prevent bleeding in patients with promyelocytic and myeloid leukemia who have enhanced fibrinolysis. However, a placebo-controlled trial using TA in patients with aplastic anemia or myelodysplasia failed to demonstrate any reduction in bleeding.[84]

The antifibrinolytics can be administered orally or intravenously. The suggested intravenous dose of TA is 10 mg/kg three or four times a day. It is suggested that it be infused over at least 1 hr. The suggested intravenous dose of EACA is 4 to 5 g in 250 ml over the first hour and then 1 g/hr in 50 ml administered continuously for 8 hr or until the bleeding is controlled.[72] The most common adverse effects of these medications are gastrointestinal and occur in 25% of cases.[71] These reactions include nausea, vomiting, and diarrhea and appear to be dose-dependent. The major theoretical risk of these agents is thromboembolism. Fortunately, this complication appears to be uncommon.[85,86] It must be noted that the urinary excretion of these agents is impaired in patients with decreased renal function. They should therefore be used in smaller doses and at longer intervals in these patients.

Transfusion therapy (platelets, whole blood, and plasma)

The bleeding time increases linearly as the platelet counts fall from 100,000 to 10,000/μl. The frequency and severity of hemorrhages also increase as the platelet count declines below 20,000/μl.[87] A recommended threshold of 20,000/μl is often proposed for the administration of prophylactic platelet transfusions. However, the use of such transfusions by strict cutoff criteria has been criticized in the areas of oncological care[87,88] and palliative care.[89] One major factor that limits the usefulness of platelet transfusions is their very limited life span, especially when thrombocytopenia is severe. Although normal autologous platelets survive for an average 9.6 ± 0.6 days, there is a direct relationship between platelet count and survival at platelet counts below 100,000/μ. When platelets counts are below 50,000/μl, platelet survival averages 5.1 ± 1.9 days and is even less at 20,000/μl and below. Therefore, platelet transfusions may be required several times a week in a patient with severe thrombocytopenia. In advanced cancer patients the aim is to control symptoms, and transfusion of platelets should be considered only when symptoms such as mucosal bleeding or epistaxis are distressing. Lassauniere and colleagues have proposed some criteria for platelet transfusions in patients with advanced hematological malignancies.[89] These criteria include continuous bleeding of the mouth or gum, epistaxis, extensive and painful hematomas, severe headaches or disturbed vision of recent onset, and continuous bleeding through the gastrointestinal, gynecological, or urinary systems. Although specifically described in patients with hematological malignancies, these criteria may serve as guidelines for thrombocytopenic patients with others malignancies.

A single unit of platelets should increase the peripheral platelet count in a 75-kg recipient by approximately 6000–10,000/μl. This estimate assumes normal splenic pooling. The transfusion of 4 to 6 units of platelet concentrates should be adequate to control bleeding in most patients. The topical use of platelets has been described when one cannot establish venous access for transfusions, but this approach is problematic on both practical and physiological grounds.[90] Platelet transfusions are often given from random donors, and a significant number of recipients who require repeated such transfusions may develop antibodies to human leukocyte antigens on the donor platelets, resulting in a febrile reaction and a poor responses to the transfusion.

When it appears that the thrombocytopenia is ongoing and irreversible, the limited role of platelet transfusions should be discussed with the patient and family. The discontinuation of further transfusions needs to be accompanied by psychological support of the patient and family.

The use of packed cell transfusions in hemorrhaging patients is limited to those who present with chronic bleeding resulting in anemia.[91,92] In palliative care, its use for resuscitation of patients in hypovolemic shock cannot generally be supported. Fresh–frozen plasma is reserved for a very select group of patients in whom specific deficiencies of certain coagulation factors have been identified; in patients in whom the effects of warfarin need to be reversed urgently; and, when appropriate, in the treatment of DIC.

Disseminated intravascular coagulation

Disseminated intravascular coagulation (DIC) is characterized, as previously discussed, primarily by coagulation, often with depletion of clotting factors and platelets, followed by fibrinolysis and the formation of fibrin degradation products, which in turn contribute to anticoagulation. DIC is, therefore, a cyclical process that eventually depletes clotting factors, leading to hemorrhage. Bleeding from DIC is seen most frequently in prostate carcinoma, but it is also commonly associated with carcinoma of the stomach, colon, breast, ovary, lung, and gallbladder and with melanoma. Infection can precipitate DIC, particularly gram-negative sepsis with release of endotoxin. The primary treatment of DIC associated with a neoplastic disorder includes treatment of the underlying malignancy and administration of heparin and fresh–frozen plasma (if the DIC is associated with liver failure). Antifibrinolytic drugs such as TA or EACA should not be used to treat the fibrinolytic phase of DIC without full heparinization. Again, the treatment needs to be highly individualized, depending on the overall medical condition of the patient. Management in the palliative care setting is often limited to comfort measures.

Conclusion

Bleeding, although relatively uncommon in patients with advanced cancer, is very stressful for both patients and their caregivers. These episodes require an individualized approach based on the specific needs of the patient and family, including the level of distress, the stage of disease, and the expertise available. A multidisciplinary approach using various treatment modalities may be required. Treatments range from simple hemostatic techniques to more invasive and sophisticated modalities. Minimal management requires identification of the patients at risk and preparatory measures to empower caregivers to deal appropriately with the situation if and when it arises.

References

1. DeVita VT, Hellman S, Rosenberg SA, eds. *Cancer. Principles and Practice of Oncology*, 4th ed. Philadelphia: J.B. Lippincott Co., 1993.
2. Smith AM. Emergencies in palliative care. *Ann Acad Med* 1992; 23(2):186–190.
3. Hoskin P, Makin W, eds. *Oncology for Palliative Medicine*. Oxford: Oxford University Press, 1998:229–234.
4. Gagnon B, Mancini I, Pereira J, et al. Palliative management of bleeding events in advanced cancer patients. *J Palliat Care* 1998; 14:50–54.
5. Pereira J, Bruera E. Miscellaneous aspects of decision making in palliative care. In: Pereira J, Bruera E, eds. *The Edmonton Aid to Palliative Care*. Edmonton: University of Alberta Press, 1996:3–6.
6. Dutcher JP. Hematologic abnormalities in patients with nonhematologic malignancies. *Hematol/Oncol Clin North Am* 1987; 1(2):281.
7. Hasegawa DK, Bloomfield CD. Thrombotic and hemorrhagic manifestations of malignancy. *Oncol Emerg* 1981; :141–193.

8. Hoskin P, Makin W, eds. *Oncology for Palliative Medicine.* Oxford: Oxford University Press, 1998:229–234.

9. Johnson MJ. Problems of anticoagulation within a palliative care setting: an audit of hospice patients taking warfarin. *Palliat Med* 1997; 11:306–312.

10. Johnson MJ. Problems of anticoagulation within a palliative care setting—correction. *Palliat Med* 1998; 12:463.

11. Weitz JI. Low molecular weight heparins. *N Engl J Med* 1997; 337:688–698.

12. Johnson MJ, Sherry K. How do palliative physicians manage venous thromboembolism? *Palliat Med* 1997; 11:462–468.

13. Pereira J, Bruera E. Emergencies in palliative care. In: Pereira J, Bruera E, eds. *The Edmonton Aid to Palliative Care.* Edmonton: University of Alberta Press, 1996:78.

14. Wright SW, Chudnofsky CR, Dronen SC, et al. Comparison of midazolam and diazepam for conscious sedation in the emergency department. *Ann Emerg Med* 1993; 22(2):201–205.

15. Hemostasis and blood loss replacement. In: Atkinson LJ, Fortunato NH, eds. *Operating Room Technique,* 8th ed. St. Louis:Mosby 1996:469–89.

16. Pringle MB, Beasley P, Brightwell AP. The use of merocel nasal packs in the treatment of epistaxis. *J Laryngol Otol* 1996; 110(6):543–546.

17. Patsner B. Topical acetone for control of life-threatening vaginal hemorrhage from recurrent vaginal gynaecological cancer. *Eur J Gynaecol Ca* 1993; 14(1):33–35.

18. *Gelfoam Preparations. Compendium of Pharmaceuticals and Specialties.* Ottawa: Canadian Pharmacists Association, 1996; 31:575.

19. *Thrombostat. Compendium of Pharmaceuticals and Specialties.* Ottawa: Canadian Pharmacists Association, 1997; 32:1587.

20. Hemostasis and blood loss replacement. In: Atkinson LJ, Fortunato NH, eds. *Operating Room Technique,* 8th ed. St. Louis: Mosby, 1996:469–489.

21. Woodruff R. Haematological problems. In: Woodruff R, ed. *Palliative Medicine: Symptomatic and Supportive Care for Patients with Advanced Cancer and AIDS.* Melbourne: Aperula Pty Ltd., 1993:228–252.

22. Tisseel Kit VH. *Compendium of Pharmaceuticals and Specialties.* Ottawa: Canadian Pharmacists Association, 1996; 31:1479–1480.

23. Russo P. Urologic emergencies. In: Devita VT Jr, Hellman S, Rosenberg SA, eds. *Cancer: Principles and Practice of Oncology.* Philadelphia: J.B. Lippincott Co., 1993:2159–2160.

24. Biswal BM, Lal P, Rath GK, et al. Intrarectal formalin application, an effective treatment for grade III haemorrhagic radiation proctitis. *Radiother Oncol* 1995; 35(3):212–215.

25. Roche B, Chautems R, Marti MC. Application of formaldehyde for treatment of hemorrhagic radiation-induced proctitis. *World J Surg* 1996; 20(8):1092–1094.

26. Vijan SR, Keating MA, Althausen AF. Ureteral stenosis after silver nitrate instillation in the treatment of essential hematuria. *J Urol* 1988; 139(5):1015–1016.

27. Brundage MD, Bezjak A, Dixon P, et al. The role of palliative thoracic radiotherapy in non-small cell lung cancer. *Can J Oncol (Suppl)* 1996; 6(1):25–32.

28. Anonymous. A Medical Research Council (MRC) randomised trial of palliative radiotherapy with two fractions or a single fraction in patients with inoperable non-small cell lung cancer (NSCLC) and poor performance status. Medical Research Council Lung Cancer Working Party. *Br J Cancer* 1992; 65:934–941.

29. Srinivasan V, Brown CH, Turner AG. A comparison of two radiotherapy regimens for the treatment of symptoms from advanced bladder cancer. *Clin Oncol* 1994; 6: 11–13.

30. Hoskin PJ. Radiotherapy in symptom management. In: Doyle D, Hanks GWC, eds. *Oxford Textbook of Palliative Medicine*. Oxford: Oxford University Press, 1993:Ch. 4:117–127.

31. Biswall BM, Lal P, Rath GK, et al. Hemostatic radiotherapy in carcinoma of the uterine cervix. *Int J Gynaecol Obstet* 1995; 50(3):281–285.

32. Miller CM, O'Neill A, Mortimer PS. Skin problems in palliative care: nursing aspects. In: Doyle D, Hanks GWC, eds. *Oxford Textbook of Palliative Medicine*. Oxford: Oxford University Press, 1993:Ch. 4:395–407.

33. MacDougall RH, Munro AJ, Wilson JA. Palliation in head and neck cancer. In: Doyle D, Hanks GWC, eds. *Oxford Textbook of Palliative Medicine*. Oxford: Oxford University Press, 1993:Ch. 4:422–433.

34. Loftus EV, Alexander GL, Ahlquist DA, et al. Endoscopic treatment of major bleeding from advanced gastroduodenal malignant lesions. *Mayo Clin Proc* 1994; 69:736–740.

35. Loscos JM, Calvo E, Alvarez-Sala JL. Treatment of dysphagia and massive hemorrhage in esophageal carcinoma by ethanol injection. *Endoscopy* 1993; 25(8):544.

36. Gupta PK, Fleischer DE. Nonvariceal upper gastrointestinal bleeding. *Med Clin North Am* 1993; 77(5):973–991.

37. Tajika M, Kato T, Magaki M. Endoscopic injection of gelatin solution for server. *Gastrointest Endosc* 1996; 43(3):247–250.

38. Savides TJ, Jensen DM, Cohen J. Severe upper gastrointestinal tumor bleeding: endoscopic findings, treatment, and outcome. *Endoscopy* 1996; 28:244–248.

39. Suzuki H, Miho O, Watanabe Y, et al. Endoscopic laser therapy in the curative and palliative treatment of upper gastrointestinal cancer. *World J Surg* 1989; 13:158–164.

40. Mathus-Vliegen EMH, Tytgat GNJ. Analysis of failures and complications of neodymium-YAG laser photocogulation in Gastrointestinal tract tumors. *Endoscopy* 1990; 22:17–23.

41. Burnett DA, Rikkers LF. Nonoperative emergency treatment of variceal hemorrhage. *Surg Clin North Am* 1990; 70(2):291–306.

42. Jutabha R, Jensen DM. Management of upper gastrointestinal bleeding in the patient with chronic liver disease. *Med Clin North Am* 1996; 80(5):1035–1068.

43. Stein C, Korula J. Variceal bleeding. *Postgrad Med* 1995; 98(6):143–152.

44. Bono MJ. Lower gastrointestinal tract bleeding. *Emerg Med Clin North Am* 1996; 14(3):547–556.

45. Schulze S, Lyng KM. Palliation of rectosigmoid neoplasms with Nd:YAG I. *Dis Colon Rectum* 1994; 37(9):882:4.

46. Schrock TR. Colonoscopic diagnosis and treatment of lower gastrointestinal bleeding. *Surg Clin North Am* 1989; 69(6):1309–1325.

47. MacKinnon KJ, Norman RW. Genitourninary disorders in palliative medicine. In: Doyle D, Hanks GWC, eds. *Oxford Textbook of Palliative Medicine*. Oxford: Oxford University Press, 1993:Ch. 4:415–422.

48. Knott-Craig CJ, Oostuizen JG, Rossouw G. Management and prognosis of massive hemoptysis. *J Thorac Cardiovasc Surg* 1993; 105(3):394–397.

49. Canellos GP, Cohen G, Posner M. Pulmonary emergencies in neoplastic disease. *Oncol Emerg* 1981: 301–322.

50. Patel U, Pattison CW, Raphael M. Management of massive haemoptysis. *Br J Hosp Med* 1994; 52(2–3):74, 76–78.

51. Kato R, Sawafuji M, Kawamura M, et al. Massive hemoptysis successfully treated by modified bronchoscopic balloon tamponade technique. *Chest* 1996; 109(3):842–843.

52. Broadley KE, Kurowska A, Dick R, et al. The role of embolization in palliative care. *Palliat Med* 1995; 9:331–335.

53. Morrissey DD, Andersen PE, Nesbit GM, et al. Endovascular management of hemorrhage in patients with head and neck cancer. *Arch Otolaryngol* 1997; 123(1): 15–19.

54. Wells I. Internal iliac artery embolization in the management of pelvic bleeding. *Clin Radiol* 1996; 51(12):825–827.

55. Yamashita Y, Harada M, Yamamoto H, et al. Transcatheter arterial embolization of obstetric and gynaecological bleeding: efficacy and clinical outcome. *Br J Radiol* 1994; 67(798):530–534.

56. Hays MC, Wilson NM, Page A, et al. Selective embolization of bladder tumors. *Br J Urol* 1996; 78(2):311–312.

57. Jenkins CN, McIvor J. Survival after embolization of the internal iliac arteries in ten patients with severe haematuria due to recurrent pelvic carcinoma. *Clin Radiol* 1996; 51(12):865–868.

58. Baum M, Breach NM, Shepherd JH, et al. Surgical palliation. In: Doyle D, Hanks GWC, eds. *Oxford Textbook of Palliative Medicine.* Oxford: Oxford University Press, 1993:Ch. 4:129–140

59. Allurn WH, Brearley S, Wheatley KE, et al. Acute haemorrhage from gastric malignancy. *Br J Surg* 1990; 77(1):19–20.

60. Mercadante S. The role of octreotide in palliative care. *J Pain Symptom Manage* 1994; 9(6):406–411.

61. Lin HJ, Perng CL, Wang K, et al. Octreotide for arrest of peptic ulcer hemorrhage—a prospective, randomized controlled trial. *Hepato-Gastroenterology* 1995; 42(6): 856– 860.

62. Hanisch E, Doertenbach J, Usadel KH. Somatostatin in acute bleeding oesophageal varices. *Drugs* 1992; Suppl 44(2):24– 35.

63. Avgerinos A, Armonis A, Raptis S. Somatostatin and octreotide in the management of acute variceal hemorrhage. *Hepato-Gastroenterology* 1995; 42(2):145–150.

64. Sommerville KW, Henry DA, Davies JG, et al. Somatostatin in treatment of haematemesis and melaena. *Lancet* 1985; 1:130–132.

65. Christiansen J, Ottenjann R, Art FV, et al. Placebo-controlled trial with the somatostatin analogue. SMS 201-995 in peptic ulcer bleeding. *Gastroenterolgoy* 1989; 97:568–574.

66. Torres AJ, Landa I, Hernandez Jover JM, et al. Somatostatin in the treatment of severe upper gastrointestinal bleeding: a multicentre controlled trial. *Br J Surg* 1986; 73:786–789.

67. Magnusson I, Ihre T, Hohansson C, et al. Randomized double blind trial of somatostatin in the treatment of massive upper gastrointestinal haemorrhage. *Gut* 1985; 26:221–226.

68. Lamberts SWJ, Van Der Lely AJ, De Herder WW, et al. Octreotide. *N Engl J Med* Vol 333(4): 1996; 246–254.
69. Burroughs AK, McCormick PA, Hughes MD, et al. Randomized, double-blind, placebo-controlled trial of somatostatin for variceal bleeding: emergency control and prevention of early variceal rebleeding. *Gastroenterology* 1990; 99:1388–1395.
70. Dean A, Tuffin P. Fibrinolytic inhibitors for cancer-associated bleeding problems. *J Pain Symptom Manage* 1997; 13(1):20–24.
71. Cada DJ, ed. *Drug Facts and Comparisons.* St Louis: 1997:91
72. Herfindal ET, Gourley DR, eds. *Textbook of Therapeutics: Drug and Disease Management,* 6th ed. Baltimore: Williams & Wilkins, 1996.
73. Ramstrom G, Sindet-Pedersen S, Hall G, et al. Prevention of post-surgical bleeding in oral surgery using tranexamic acid without dose modification or oral anticogulants. *J Oral Maxillofac Surg* 1993; 51:1211–1216.
74. Chandra B. Treatment of subarachnoid haemorrhage from ruptured intracranial aneurysm with tranexamic acid: a double blind clinical trial. *Ann Neurol* 1978; 3:502–504.
75. Biggs JC, Hugh TB, Dodds AJ. Tranexamic acid and upper gastrointestinal haemorrhage: a double blind trial. *Gut* 1976; 17:729–734.
76. De Boer WA, Koolen MGJ, Roos CM, et al. Tranexamic acid treatment of haemothorax in two patients with malignant mesothelioma. *Chest* 1991; 100:847–848.
77. Kaufman B, Wise A. Antifibrinolytic therapy for haemoptysis related to bronchial carcinoma. *Postgrad Med J* 1993; 69:80–81.
78. Cooper DL, Sandler AB, Wilson LD, et al. Disseminated intravascular coagulation and excessive fibrinolysis in a patient with metastatic prostate cancer: response to epsilon-aminocaproic acid. *Cancer* 1992; 70:656–658.
79. Shpilberg O, Blumenthal R, Sofer O, et al. A controlled trial of tranexamic acid therapy for the reduction of bleeding during treatment of acute myeloid leukemia. *Leukemia Lymphoma* 1995; 19(1–2):141–144.
80. Avvisat G, Buller HR, Cate JWT, et al. Tranexamic acid for control of haemorrhage in acute promyelocytic leukaemia. *Lancet* 1989; 2(8655):122–124.
81. Hashimoto S, Koike T, Tatewaki W, et al. Fatal thromboembolism in acute promyelocytic leukemia during All-trans retinoic acid therapy combined with antifibrinolytic therapy for prophylaxis of hemorrhage. *Leukemia* 1994; 8:1113–1115.
82. McElligot E, Quigley C, Hanks GW. Tranexamic acid and rectal bleeding. *Lancet* 1991; 337:431.
83. Garewal HS, Durie BG. Anti-fibrinolytic therapy with aminocaproic acid for the control of bleeding in thrombocytopenic patients. *Scand J Haematol* 1985; 35:497–500.
84. Fricke W, Alling D, Kimball J, et al. Lack of efficacy of tranexamic acid in thrombocytopenic bleeding. *Transfusion* 1991; 31(4):345–348.
85. Woo KS, Tse LKK, Woo JLF, et al. Massive pulmonary thromboembolism after tranexamic acid antifibrinolytic therapy. *Br J Clin Pract* 1989; 43(12):465–466.
86. Hashimoto S, Koike T, Tatewaki W, et al. Fatal thromboembolism in acute promyelocytic leukemia during all-trans retinoic acid therapy combined with antifibrinolytic therapy for prophylaxis of hemorrhage. *Leukemia* 1994; 8:1113–1115.
87. Aderka D, Praff G, Santo M, et al. Bleeding due to thrombocytopenia in acute leukemias and reevaluation of the prophylactic platelet tranfusion policy. *Am J Med Sci* 1986; 291:147.

88. Pisciotto PT, Benson K, Hume AB, et al. Prophylactic versus therapeutic platelet transfusion practices in hematology and/or oncology patients. *Tranfusion* 1995; 35(6):498–502.

89. Lassauniere JM, Bertolino M, Hunault M, et al. Platelet tranfusions in advanced hematological malignancies: a position paper. *J Palliat Care* 1996; 12(1):38–41.

90. Friedberg RC. Issues in transfusion therapy in the patient with malignancy. *Hematol-Oncol Clin North Am* 1994; 8(6):1223–1253.

91. Gleeson C, Spencer D. Blood transfusion and its benefits in palliative care. *Palliat Med* 1995; 9:307–313.

92. Monti M, Castellani L, Berlusconi A, et al. Use of red blood cell transfusions in terminally ill cancer patients admitted to a palliative care unit. *J Pain Symptom Manage* 1996; 12(1):18–22.

10

The Use of Heparin, Low Molecular Weight Heparin, and Oral Anticoagulants in the Management of Thromboembolic Disease

GRAHAM F. PINEO AND RUSSELL D. HULL

Patients with cancer, regardless of the site of origin, are prone to develop venous thromboembolic disease. Cancer has been known to be a risk factor for the development of thromboembolism since the time of the original publication by Trousseau.[1] Patients presenting with idiopathic venous thrombosis who do not have cancer at presentation are at risk for the development of cancer later on.[2-4] The incidence of cancer in patients with recurrent idiopathic venous thrombosis is higher than in patients with secondary venous thrombosis.[5] Cancer is also a significant cause of death during follow-up in patients who present with deep vein thrombosis or pulmonary embolism.[6]

At present, the benefit of a search for cancer in a patient with idiopathic venous thromboembolism is uncertain.[2,3] Apart from an adequate history, physical examination, routine laboratory tests, and a chest X-ray, a more thorough search for an underlying cancer at presentation is unjustified. However, in patients who have recurrent venous thrombosis or whose thrombosis is difficult to control with anticoagulants, a more thorough search for an underlying malignancy is justified.

The association of thrombotic disorders and cancer has been the subject of a number of reviews,[7-10] and the effect of heparin in cancer both in vitro and in vivo has recently been reviewed.[11] These associations will not be reviewed here. This review will be devoted to the role of heparin, low molecular weight heparin (LMWH), and warfarin sodium in the management of venous thromboembolism, with particular reference to the cancer patient.

Treatment of Venous Thromboembolism

The objectives of treatment in patients with venous thromboembolism are to prevent (1) death from pulmonary embolism, (2) recurrent venous thromboembolism, and (3) the postphlebitic syndrome. The anticoagulant drugs heparin, LMWH, and warfarin are the mainstay of treatment of venous thrombosis. The use of graduated compression stockings for 24 months significantly decreases the incidence of the postthrombotic syndrome.[12] Furthermore, the incidence of the postthrombotic syndrome has been decreasing in recent years, suggesting that the more efficient treatment of venous thromboembolism and the prevention of recurrent deep vein thrombosis are having a positive impact on this complication.

Heparin therapy

The anticoagulant activity of unfractionated heparin depends on a unique pentasaccharide that binds to antithrombin III (ATIII) and potentiates the inhibition of thrombin and activated factor X (Xa) by ATIII.[13,14] About one-third of all heparin molecules contain the unique pentasaccharide sequence, regardless of whether they are low or high molecular weight fractions.[14–18] It is the pentasaccharide sequence that confers molecular high affinity for ATIII.[14–18] In addition, heparin catalyzes the inactivation of thrombin by another plasma cofactor (cofactor II), which acts independently of ATIII.[19]

Heparin has a number of other effects, including release of tissue factor pathway inhibitor[20]; binding to numerous plasma and platelet proteins, endothelial cells, and leukocytes[13,18]; suppression of platelet function[17]; and an increase in vascular permeability.[21] The anticoagulant response to a standard dose of heparin varies widely among patients. This makes it necessary to monitor the response, using either the activated partial thromboplastin time (APTT) or heparin levels, and to titrate the dose to the individual patient.

The accepted anticoagulant therapy for venous thromboembolism is a combination of continuous intravenous heparin and oral warfarin. The initial intravenous heparin therapy period has been reduced to 5 days, shortening the hospital stay and leading to significant cost savings.[22,23] The simultaneous use of initial heparin and warfarin has become standard clinical practice for all patients with venous thromboembolism who are medically stable.[22–24] Exceptions include patients who require immediate medical or surgical intervention, such as with thrombolysis or insertion of a vena cava filter, or patients at very high risk of bleeding. Heparin is continued until the International Normalized Ratio (INR) is within the therapeutic range (2 to 3) for 2 consecutive days.[24]

It has been established from experimental studies and clinical trials that the efficacy of heparin therapy depends on achieving a critical therapeutic level of heparin within the first 24 hr of treatment.[25–27] This finding was recently challenged in an overview of the relevant literature when the authors were unable to find convincing evidence that the risk of recurrent venous thromboembolism was dependent on achieving a therapeutic APTT result at 24 to 48 hr.[28] However, data from three consecutive double-blind clinical trials indicate that failure to achieve the therapeutic APTT threshold by 24 hr was associated with a 23.3% subsequent recurrent venous thromboembolism rate compared with a rate of 4–6% for the patients who were therapeutic at 24 hr.[28] The recurrences occurred throughout the 3-month follow-up period and could not be attributed to inadequate oral anticoagulant therapy.[25,26] The critical therapeutic level of heparin, as measured by the APTT, is 1.5 times the mean of the control value or the upper limit of the normal APTT range.[25] This corresponds to a heparin blood level of 0.2 to 0.4 U/ml by the protamine sulfate titration assay and 0.35 to 0.70 U/ml by the anti-factor Xa assay.

However, there is a wide variation in the APTT and heparin blood levels with different reagents and even with different batches of the same reagent.[29] It is, therefore, vital for each laboratory to establish the minimal therapeutic level of heparin, as measured by the APTT, that will provide a heparin blood level of at least 0.35 U/ml by the anti-factor Xa assay for each batch of thromboplastin reagent being used, particularly if the reagent is provided by a different manufacturer.[29]

Although there is a strong correlation between subtherapeutic APTT values and recurrent thromboembolism, the relationship between supratherapeutic APTT values and bleeding (an APTT ratio of 2.5 or more) is less definite.[25] Indeed, bleeding during heparin therapy is more closely related to underlying clinical risk factors than to APTT elevation above the therapeutic range.[25] Recent studies confirm that weight and age above 65 are independent risk factors for bleeding while on heparin therapy.[30,31]

Numerous audits of heparin therapy indicate that administration of intravenous heparin is fraught with difficulty and that the clinical practice of using an ad hoc approach to heparin dose titration frequently results in inadequate therapy.[32,33] For example, an audit of physician practices at three university-affiliated hospitals found that 60% of patients failed to achieve an adequate APTT response (ratio of 1.5) during the initial 24 hr of therapy and, further, that 30–40% of patients remained subtherapeutic over the next 3 to 4 days.[33]

The use of a prescriptive approach or protocol for administering intravenous heparin therapy has been evaluated in two prospective studies in patients with venous thromboembolism.[25,34]

In one clinical trial for the treatment of proximal venous thrombosis, patients were given either intravenous heparin alone, followed by warfarin, or intravenous heparin and warfarin simultaneously.[25] The heparin nomogram is summarized in Tables 10.1 and 10.2. Only 1% and 2% of the patients were undertreated for more than 24 hr in the heparin and heparin-warfarin groups, respectively. Recurrent venous thromboembolism (objectively documented) occurred infrequently in both groups (7%), at rates similar to those previously reported. These findings demonstrated that subtherapy was avoided in most patients and that the heparin protocol resulted in effective delivery of heparin therapy in both groups.

Table 10.1. Heparin protocol

1. Administer an initial intravenous heparin bolus: 5000 U.

2. Administer a continuous intravenous heparin infusion: commence at a rate of 42 ml/hr of 20,000
   U (1680 U/hr) in 500 ml of two-thirds dextrose and one-third saline (a 24-hr heparin dose of
   40,320 U), except for the following patients, in whom heparin infusion is commenced at a rate
   of 31 ml/hr (1240 U/hr, a 24-hr dose of 29,760 U):

   a. Patients who have undergone surgery within the previous 2 weeks.

   b. Patients with a previous history of peptic ulcer disease or gastrointestinal or genitourinary
      bleeding.

   c. Patients with recent stroke (i.e., thrombotic stroke within the previous 2 weeks).

   d. Patients with a platelet count <150 · 10⁹/l.

   e. Patients with miscellaneous reasons for a high risk of bleeding (e.g., hepatic failure, renal
      failure, or vitamin K deficiency)

3. Adjust the heparin dose using the adjusted partial thromboplastin time (APTT). The APTT test is
   performed in all patients as follows:

   a. Four to 6 hr after commencing heparin therapy; the heparin dose is then adjusted.

   b. Four to 6 hr after the first dosage adjustment.

   c. Then, as indicated by the nomogram for the first 24 hr of therapy.

   d. Thereafter, once daily unless the patient is subtherapeutic,* in which case the aPTT test is
      repeated 4–6 hr after the heparin dose is increased.

*Subtherapeutic = aPTT <1.5 times the mean normal control value for the thromboplastin reagent being used.
Source: Adopted from Reference 25 with permission.

In the other clinical trial, a weight-based heparin dosage nomogram was
compared with a standard-care nomogram[34] (Table 10.3). Patients on the weight-
adjusted heparin nomogram received a starting dose of 80 U/kg as a bolus and 18
U/kg/hr as an infusion. The heparin dose was adjusted to maintain an APTT of
1.5 to 2.3 times the control value. In the weight-adjusted group, 89% of patients
achieved the therapeutic range within 24 hr compared with 75% in the standard-
care group. The risk of recurrent thromboembolism was more frequent in the
standard-care group, supporting the previous observation that subtherapeutic
heparin during the initial 24 hr is associated with a higher incidence of recurrences. This study included patients with unstable angina and arterial thromboembolism in addition to venous thromboembolism, which suggests that the
principles applied to a heparin nomogram for the treatment of venous thromboembolism may be generalizable to other clinical conditions. Continued use of
the weight-based nomogram has been similarly effective.[35]

Complications of heparin therapy

The main adverse effects of heparin therapy include bleeding, thrombocytopenia,
and osteoporosis. Patients at particular risk are those who have had recent surgery
or trauma, or who have other clinical conditions that predispose them to bleeding

Table 10.2. Intravenous heparin dose titration nomogram according to the adjusted partial thromboplastin time (APTT)

APTT (sec)	Rate change (ml/hr)	Dose change (IU/24 hr)°	Additional action
#45	+6	+5760	Repeated APTT[†] in 4–6 hr
46–54	+3	+2880	Repeated APTT in 4–6 hr
55–85	0	0	None[‡]
86–110	−3	−2880	Stop heparin sodium treatment for 1 hr; repeated APTT 4–6 hr after restarting heparin treatment
>110	−6	−5760	Stop heparin treatment for 1 hr; repeated APTT 4–6 hr after restarting heparin treatment

° Heparin sodium concentration 20,000 IU in 500ml = 40 IU/ml

† With the use of Actin-FS thromboplastin reagent (Dade, Mississauga, Ontario, Canada)

‡ During the first 24h, repeated APTT in 4-6h. Thereafter, the APTT Will be determined once daily, unless subtherapeutic.

Source: Adopted from Reference 25 with permission.

on heparin therapy, such as peptic ulcer, occult malignancy, liver disease, hemostatic defects, low body weight, age above 65 years, and female gender.

The management of bleeding with heparin therapy depends on the location and severity of bleeding, the risk of recurrent venous thromboembolism, and the APTT. Heparin should be discontinued temporarily or permanently. Patients with recent venous thromboembolism may be candidates for insertion of an

Table 10.3. Weight-based nomogram for initial intravenous heparin therapy (figures in parentheses show comparison with control values)

	Dose (IU/kg)
Initial dose	80 bolus, then 18/hr
APTT <35 sec (<1.2×)	80 bolus, then 4/hr
APTT 35–45 sec (1.2–1.5×)	40 bolus, then 2/hr
APTT 46–70 sec (1.5–2.3×)	No change
APTT 71–90 sec (2.3–3.0×)	Decrease infusion rate by 2/hr
APTT >90 sec (>3.0×)	Hold infusion for 1 hr, then decrease infusion rate by 3/hr

APTT = activated partial thromboplastin time.
Source: Adopted from Reference 34 with permission.

inferior vena cava filter. If urgent reversal of the heparin effect is required, protamine sulfate can be administered.[36]

Heparin-induced thrombocytopenia is a well-recognized complication of heparin therapy, usually occurring within 5–10 days after heparin treatment has started.[37-41] Approximately 1–2% of patients receiving unfractionated heparin experience a fall in the platelet count to less than the normal range or a 50% fall in the platelet count within the normal range. In the majority of cases, this mild to moderate thrombocytopenia appears to be a direct effect of heparin on platelets and is of no consequence. However, approximately 0.1–0.2% of patients receiving heparin develop an immune thrombocytopenia mediated by immunoglobulin G (IgG) antibody directed against a complex of platelet factor-4 (PF4) and heparin.[38,42]

The development of thrombocytopenia may be accompanied by arterial or venous thrombosis, which may lead to serious consequences such as death or limb amputation.[43] The diagnosis of heparin-induced thrombocytopenia, with or without thrombosis, must be made on clinical grounds because the assays with the highest sensitivity and specificity are not readily available and have a slow turn-around time.

When the diagnosis of heparin-induced thrombocytopenia is made, heparin therapy in all forms must be stopped immediately. In patients requiring ongoing anticoagulation, several alternatives exists.[43] Recently, the agents most extensively used include the heparinoid Danaproid,[40] hirudin,[44] and, most recently, the specific antithrombin argatroban.[45] Danaproid and hirudin are available for limited use on compassionate grounds and are currently under review for approval by regulatory agencies. Warfarin may be used, but it probably should not be started until one of the above agents has been used for 3 or 4 days to suppress thrombin generation. The defibrinogenating snake venom Arvin[46] was used extensively in the past but will probably be replaced by other agents, as will the use of plasmapheresis and intravenous gamma globin infusion. Insertion of an inferior vena cava filter is often indicated.

Osteoporosis has been reported in patients receiving unfractionated heparin in dosages of 20,000 U/day (or more) for more than 6 months. Demineralization can progress to the fracture of vertebral bodies or long bones, and the defect may not be entirely reversible.[36]

Low molecular weight heparin

Heparin currently in use clinically is polydispersed unmodified heparin, with a mean molecular weight ranging from 10 to 16 kD. In recent years, low molecular weight derivatives of commercial heparin have been prepared that have a mean molecular weight of 4–5 kD.[47-53]

The commercially available LMWHs are made by different processes (such as nitrous acid, alkaline, or enzymatic depolymerization), and they differ both chemically and pharmacokinetically.[47-53] The clinical significance of these differences, however, is unclear, and there have been very few studies comparing different LMWHs with respect to clinical outcomes.[53] The doses of the different LMWHs have been established empirically and are not necessarily interchangeable. Therefore, at this time, the effectiveness and safety of each of the LMWHs must be tested separately.[53]

The LMWHs differ from unfractionated heparin in numerous ways. Of particular importance are the following: increased bioavailability[47,49] (>90% after subcutaneous injection); prolonged half-life[47,49,50] and predictable clearance, enabling once or twice daily injection[49,54]; and a predictable antithrombotic response based on body weight, permitting treatment without laboratory monitoring.[51,52] Other possible advantages are the ability of LMWHs to inactivate platelet-bound factor Xa,[54] resistance to inhibition by platelet factor IV,[17] and their decreased effect on platelet function[17] and vascular permeability[21] (possibly accounting for less hemorrhagic effects at comparable antithrombotic doses).[55–57]

It has been hoped that the LMWHs will have fewer serious complications, such as bleeding,[55–58] osteoporosis,[59–62] and heparin-induced thrombocytopenia,[41] compared with unfractionated heparin. Evidence is accumulating that these complications are indeed less serious and less frequent with the use of LMWHs. The LMWHs all cross-react with unfractionated heparin and, therefore, cannot be used as alternative therapy in patients who develop heparin-induced thrombocytopenia. The heparinoid Danaparoid possesses 10–20% cross-reactivity with heparin, and it can be safely used in patients who have no cross-reactivity.

Several different LMWHs and one heparinoid are available for the prevention and treatment of venous thromboembolism in various countries. Four LMWHs are approved for clinical use in Canada, and three LMWHs and one heparinoid have been approved for use in the United States.

In a number of early clinical trials (some of which were dose finding), LMWH given by subcutaneous or intravenous injection was compared with continuous intravenous unfractionated heparin, with repeat venography at days 7–10 being the primary endpoint.[63–67] These studies demonstrated that LMWH was at least as effective as unfractionated heparin in preventing extension or increasing resolution of thrombi on repeat venography.

Subcutaneous unmonitored LMWH has been compared with continuous intravenous heparin in a number of clinical trials for the treatment of proximal venous thrombosis, using long-term follow-up as an outcome measure[68–73] (Table 10.4). These studies have shown that LMWH is at least as effective and safe as unfractionated heparin in the treatment of proximal venous thrombosis.[68–73] When the mortality data for patients with cancer in two of the studies were reported,[68,69] a striking decrease in mortality was found for patients receiving LMWH compared with those receiving unfractionated heparin.[74] Most of the abrupt deaths that did occur could not be attributed to thromboembolic events,[68] suggesting that the benefits of LMWH may not be entirely related to thrombotic events. A recent review of all of the clinical trials comparing LMWH with heparin showed that in the initial treatment of venous thromboembolism, the risk of

Table 10.4. Randomized trials of LMWH vs. unfractionated heparin for the in-hospital treatment of proximal deep vein thrombosis or acute pulmonary embolism: results of long-term follow-up

Reference	Treatment	Recurrent venous thromboembolism No. (%)	Major bleeding No. (%)	Mortality No. (%)
Hull et al.[68]	Tinzaparin	6/213 (2.8)	1/213 (0.5)	10/213 (4.7)
	Heparin	15/219 (6.8)	11/219 (5.0)	21/219 (9.6)
Prandoni et al.[69]	Nadroparin	6/85 (7.1)	1/85 (1.2)	6/85 (7.1)
	Heparin	12/85 (14.1)	3/85 (3.8)	12/85 (14.1)
Lopaciuk et al.[70]	Nadroparin	0/74 (0)	0/74	0/74
	Heparin	3/72 (4.2)	1/72 (1.4)	1/72 (1.4)
Simonneau et al.[71]	Enoxaparin	0/67	0/67	3/67 (4.5)
	Heparin	0/67	0/67	2/67 (3.0)
Lindmarker et al.[72]	Dalteparin	5/101 (5.0)	1/101	2/101 (2.0)
	Heparin	3/103 (2.9)	0/103	3/103 (2.9)
Simonneau et al.[79]	Tinzaparin	5/304 (1.6)	3/304 (1.0)	12/304 (3.9)
	Heparin	6/308 (1.9)	5/308 (1.6)	14/308 (4.5)
Decousus et al.[73]	Enoxaparin	10/195 (5.1)	7/195 (3.6)	10/195 (5.1)
	Heparin	12/205 (5.0)	8/205 (3.9)	15/205 (7.3)

recurrent venous thromboembolism major bleeding, and death were all less in patients receiving LMWH. The proportion of cancer patients in these studies had a statistically significant effect on the incidence of recurrent venous thromboembolism ($p = .03$) and mortality ($p = .002$) but no influence on the estimated treatment effect of LMWH.[75] Both the type of treatment and the interaction between treatment type and proportion of cancer patients had no statistically significant relationship with the incidence of all three outcome events.

More recent studies indicate that LMWH used predominantly outside of the hospital was as effective and safe as intravenous unfractionated heparin given in the hospital[76–78] (Table 10.5), and two clinical trials showed that LMWM was as effective as intravenous heparin in the treatment of patients presenting with pulmonary embolism.[78,79] Economic analysis of treatment with LMWH versus intravenous heparin demonstrated that LMWH was cost-effective for treatment in the hospital[80] as well as outside of the hospital.[81] As these agents become more widely available for treatment, they will undoubtedly replace intravenous unfractionated heparin in the initial management of patients with venous thromboembolism.

Warfarin therapy is started on day 1 or 2, with the LMWH therapy for 4 or 5 days or until the INR is therapeutic for 2 consecutive days. Protamine sulfate has been shown to reduce clinical bleeding if patients bleed while receiving LMWHs,

Table 10.5. Predominantly outpatient treatment of proximal deep vein thrombosis (DVT) with LMWH vs. inpatient treatment with intravenous heparin

Study	Treatment	Recurrent DVT	Major bleeding
Levine et al.[11]	Enoxaparin	13/247 (5.3%)	5/247 (2.0%)
	vs. heparin	17/253 (6.7%)	3/253 (1.2%)
Koopman et al.[76]	Nadroparin	14/202 (6.9%)	1/202 (0.5%)
	vs. heparin	17/198 (8.6%)	4/198 (2.0%)
Columbus Study[78]	Reviparin	27/510 (5.3%)	16/510 (3.1%)
	vs. heparin	24/511 (4.9%)	12/511 (2.3%)

presumably by neutralizing high molecular fractions of heparin, which are thought to be most responsible for bleeding.

Upper extremity deep vein thrombosis

The treatment of upper extremity deep vein thrombosis is the same as for proximal venous thrombosis: heparin or LMWH plus warfarin for at least 3 months.[82] Patients with upper extremity deep vein thrombosis of recent onset have been treated with thrombolytic agents, but there is no evidence from clinical trials that this decreases long-term sequelae. The rare patient with thoracic outlet obstruction may benefit from surgery.

Oral Anticoagulant Treatment

There are two distinct chemical groups of oral anticoagulants: the 4-hydroxy coumarin derivatives (e.g., warfarin sodium) and the indane-1,3-dione derivatives (e.g., phenindione).[83] The coumarin derivatives are the oral anticoagulants of choice because they are associated with fewer nonhemorrhagic side effects than are the indanedione derivatives.

The anticoagulant effect of warfarin is mediated by the inhibition of the vitamin K–dependent gamma-carboxylation of coagulation factors II, VII, IX, and X.[83,84] This results in the synthesis of immunologically detectable but biologically inactive forms of these coagulation proteins. Warfarin also inhibits the vitamin K–dependent gamma-carboxylation of proteins C and S.[85] Protein C circulates as a proenzyme that is activated on endothelial cells by the thrombin/thrombomodulin complex to form activated protein C. Activated protein C in the presence of protein S inhibits activated factor VIII and activated factor V activity.[85] Therefore, vitamin K antagonists such as warfarin create a biochemical paradox by producing an anticoagulant effect due to the inhibition of procoagulants (factors II, VII, IX, and X) and a potentially thrombogenic effect by impairing the synthesis of naturally occurring inhibitors of coagulation (proteins C and S).[85] Heparin and warfarin treatment should overlap by 4 to 5 days when warfarin treatment is initiated in patients with thrombotic disease.

The anticoagulant effect of warfarin is delayed until the normal clotting factors are cleared from the circulation, and the peak effect does not occur until 36 to 72 hr after drug administration.[86] During the first few days of warfarin therapy, the prothrombin time (PT) reflects mainly the depression of factor VII, which has a half-life of 5 to 7 hr. Equilibrium levels of factors II, IX, and X are not reached until about 1 week after the initiation of therapy. The use of small initial daily doses (e.g., 5 to 10 mg) is the preferred approach for initiating warfarin treatment. The dose-response relationship to warfarin therapy varies widely among individuals; therefore, the dose must be carefully monitored to prevent overdosing or underdosing. A number of drugs interact with warfarin. Critical appraisal of the literature reporting such interactions indicates that the evidence substantiating many of the claims is limited.[87] Nonetheless, patients must be warned against taking any new drugs without the knowledge of their attending physician.

Laboratory monitoring and therapeutic range

The laboratory test most commonly used to measure the effects of warfarin is the one-stage PT test. The PT is sensitive to reduced activity of factors II, VII, and X but is insensitive to reduced activity of factor IX. Confusion about the appropriate therapeutic range has occurred because the different tissue thromboplastins used to measure the PT vary considerably in sensitivity to the vitamin K–dependent clotting factors and in response to warfarin.[88] Rabbit brain thromboplastin, which is widely used in North America, is less sensitive than standardized human brain thromboplastin, which is widely used in the United Kingdom and other parts of Europe. A PT ratio of 1.5 to 2.0 using rabbit brain thromboplastin (i.e., the traditional therapeutic range in North America) is equivalent to a ratio of 4.0 to 6.0 using human brain thromboplastin.[88] Conversely, a 2- to 3-fold increase in the PT using standardized human brain thromboplastin is equivalent to a 1.25- to 1.5-fold increase in the PT using a rabbit brain thromboplastin such as Simplastin or Dade-C.[88]

In order to promote standardization of the PT for monitoring oral anticoagulant therapy, the World Health Organization (WHO) developed an international reference thromboplastin from human brain tissue and recommended that the PT ratio be expressed as the International Normalized Ratio (INR).[84] The INR is the PT ratio obtained by testing a given sample using the WHO reference thromboplastin. For practical clinical purposes, the INR for a given plasma sample is equivalent to the PT ratio obtained with a standardized human brain thromboplastin known as the Manchester Comparative Reagent, which is widely used in the United Kingdom.

Warfarin is administered in an initial dose of 5 to 10 mg/day for the first 2 days, and the daily dose is then adjusted according to the INR. Heparin or LMWH therapy is discontinued on the fourth or fifth day following initiation of warfarin therapy, provided that the INR is within the recommended therapeutic range (INR 2.0 to 3.0) for at least 2 consecutive days (84). Because some individuals are either fast or slow metabolizers of the drug, the correct dosage of warfarin must be individualized. Therefore, frequent INR determinations are required initially to establish therapeutic anticoagulation.

Once the anticoagulant effect and patient's warfarin dose requirements are stable, the INR should be monitored every 1 to 2 weeks throughout the course of warfarin therapy for venous thromboembolism. However, if there are factors that may produce an unpredictable response to warfarin (e.g., contamitant drug therapy),[87] the INR should be monitored more frequently to minimize the risk of complications due to poor anticoagulant control.

Long-term treatment of venous thromboembolism

Patients with established venous thrombosis or pulmonary embolism require long-term anticoagulant therapy to prevent recurrent disease.[88] Warfarin therapy is highly effective and is preferred in most patients.[88] In patients with proximal vein thrombosis, long-term therapy with warfarin reduces the frequency of objectively documented recurrent venous thromboembolism from 47% to 2%.[89] The use of a less intense warfarin regimen (INR of 2.0 to 3.0) markedly reduces the risk of bleeding from 20% to 4%, without loss of effectiveness in comparison with more intense warfarin therapy.[88] With the improved safety of oral anticoagulant therapy using a less intense warfarin regimen, there has been renewed interest in evaluating the long-term treatment of thrombotic disorders. In clinical trials involving patients with atrial fibrillation, it has been shown that oral anticoagulant treatment can be given safely, with a low risk of major bleeding complications (1–2% per year).[90] In trials such as these, the safety of oral anticoagulant treatment depends heavily on the maintenance of a narrow therapeutic INR range. When the INR falls below the therapeutic range, the incidence of thrombotic stroke increases, and when the INR exceeds 3.5 to 5.0, the incidence of major hemorrhage markedly increases. These and other studies have emphasized the importance of maintaining careful control of oral anticoagulant therapy, particularly with the use of anticoagulant management clinics if oral anticoagulants will be used for extended periods of time.

Data from clinical trials indicating an unacceptably high incidence of recurrent venous thromboembolism, including fatal pulmonary embolism in clinical trials on the long-term clinical course of patients with proximal deep vein thrombosis who were treated according to the current practice with intravenous heparin for several days, followed by oral anticoagulant treatment for 3 to 6 months, are further reasons for renewed interest in longer-term treatment of venous thromboembolism.[5,88,91–94] These studies indicate that patients with deep vein thrombosis who are treated according to current clinical practice have an unfavorable long-term prognosis. Three groups of patients who have a particularly poor prognosis have been identified: patients with idiopathic, recurrent venous thromboembolism; patients who carry genetic mutations that predispose them to venous thromboembolism, such as the factor V Leiden mutation; and patients with cancer.[95,96]

Optimal Duration of Oral Anticoagulant Treatment After the First Episode of Deep Vein Thrombosis

It has been recommended that all patients with a first episode of venous thromboembolism receive warfarin therapy for 12 weeks. Attempts to decrease the treatment to 4 weeks[97,98] or 6 weeks[93] resulted in higher rates of recurrent thromboembolism in comparison with either 12 or 26 weeks of treatment (11–18% recurrence of thromboembolism in the following 1 to 2 years). Most of the recurrent thromboembolic events occurred in the 6 to 8 weeks immediately after anticoagulant treatment was stopped, and the incidence was higher in patients with continuing risk factors such as cancer and immobilization.[93,98] Treatment with oral anticoagulants for 6 months reduced the incidence of recurrent thromboembolic events, but there was a cumulative incidence of recurrent events at 2 years (11%) and an ongoing risk of recurrent thromboembolism of approximately 5–6% per year.[93] In patients with a first episode of idiopathic venous thromboembolism treated with intravenous heparin followed by warfarin for 3 months, continuation of warfarin for 24 months led to a significant reduction in the incidence of recurrent venous thromboembolism when compared with placebo.[99] This continued risk of recurrent thromboembolism even with 6 months of treatment after a first episode of deep vein thrombosis has encouraged the development of clinical trials evaluating the effectiveness of long-term anticoagulant treatment beyond 6 months.

Optimal Duration of Oral Anticoagulant Treatment in Patients with Recurrent Deep Vein Thrombosis

In a multicenter clinical trial, Schulman et al. randomized patients with a first recurrent episode of venous thromboembolism to receive oral anticoagulants for either 6 months or indefinitely, with a targeted INR of 2.0 to 2.85.[93] The analysis was reported at 4 years. In the patients receiving anticoagulants for 6 months, recurrent thromboembolism occurred in 20.7%, compared with 2.6% of patients on the indefinite treatment ($p < .001$). However, the rates of major bleeding were 2.7% in the 6-month group compared with 8.6% in the indefinite group. In the indefinite group, two of the major hemorrhages were fatal, whereas there were no fatal hemorrhages in the 6-month group. This study showed that extending the duration of oral anticoagulant therapy for approximately 4 years resulted in a significant decrease in the incidence of recurrent venous thromboembolism, but with a higher incidence of major bleeding. With no mortality difference, the risk of hemorrhage versus the benefit of decreased recurrent thromboembolism with the use of extended warfarin treatment remains uncertain and will require further clinical trials.

For patients experiencing a first episode of venous thromboembolism, long-term anticoagulant therapy should be continued for at least 3 months, using warfarin to prolong the PT to an INR of 2.0 to 3.0 (248). For patients with recurrent venous thromboembolism or a continuing risk factor such as immobilization, heart failure, or cancer, anticoagulants should be continued for a longer period of time, and possibly indefinitely, particularly for those patients with more than one recurrent episode of thrombosis.[24] For patients with genetic mutations predisposing them to venous thromboembolism, such as the factor IV Leiden mutation, ATIII, protein C or protein S deficiency, or the presence of a lupus anticoagulant, anticoagulant treatment may be required for more than 3 months. However, until further information from randomized clinical trials is available, firm recommendations cannot be made.[24]

Adverse effects

The major side effect of oral anticoagulant therapy is bleeding.[100] Bleeding during well-controlled oral anticoagulant therapy is usually due to surgery or other forms of trauma, or to local lesions such as peptic ulcer or carcinoma.[100] Spontaneous bleeding may occur if warfarin sodium is given in an excessive dose, resulting in marked prolongation of the INR; this bleeding may be severe and even life-threatening. The risk of bleeding can be substantially reduced by adjustment of the warfarin dose to achieve a less intense anticoagulant effect than has traditionally been used in North America (INR, 2.0 to 3.0; PT, 1.25 to 1.5 times the control value obtained using a rabbit brain thromboplastin, such as Simplastin or Dade-C).[88]

Nonhemorrhagic side effects of oral anticoagulant therapy differ according to whether coumarin derivatives (e.g., warfarin sodium) or indanediones are administered. Such side effects are uncommon with coumarin anticoagulants, and the coumarins are therefore the oral anticoagulants of choice.

Coumarin-induced skin necrosis is a rare but serious complication that requires immediate cessation of oral anticoagulant therapy.[101,102] It usually occurs 3 to 10 days after therapy has commenced, is more common in women than in men, and most often involves areas of abundant subcutaneous tissues, such as the abdomen, buttocks, thighs, and breast. The mechanism of coumarin-induced skin necrosis, which is associated with microvascular thrombosis, is uncertain but appears to be related, at least in some patients, to reduction of the protein C level. Patients with congenital deficiencies of protein C may be particularly prone to the development of coumarin skin necrosis.

Antidote to oral anticoagulant agents

The antidote to the vitamin K antagonists is vitamin K_1. If an excessive increase in the INR occurs, the treatment depends on the degree of the increase and whether or not the patient is bleeding. If the increase is mild and the patient is not bleeding, no specific treatment is necessary other than reduction of the warfarin dose. The INR is expected to decrease during the next 24 hr with this approach. With a more marked INR increase in patients who are not bleeding, treatment with small doses of vitamin K_1, given either orally or by subcutaneous injection (1 mg), may be considered. With a very marked increase in the INR, particularly in a patient who is either actively bleeding or at risk of bleeding, the coagulation defect should be corrected.

Reported side effects of vitamin K include flushing, dizziness, tachycardia, hypotension, dyspnea, and sweating.[84] Intravenous administration of vitamin K_1 should be performed with caution to avoid inducing an anaphylactoid reaction. The risk of this reaction can be reduced by administration of vitamin K_1 at a rate of no more than 1 mg/min. In most patients, intravenous administration of vitamin K_1 produces a demonstrable effect on the INR within 6 to 8 hr and corrects the increased INR within 12 to 24 hr. Because the half-life of vitamin K_1 is less than that of warfarin sodium, a repeat course of vitamin K_1 may be necessary. If bleeding is very severe and life-threatening, vitamin K therapy can be supplemented with concentrates of factors II, VII, IX, and X.

Alternatives to warfarin for long-term treatment

For patients in whom anticoagulant therapy is contraindicated because of active bleeding or in whom the potential for major bleeding is high, an inferior vena cava filter may be inserted. The use of this filter for the prevention of pulmonary embolism is not justified.[73]

For patients who have recurrent venous thromboembolism while receiving adequate warfarin treatment or in whom control becomes difficult or impossible, long-term LMWH by a daily subcutaneous injection may be used as an alternative to oral anticoagulants. In case series,[103,104] LMWH has been shown to be an effective and safe alternative to warfarin, and in randomized studies, prophylactic doses of LMWH have been as effective and safe as warfarin for the long-term treatment of venous thromboembolism.[105] Studies are currently underway to determine if therapeutic doses of LMWH are superior to warfarin for the prevention of recurrent thromboembolism and death in cancer patients with acute venous thromboembolism.[106]

Conclusion

Knowledge of the appropriate management of venous thromboembolism has been revolutionized by the results of a large number of Level 1 clinical trials.

Although questions remain, the clinician is in a much better position to manage venous thromboembolism in a safe, effective manner, and this will undoubtedly lead to improved patient care and a decreased threat of medical liability. LMWH for the treatment of venous thromboembolism is an effective, safe, and convenient alternative to intravenous heparin and permits outpatient management of many patients with venous thromboembolism, resulting in better use of hospital beds, increased patient satisfaction, and considerable cost savings for the health care system. Long-term LMWH is an acceptable alternative to warfarin, particularly for patients with cancer who have recurrent venous thromboembolism with warfarin therapy or in whom warfarin control becomes difficult. Studies are currently underway to determine if long-term LMWH use is superior to warfarin for the prevention of death and recurrent venous thromboembolism, particularly in patients with cancer.

References

1. Trousseau A. Phlegmaia alba dolens. In: *Clinique Medical de l-Hotel-Dieu de Paris,* Vol 3. Paris: Bailliere, 1865:654–712.
2. Baron JA, Gridley G, Weiderpass E, et al. Venous thromboembolism and cancer. *Lancet* 1998; 351:1077–1080.
3. Nordstrom M, Lindbald B, Anderson H, et al. Deep venous thrombosis and occult malignancy: an epidemiological study. *BMJ* 1994; 308:891–894.
4. Sorenson HT, Mellemkjaer L, Steffensen FH, et al. The risk of a diagnosis of cancer after primary deep venous thrombosis or pulmonary embolism. *N Engl J Med* 1998; 338:1169–1173.
5. Prandoni P, Lensing AWA, Cogo A, et al. The long-term clinical course of acute deep venous thrombosis. *Ann Intern Med* 1996; 125:1–7.
6. Carson JL, Kelley MA, Duff A, et al. The clinical course of pulmonary embolism. *N Engl J Med* 1992; 326(19):1240–1244.
7. Rickles FR, Edwards RL. Activation of blood coagulation in cancer: Trousseau's syndrome revisited. *Blood* 1963; 62:14–31.
8. Edwards RL, Silver J, Rickles FR. Human tumour procoagulants. Registry of the Subcommittee on Haemostasis and Malignancy of the Scientific and Standardisation Subcommittee, International Society on Thrombosis and Haemostasis. *Thromb Haemost* 1993; 69:205–213.
9. Karpatkin S, Pearlstein E. Role of platelets in tumour cell metastases. *Ann Intern Med* 1981; 95:636–641.
10. Kakkar AK, De Lorenzo E, Pineo GF, et al. Venous thromboembolism and cancer. *Bailliere's Clin Haematol* 1998; 11(3):675–687.
11. Zacharski LR, Ornstein DL. Heparin and cancer. *Thromb Haemost* 1988; 80:10–23.
12. Brandjes DPM, Buller HR, Heijboer H, et al. Randomised trial of effect of compression stockings in patients with symptomatic proximal vein thrombosis. *Lancet* 1997; 349:759–762.
13. Lane DA. Heparin binding and neutralising protein. In: Lane DA, Lindahl U, eds. *Heparin, Chemical and Biological Properties, Clinical Applications.* London: Edward Arnold, 1989:363–391.

14. Lindahl U, Thunberg L, Backstrom G, et al. Extension and structural variability of the antithrombin-binding sequence in heparin. *J Biol Chem* 1984; 259:12368–12376.

15. Casu B, Oreste P, Torri G, et al. The structure of heparin oligosaccharide fragments with high anti-(factor X_a) activity containing the minimal antithrombin III-binding sequence. *Biochem J* 1986; 197:599–609.

16. Rosenberg RD, Lam L. Correlation between structure and function of heparin. *Proc Natl Acad Sci USA* 1979; 76:1218–1222.

17. Salzman EW, Rosenberg RD, Smith MH, et al. Effect of heparin and heparin fractions on platelet aggregation. *J Clin Invest* 1980; 65:64–73.

18. Weitz JI, Huboda M, Massel D, et al. Clot-bound thrombin is protected from inhibition by heparin-antithrombin III but is suspectible to inactivation by antithrombin III-independent inhibitors. *J Clin Invest* 1990; 86:385–391.

19. Rollefsen DM, Majerus DW, Blank MK. Heparin cofactor II. Purification and properties of a heparin-dependent inhibitor of thrombin in human plasma. *J Biol Chem* 1982; 257(5):2162–2169.

20. Hoppensteadt D, Walenga JM, Fasanella A, et al. TFPI antigen levels in normal human volunteers after intravenous and subcutaneous administration of unfractionated heparin and low molecular weight heparin. *Thromb Res* 1995; 77(2):175–185.

21. Blajchman MA, Young E, Ofosu FA. Effects of unfractionated heparin, dermatan sulfate and low molecular weight heparin on vessel wall permeability in rabbits. *Ann NY Acad Sci* 1989; 556:245–254.

22. Gallus A, Jackaman J, Tillett J, et al. Safety and efficacy of warfarin started early after submassive venous thrombosis or pulmonary embolism. *Lancet* 1986; I2I:1293–1296.

23. Hull RD, Raskob GE, Rosenbloom D, et al. Heparin for 5 days as compared with 10 days in the initial treatment of proximal venous thrombosis. *N Engl J Med* 1990; 322:1260–1264.

24. Hyers TN, Agnelli G, Hull RD, et al. Antithrombotic therapy for venous thromboembolic disease. *Chest* 1998; 114(5) Suppl:561S–578S.

25. Hull RD, Raskob GE, Rosenbloom DR, et al. Optimal therapeutic level of heparin therapy in patients with venous thrombosis. *Arch Intern Med* 1992; 152:1589–1595.

26. Hull RD, Raskob GE, Brant RF, et al. The importance of initial heparin treatment on long-term clinical outcomes of antithrombotic therapy. *Arch Intern Med* 1997; 157:2317–2321.

27. Hull RD, Raskob GE, Brant RF, et al. Relation between the time to achieve the lower limit of the APTT therapeutic range and recurrent venous thromboembolism during heparin treatment for deep vein thrombosis. *Arch Intern Med* 1997; 157:2562–2568.

28. Anand S, Ginsberg JS, Kearon C, et al. The relation between the activated partial thromboplastin time response and recurrence in patients with venous thrombosis treated with continuous intravenous heparin. *Arch Intern Med* 1996; 156:1677–1681.

29. Brill-Edwards P, Ginsberg S, Johnston M, et al. Establishing a therapeutic range for heparin therapy. *Ann Intern Med* 1993; 119:104–109.

30. Campbell N, Hull RD, Brant R, et al. Aging and heparin-related bleeding. *Arch Intern Med* 1996; 156:857–860.

31. White TH, Zhou H, Woo L, et al. Effect of weight, sex, age, clinical diagnosis and thromboplastin reagent on steady-state intravenous heparin requirements. *Arch Intern Med* 1997; 157:2468–2472.

32. Fennerty A, Thomas P, Backhouse G, et al. Audit of control of heparin treatment. *BMJ* 1985; 290:27–28.

33. Wheeler AP, Jaquiss RD, Newman JH. Physician practices in the treatment of pulmonary embolism and deep venous thrombosis. *Arch Intern Med* 1988; 148: 1321–1325.

34. Raschke RA, Reilly BM, Guidry JR, et al. The weight-based heparin dosing nomogram compared with a "standard care" nomogram. *Ann Intern Med* 1993; 119: 874–881.

35. Raschke R, Gollihare B, Pierce JC. The effectiveness of implementing one weight based heparin nomogram as a practice guideline. *Arch Intern Med* 1996; 156: 1645–1649.

36. Hirsh J, Warkentin TE, Raschke R, et al. Heparin and low-molecular-weight heparin: mechanisms of action, pharmacokinetics, dosing considerations, monitoring, efficacy, and safety. *Chest* 1998; 114(S)Suppl:489 S–510S.

37. Kelton JG. Heparin-induced thrombocytopenia. *Haemostasis* 1986; 16(2):173–186.

38. Greinacher A, Michel I, Kiefel V, et al. A rapid and sensitive test for diagnosis heparin-associated thrombocytopenia. *Thromb Haemost* 1991; 66:734–736.

39. Boshkov LK, Warkentin TE, Hayward CPM, et al. Heparin induced thrombocytopenia and thrombosis: clinical and laboratory studies. *Br J Haematol* 1993; 84: 322–328.

40. Magnani HN. Heparin-induced thrombocytopenia (HIT): an overview of 230 patients treated with organon (Org 10172). *Thromb Haemost* 1993; 70:554–561.

41. Warkentin TE, Levine MN, Hirsh J, et al. Heparin induced thrombocytopenia in patients treated with low molecular weight heparin or unfractionated heparin. *N Engl J Med* 1995; 332(20):1330–1335.

42. Arepally G, Reynolds C, Tomaski A, et al. Comparison of PF4/heparin ELISA assay with the (^{14}C) serotonin release assay in the diagnosis of heparin-induced thrombocytopenia. *Am J Clin Pathol* 1995; 104 (6):648–654.

43. Warkentin TE, Chong BH, Greinacher A. Heparin-induced thrombocytopenia: towards consensus. *Thromb Haemost* 1998; 79:1–7.

44. Greinacher A, Volpel H, Porzsch B. Recombinant hirudin in the treatment of patients with heparin-induced thrombocytopenia (HIT). *Blood* 1996; 88:281a.

45. Matsuo T, Kario K, Chikahira Y, et al. Treatment of heparin-induced thrombocytopenia by use of argatroban, a synthetic thrombin inhibitor. *Br J Haematol* 1992; 82:627–629.

46. Demers C, Ginsberg JS, Brill-Edwards P, et al. Rapid anticoagulation using ancrod for heparin-induced thrombocytopenia. *Blood* 1991; 78:2194–2197.

47. Anderson L-O, Barrowcliffe TW, Holmer E, et al. Molecular weight dependency of the heparin potentiated inhibition of thrombin and activated factor X. Effect of heparin neutralisation in plasma. *Thromb Res* 1979; 115:531–538.

48. Holmer E, Soderberg K, Bergqvist D, et al. Heparin and its low molecular weight derivatives: anticoagulant and antithrombotic properties. *Haemostasis* 1986; 16 (Suppl 2): 1–7.

49. Barrowcliffe TW, Curtis AD, Johnson EA, et al. An international standard for low molecular weight heparin. *Thromb Haemost* 1988; 60:1–7.

50. Fareed J, Walenga JM, Racanelli A, et al. Validity of the newly established low molecular weight herapin standard in cross referencing low molecular weight heparins. *Haemostasis* 1988; 3 (Suppl):33–47.

51. Hirsh J, Levine MN. Low molecular weight heparin. *Blood* 1992; 79:1–17.

52. Weitz JI. Low molecular weight heparins. *N Engl J Med* 1997; 337:688–698.

53. Fareed J, Hoppensteadt D, Jeske W, et al. The available low molecular weight heparin preparations are not the same. *Thromb Haemost* 1997; 3(Suppl 1):S38–S52.

54. Boneu B, Caranobe C, Cadroy Y, et al. Pharmacokinetic studies of standard unfractionated heparin and low molecular weight heparins in the rabbit. *Semin Thromb Hemost* 1988; 14:18–27.

55. Andriuoli G, Mastacchi R, Barnti M, et al. Comparison of the antithrombotic and hemorrhagic effects of heparin and a new low molecular weight heparin in the rat. *Haemostasis* 1985; 15:324–330.

56. Carter CJ, Kelton JG, Hirsh J, et al. The relationship between the hemorrhagic and antithrombotic properties of low molecular weight heparins and heparin. *Blood* 1982; 59:1239–1245.

57. Cade JF, Buchanan MR, Boneu B, et al. A comparison of the antithrombotic and haemorrhagic effects of low molecular weight heparin fractions: the influence of the method of preparation. *Thromb Res* 1984; 35:613–625.

58. Lensing AW, Prins MH, Davidson BL, et al. Treatment of deep venous thrombosis with low molecular weight heparins. *Arch Intern Med* 1995; 155:601–607.

59. Matzsch T, Bergqvist D, Hedner U, et al. Effects of low molecular weight heparin and unfragmented heparin on induction of osteoporosis in rats. *Thromb Haemost* 1990; 63:505–509.

60. Monreal M, Lafoz E, Salvador R, et al. Adverse effects of three different forms of heparin therapy. Thrombocytopenia, increased transaminases, and hyperkalaemia. *Eur J Clin Pharmacol* 1989; 37:415–418.

61. Monreal M, Vinas L, Monreal L, et al. Heparin related osteoporosis in rats. A comparative study between unfractionated heparin and a low molecular weight heparin. *Haemostasis* 1990; 20:204–207.

62. Shaughnessy SG, Young E, Deschamps P, et al. The effects of low molecular weight and standard heparin on calcium loss from fetal rat calvaria. *Blood* 1995; 86:1368–1373.

63. Bratt G, Tornebohm E, Granqvist S, et al. A comparison between low molecular weight heparin (KABI 2165) and standard heparin in the intravenous treatment of deep venous thrombosis. *Thromb Haemost* 1985; 54:813–817.

64. Holm HA, Ly B, Handeland GF, et al. Subcutaneous heparin treatment of deep venous thrombosis. A comparison of unfractionated and low molecular weight heparin. *Haemostasis* 1986; 16:30–37.

65. Siegbahn A, Y-Hassan S, Boberg J, et al. Subcutaneous treatment of deep venous thrombosis with low molecular weight heparin. A dose finding study with LMWH-Novo. *Thromb Res* 1989; 326:975–988.

66. Albada J, Nieuwenhuis HK, Sixma JJ. Treatment of acute venous thromboembolism with low molecular weight heparin (Fragmin): results of a double-blind randomised study. *Circulation* 1989; 80:935–940.

67. Harenberg J, Huck K, Bratsch H, et al. Therapeutic application of subcutaneous low

molecular weight heparin in acute venous thrombosis. *Haemostasis* 1990; 20 (Suppl 1):205–219.

68. Hull RD, Raskob GE, Pineo GF, et al. Subcutaneous low molecular weight heparin compared with continuous intravenous heparin in the treatment of proximal vein thrombosis. *N Engl J Med* 1992; 326:975–988.

69. Prandoni P, Lensing AW, Buller HR, et al. Comparison of subcutaneous low molecular weight heparin with intravenous standard heparin in proximal deep vein thrombosis. *Lancet* 1992; 339:441–445.

70. Lopaciuk S, Meissner AJ, Filipecki S, et al. Subcutaneous low molecular weight heparin versus subcutaneous unfractionated heparin in the treatment of deep vein thrombosis. A Polish multicentre trial. *Thromb Haemost* 1992; 68:14–18.

71. Simonneau G, Charbonnier B, Decousus H, et al. (1993). Subcutaneous low molecular weight heparin compared with continuous intravenous unfractionated heparin in the treatment of proximal deep vein thrombosis. *Arch Intern Med* 1993; 153: 1541–1566.

72. Lindmarker P, Holmstrom M, Granqvist S, et al. Comparison of once-daily subcutaneous Fragmin with continuous intravenous unfractionated heparin in the treatment of deep venous thrombosis. *Thromb Haemost* 1994; 72:186–190.

73. Decousus H, Leizorovicz A, Parent F, et al. A clinical trial of vena caval filters in the prevention of pulmonary embolism in patients with proximal deep vein thrombosis. *N Engl J Med* 1998; 338:409–415.

74. Green D, Hull RD, Brant R, et al. Lower mortality in cancer patients treated with low-molecular-weight heparin versus standard heparin. *Lancet* 1992; 339:1476.

75. Hettiarachichi JK, Prins MH, Lensing WA, et al. Low molecular weight heparin versus unfractionated heparin in the initial treatment of venous thromboembolism. *Curr Opin Pulmon Med* 1998; 4:220–225.

76. Koopman MMW, Prandoni P, Piovella F, et al. Treatment of venous thrombosis with intravenous unfractionated heparin administered in the hospital as compared with subcutaneous low molecular weight heparin administered at home. *N Engl J Med* 1996; 334:682–687.

77. Levine M, Gent M, Hirsh J, et al. A comparison of low molecular weight heparin administered primarily at home with unfractionated heparin administered in the hospital for proximal deep vein thrombosis. *N Engl J Med* 1996; 334:677– 681.

78. Columbus Investigators. Low molecular weight heparin in the treatment of patients with venous thromboembolism. *N Engl J Med* 1997; 337:657–662.

79. Simonneau G, Sors H, Charbonnier B, et al. A comparison of low molecular weight heparin with unfractionated heparin for acute pulmonary embolism. *N Engl J Med* 1997; 337:663–669.

80. Hull RD, Raskob GE, Rosenbloom D, et al. Treatment of proximal vein thrombosis with subcutaneous low molecular weight heparin vs. intravenous heparin. An economic perspective. *Arch Intern Med* 1997; 157:289–294.

81. Van den Belt AGM, Bossuyt PMM, Prins MH, et al. Replacing inpatient care by outpatient care in the treatment of deep vein thrombosis. An economic evaluation. *Thromb Haemost* 1998; 79:259–263.

82. Prandoni P, Polistena P, Bernardi E, et al. Upper-extremity deep vein thrombosis. *Arch Intern Med* 1997; 157:57–62.

83. Freedman MD. Oral anticoagulants: pharmacodynamics, clinical indications and adverse effects. *J Clin Pharmacol* 1992; 32:196–209.

84. Hirsh J, Dalen JE, Anderson D, et al. Oral anticoagulants; mechanism of action, clinical effectiveness, and optimal therapeutic range. *Chest* 1998; 114(S):445S–469S.

85. Clouse LH, Comp PC. The regulation of haemostasis: the protein C system. *N Engl J Med* 1986; 14:1298–1304.

86. O'Reilly RA, Aggeler PM. Studies on coumarin anticoagulant drugs: initiation of warfarin therapy without a loading dose. *Circulation* 1968; 38:169–177.

87. Wells PS, Holbrook AM, Crowther R, et al. Warfarin and its drug/food interactions; a critical appraisal of the literature. *Ann Intern Med* 1994; 121:676–683.

88. Hull R, Hirsh J, Jay R, et al. Different intensities of oral anticoagulant therapy in the treatment of proximal-vein thrombosis. *N Engl J Med* 1982; 307:1676–1681.

89. Hull R, Delmore T, Genton E. Warfarin sodium vs low dose heparin in the long-term treatment of venous thrombosis. *N Engl J Med* 1979; 301:855–858.

90. Laupacis A, Albers G, Dalen J, et al. Antithrombotic therapy in atrial fibrillation. *Chest* 1995; 108:352S–359S.

91. Beyth RJ, Cohen AM, Landefeld CS. Long-term outcomes of deep vein thrombosis. *Arch Intern Med* 1995; 155:1031–1037.

92. Franzeck UK, Schaich I, Jager KA, et al. Prospective 12 year follow-up study of clinical and hemodynamic sequelae after deep vein thrombosis in low-risk patients (Zurich study). *Circulation* 1996; 93:74–79.

93. Schulman S, Rhedin AS, Lindmarker P, et al. A comparison of six weeks with six months of oral anticoagulation therapy after a first episode of venous thromboembolism. *N Engl J Med* 1995; 332:1661–1665.

94. Schulman S, Granqvist S, Holmstrom M, et al. The duration of oral anticoagulant therapy after a second episode of venous thromboembolism. *N Engl J Med* 1997; 336:393–398.

95. Prandoni P, Lensing A, Buller H, et al. Deep vein thrombosis and the incidence of subsequent symptomatic cancer. *N Engl J Med* 1992; 327:1128–1133.

96. Simioni P, Prandoni P, Lensing AWA, et al. The risk of recurrent venous thromboembolism in patients with an Arg[506]:T0 Gin mutation in the gene for factor V (factor V Leiden). *N Engl J Med* 1997; 336:339–403.

97. Research Committee of the British Thoracic Society. Optimum duration of anticoagulation for deep vein thrombosis and pulmonary embolism. *Lancet* 1992; 340:873–876.

98. Levine MN, Hirsh J, Gent M, et al. Optimal duration of oral anticoagulant therapy: a randomized trial comparing four weeks with three months of warfarin in patients with proximal deep vein thrombosis. *Thromb Haemost* 1995; 74:606–611.

99. Kearon C, Gent M, Hirsh J, et al. A comparison of three months of anticoagulation with extended anticoagulation for a first episode of idiopathic venous thromboembolism [see comments]. *N Engl J Med* 1999. Mar 25; 340(12):955–956.

100. Levine MN, Raskob GE, Hirsh J. Hemorrhagic complications of long term anticoagulant therapy. *Chest* 1989; 95 (Supl 2):26S.

101. Grimaudo V, Gueissaz F, Hauert J, et al. Necrosis of skin induced by coumarin in a patient deficient in protein S. *BMJ* 1989; 298:233.

102. Becker CG. Oral anticoagulant therapy and skin necrosis: speculation on pathogenesis. *Adv Exp Med Biol* 1987; 214:217.

103. Harenberg J, Huhle G, Piazolo L, et al. Long-term anticoagulation of outpatients

with adverse events to oral anticoagulants using low-molecular-weight heparin. *Semin Thromb Haemost* 1997; 23(2):167–172.

104. Pini M. Prevention of recurrences after deep venous thrombosis: role of low-molecular-weight heparins. *Semin Thromb Haemost* 1997; 23(1):51–54.

105. Das SK, Cohen AT, Edmondson RA, et al. Low-molecular-weight heparin versus warfarin for prevention of recurrent venous thromboembolism: a randomized trial. *World J Surg* 1996; 20:521–527.

106. Hull RD, Pineo GF, Brant RF. Effect of low molecular weight heparin versus warfarin sodium on mortality in long-term treatment of proximal vein thrombosis. *Clin Appl Thromb/Hemost* 1996; 2 (Suppl):S4–S11.

11

Prophylactic Anticoagulant Therapy in the Terminally Ill Cancer Patient

MARK N. LEVINE

Thromboembolism commonly occurs in cancer patients and complicates their management. The etiology of thrombosis in malignancy is multifactorial; mechanisms include release of procoagulants by tumor cells, co-morbid predisposing factors (e.g., surgery, bed rest, infection), and anticancer drugs (chemotherapy, hormones).[1,2] Acute pulmonary embolism can result in increased mortality, and the symptoms of pulmonary embolism (e.g., dyspnea) and deep vein thrombosis (pain and swelling) can have a substantial impact on the patient's quality of life. In addition, if thromboembolism develops, patients require anticoagulant therapy, with the associated risk of bleeding and the inconvenience of laboratory monitoring. For these reasons it seems worthwhile to prevent such complications.

Cancer patients thought to be at high risk of venous thromboembolism include (1) those undergoing surgery (hip, abdominal, thoracic, brain); (2) those with prolonged immobilization; (3) those with central venous catheters; and (4) those with previous thromboembolic complications (Table 11.1).

There is abundant literature on the use of antithrombotic agents and mechanical methods to prevent venous thromboembolism in patients undergoing surgery. There are limited data, if any, on prophylaxis in the terminally ill cancer patient. In this chapter, prophylactic approaches in cancer surgery and in medically managed cancer patient will be considered, followed by a discussion of an approach to thrombosis prophylaxis in the terminally ill patient.

Surgical Patients

Cancer patients undergoing major general surgery are considered to be at greater risk of postoperative venous thromboembolism than patients with benign dis-

Table 11.1. Groups at high risk of venous thromboembolism

Cancer patients undergoing surgery (hip, abdominal, thoracic, brain)

Cancer patients with prolonged immobilization

Cancer patients with central venous catheters

Cancer patients with previous thromboembolic complications

ease.[3,4] Clinical trials have demonstrated the efficacy of low-dose subcutaneous heparin in preventing deep vein thrombosis and pulmonary embolism in patients undergoing general surgery.[5,6] Many of the patients involved in these studies had cancer. In some of these trials, the results of antithrombotic prophylaxis were reported separately for cancer patients; low-dose heparin was effective in reducing postoperative deep vein thrombosis in this group.[6]

Standard heparin can be depolymerized to low molecular weight fragments.[7] Low molecular weight heparins (LMWHs) have a more predictable anticoagulant response than standard unfractionated heparin (UH), a longer plasma half-life, and better bioavailability when administered subcutaneously. In laboratory studies, LMWH preparations cause less bleeding with an equivalent antithrombotic effect. Standard UH is usually given three times a day, whereas LMWH can be administered once a day.

Most studies comparing UH with LMWH have demonstrated equal efficacy and safety in patients undergoing general surgery. Nurmohamed and colleagues performed a meta-analysis of studies comparing UH with LMWH in general surgery.[8] LMWH was associated with a 20% reduction in postoperative deep vein thrombosis and a 50% reduction in pulmonary embolism. There was no detectable difference in bleeding.

In a double-blind trial conducted by the Enoxacan Study Group, patients undergoing abdominal or pelvic surgery for cancer were randomized to enoxaparin LMWH 40 mg once daily or unfractionated heparin 5000 units three times daily.[9] Patients underwent postoperative venography. Fifty-eight (18.2%) of the UH patients and 46 (14.7%) of the LMWH patients experienced thromboembolism; the rates were not statistically significantly different. The rates of major bleeding were 2.9% and 4.1%, respectively.

A higher dose of LMWH might be required to achieve adequate prophylaxis in cancer patients undergoing general surgery. In a trial reported by Berqvist and colleagues in which patients undergoing general surgery were randomized to 2500 ant-Xa units versus 5000 anti-Xa units of dalteparin, the higher dose was more effective in cancer patients.[10] In another trial of prophylaxis in general surgery, 20 mg of enoxaparin was less effective than UH in cancer patients, whereas it was effective in patients without malignancy.[11]

Mechanical methods of thromboprophylaxis have also been demonstrated to be effective in surgical patients.[12] Thus, in the cancer patient undergoing major general surgery, prophylaxis should consist of low-dose UH or LMWH.[12] Graduated compression stockings should also be used.

There has been a reluctance to use low-dose heparin prophylaxis in cancer patients undergoing neurosurgery because of the concern for bleeding. Physical prophylactic methods, that is, intermittent pneumatic compression or graduated compression stockings, are effective in patients undergoing neurosurgery.[12,13] Two recent trials have compared LMWH plus graduated compression stockings to stockings alone in patients undergoing neurosurgery, many of whom had brain tumors.[14,15] LMWH improved the efficacy of stockings alone, and there was no difference in major bleeding between the groups.

Patients undergoing hip surgery are at substantial risk of postoperative deep vein thrombosis. Without prophylaxis, the risk of venographically detected deep vein thrombosis is at least 50%. Clinical trials have demonstrated the efficacy of a number of approaches, including oral anticoagulants, low-dose μH, LMWH, and external pneumatic compression, in preventing deep vein thrombosis.[12] Nurmohamed and colleagues have conducted a meta-analysis of trials compared LDH and a LMWH in orthopedic surgery.[8] LMWH was associated with a 30% reduction in deep vein thrombosis and a 50% reduction in pulmonary embolism. There was a trend toward less bleeding with LMWH. Clinical trials comparing LMWH with oral anticoagulants in hip surgery have not detected a major difference in efficacy; however, oral anticoagulants require laboratory monitoring, whereas LMWH does not.[12] Clinical trials comparing LMWH with oral anticoagulants in knee surgery have demonstrated the increased efficacy of LMWH, with no increase in bleeding.[16,17] External pneumatic compression, which is cumbersome and inconvenient for patients, has been shown to be inferior to oral anticoagulants in one hip surgery trial.[18] Thus, it would appear that LMWH is the prophylactic agent of choice to prevent venous thromboembolism in patients undergoing orthopedic surgery. Given that the focus of this chapter is the terminally ill patient, a clinical scenario that might be applicable involves the patient with widely metastatic cancer to the bone who develops a pathologic fracture of the hip and requires hip surgery to relieve pain and increase mobility.

Medical Patients

The most reliable information on the incidence of thromboembolism is available for patients with breast cancer. The rates of thromboembolism in women with early-stage breast cancer receiving adjuvant chemotherapy range from 3% to 10%.[19] The rates are highest in postmenopausal women.[19] The risk of thrombosis with tamoxifen is approximately 1%, and the combination of tamoxifen plus chemotherapy increases the thrombotic rate over that occurring with either agent alone.[19] In one report, the rate of thromboembolism in metastatic breast cancer was 17%.[20]

There are limited data on the rates of thrombosis in association with other cancers. Von Templehoff and colleagues reported a 10.6% rate of thrombosis in women with ovarian cancer receiving chemotherapy.[21] Weijl and colleagues reported an 8.7% thrombosis rate in patients with germ cell tumors receiving chemotherapy,[22] and Ottinger and colleague reported a 6.6% rate in patients receiving chemotherapy for high-grade lymphoma.[23]

Much less data are available on antithrombotic prophylaxis in ambulatory cancer patients compared to surgical patients. Levine et al. demonstrated that very-low-dose warfarin is safe and effective for prevention of thromboembolism in patients with metastatic breast cancer receiving chemotherapy.[24] The warfarin dose was 1 mg daily for 6 weeks and then was adjusted to maintain an International Normalized Ratio (INR) between 1.3 and 1.9. An economic analysis of this trial demonstrated the cost effectiveness of this approach.[25] Strategies for the prevention of venous catheter–associated thrombosis in cancer patients have also been reported. Studies of warfarin (1 mg daily) or LMWH (e.g., dalteparin sodium 2500 IU daily) have demonstrated a significant reduction in the incidence of catheter-related thrombosis.[26] Routine use of these agents in cancer patients with venous access devices may be warranted.

Few studies have evaluated antithrombotic prophylaxis in medical patients who are immobile for a prolonged period of time.[12] Some studies have demonstrated the efficacy of low-dose heparin in patients with acute myocardial infarction[12] and the efficacy of low-dose heparin and LMWH in patients with acute ischemic stroke.[12] Two more recent trials by Bergmann and Neuharth[27] and Harenberg et al.[28] have demonstrated the efficacy and safety of LMWH and low-dose heparin in patients hospitalized with acute medical illnesses. However, all of these conditions may not be analogous to that of the terminally ill, bedridden cancer patient.

Arterial Thromboembolism

Although the focus of this chapter has been on venous thromboembolism, some terminally ill patients have received long-term oral anticoagulant therapy for atrial fibrillation or prosthetic heart valves. A number of trials have demonstrated the efficacy and safety of oral anticoagulant therapy to prevent systemic embolism in patients with atrial fibrillation.[29] Oral anticoagulants with or without antiplatelet agents are used to prevent systemic embolism in patients with heart valves.[30] Bleeding on long-term oral anticoagulant therapy is related to a number of factors, including increasing patient age and intensity of anticoagulant therapy.[31]

Discussion

In order to determine an approach to antithrombotic prophylaxis in the terminally ill cancer patient, it is first necessary to define *terminally ill*. For some persons this term connotes the last few days of life, whereas for others it may mean several months. When considering the use of prophylactic antithrombotic therapy, efficacy (i.e., prevention of thrombosis) needs to be weighed against safety (i.e., bleeding), and there must be a net benefit, that is, the reduction in thrombosis outweighs the risk of bleeding. It is important to recognize that net benefit depends on where on the continuum of the natural history of the illness the patient falls.

Patients with terminal illness who undergo surgery should receive antithrombotic prophylaxis. For patients undergoing general surgery, suggested approaches include low-dose heparin plus graduated compression stockings or LMWH plus stockings. For patients undergoing orthopedic surgery, LMWH is suggested. For patients undergoing neurosurgery, LMWH plus graduated compression stockings is suggested.

In the last few days of life, when the patient may not be eating and may have a decreased mental state, the use of prophylactic anticoagulant therapy is likely to do more harm than good.

The dilemma of whether to use antithrombotic prophylaxis is greater when the patient falls between the extremes of the illness's natural history continuum described above. There is no clear-cut, correct answer, and the approach should be tailored to the individual patient. For example, consider the patient with advanced cancer who is confined to bed, but whose symptoms are well controlled and whose quality of life is stable. In this case, the use of prophylactic low-dose heparin or graduated compression stockings seem to be reasonable to prevent venous thromboembolism. Similarly, if this patient had been on long-term oral anticoagulant therapy for atrial fibrillation, it would seem reasonable to continue this medication. Any deterioration in the patient's condition would require closer monitoring of the prothrombin time and discontinuation of anticoagulants if warranted. The best approach in such situations is to discuss the pros and cons of antithrombotic prophylaxis with the patient and family.

Conclusion

There is limited information on strategies to prevent thromboembolism in the terminally ill patient. At this time, antithrombotic methods for such patients need to be extrapolated from the results of studies that, by and large, did not include terminally ill patients. Clearly, there are many unanswered questions concerning prophylaxis in this population, and further research is required. Possible studies include trials of specific antithrombotic agents in patients in the palliative care setting, and qualitative research to determine whether terminally ill patients and their families would choose to receive antithrombotic prophylaxis given the nature of the illness.

References

1. Rickles FR, Edwards RL. Activation of blood coagulation in cancer. Trousseau's syndrome revisited. *Blood* 1983; 62:14–31.

2. Levine MN, Gent M, Hirsh J, et al. The thrombogenic effect of anticancer drug therapy in women with Stage II breast cancer. *N Engl J Med* 1988; 318:404–407.

3. Gallus AS. Prevention of postoperative deep leg vein thrombosis in patients with cancer. *Thromb Hemostat* 1997; 78:126–132.

4. Kakkar VV, Howe CT, Nicolaides AN, et al. Deep vein thrombosis of the leg. Is there a high risk group? *Am J Surg* 1970; 120:527–531.

5. Collins R, Scrimgeour A, Yusuf S, et al. Reduction in fatal pulmonary embolism and venous thrombosis by perioperative administration of subcutaneous heparin. *N Engl J Med* 1988; 318:1162–1173.

6. Claggett GP, Reisch JS. Prevention of venous thromboembolism in general surgical patients. *Ann Surg* 1988; 208:227–240.

7. Hirsh J, Levine MN. Low molecular weight heparin. *Blood* 1992; 79:1–17.

8. Nurmohamed MT, Rosendal FR, Buller HR, et al. Low molecular weight heparin versus standard heparin in general and orthopedic surgery. A meta-analysis. *Lancet* 1992; 340:152–155.

9. Enoxacan Study Group. Efficacy and safety of enoxaparin versus unfractionated heparin for prevention of deep vein thrombosis in elective cancer surgery: a double-blind randomized multicentre trial with venographic assessment. *Br J Surg* 1997; 84:1099–1103.

10. Bergqvist D, Burmakk US, Flordal PA, et al. Low molecular weight heparin started before surgery as prophylaxis against deep vein thrombosis: 2,500 versus 5,000 units in 2,070 patients. *Br J Surg* 1995; 82:496–501.

11. Nurmohamed MT, Verhaege R, Haas S, et al. A comparative trial of a low molecular weight heparin (enoxaparin) versus standard heparin for the prophylaxis of postoperative deep vein thrombosis in general surgery. *Am J Surg* 1995; 169:567–571.

12. Clagett GP, Anderson FA, Geerts W, et al. Prevention of venous thromboembolism. *Chest* 1998; 114 (Suppl):531–560.

13. Turpie AGG, Hirsh J, Gent M, et al. Prevention of deep vein thrombosis in potential neurosurgical patients: a randomized trial comparing graduated compression stockings alone or graduated compression stockings plus intermittent pneumatic compression with control. *Arch Intern Med* 1989; 149:679–681.

14. Agnelli G, Piovella F, Buoncristiani P, et al. Enoxaparin plus compression stockings compared with compression stockings alone in the prevention of venous thromboembolism after elective neurosurgery. *N Engl J Med* 1998; 339:80–85.

15. Nurmohamed MT, van Riel AM, Henkens CMA, et al. Low molecular weight heparin and compression stockings in the prevention of venous thromboembolism in neurosurgery. *Thromb Haemost* 1996; 75:223–228.

16. Leclerc JR, Geerts WH, Desjardins L, et al. Prevention of venous thromboembolism after knee arthroplasty: a randomized double blind trial comparing enoxaparin with warfarin. *Ann Intern Med* 1996; 124:619–626.

17. Hull RD, Raskob GE, Pineo GF, et al. A comparison of subcutaneous low molecular weight heparin with warfarin sodium for prophylaxis against deep vein thrombosis after hip or knee implantation. *N Engl J Med* 1993; 329:1370–1376.

18. Francis CW, Pellegrini VD, Marder VJ, et al. Comparison of warfarin and external pneumatic compression in prevention of venous thrombosis after total hip replacement. *JAMA* 1992; 267:2911–2915.

19. Levine MN. Prevention of thrombotic disorders in cancer patients undergoing chemotherapy. *Thromb Haemostat* 1997; 78:133–136.

20. Goodnough LT, Saito H, Manni A, et al. Increased incidence of thromboembolism in stage IV breast cancer patients treated with a five-day chemotherapy regimen. A study of 159 patients. *Cancer* 1984; 54:1264–1268.
21. Von Templehoff GF, Dietrich M, Niemann F, et al. Blood coagulation and thrombosis in patients with ovarian malignancy. *Thromb Haemost* 1997; 77:456–461.
22. Weijl NI, Rutten M, Zwinderman AH, et al. Major thromboembolic events (MTEE's) in patients undergoing combination chemotherapy for germ cell cancer. *Proc ASCO* 1998; 17:348a.
23. Ottinger H, Belka C, Kozole G, et al. Deep venous thrombosis and pulmonary artery embolism in high-grade non Hodgkin's lymphoma: incidence, causes and prognostic relevance. *Eur J Haemotol* 1995; 54:186–194.
24. Levine M, Hirsh J, Gent M, et al. Double blind trial of very low dose warfarin for prevention of thromboembolism in stage IV breast cancer. *Lancet* 1994; 343: 886–889.
25. Rajan R, Gafni A, Levine M, et al. Very low dose warfarin prophylaxis to prevent thromboembolism in women with metastatic breast cancer receiving chemotherapy: an economic evaluation. *J Clin Oncol* 1995; 13:42–46.
26. Monreal M, Alastrue A, Rull M, et al. Upper extremity deep vein thrombosis in cancer patients with venous access devices — prophylaxis with a low molecular weight heparin (Fragmin). *Thromb Haemost* 1996; 75:251–253.
27. Bergman J, Neuhart E. A multicentre randomized double blind study of enoxaparin compared with unfractionated heparin in the prevention of venous thromboembolic disease in elderly inpatients bedridden for an acute medical illness. *Thromb Haemost* 1996; 76:529–534.
28. Harenberg J, Roebruck P, Heene D, et al. Subcutaneous low molecular weight heparin versus standard heparin and the prevention of thromboembolism in medical inpatients. *Haemostasis* 1996; 26:127–139.
29. Laupacis A, Albers GW, Dalen JE, et al. Antithrombotic therapy in atrial fibrillation. *Chest* 1998; 114:579S–589S.
30. Salem DN, Levine HJ, Pauker SG, et al. Antithrombotic therapy in valvular heart disease. *Chest* 1998; 114:590S–601S.
31. Levine M, Raskob GE, Landefeld S, et al. Hemorrhagic complications of anticoagulant treatment. *Chest* 1998; 114:511S–523S.

IV
ISSUES IN THE ASSESSMENT AND MANAGEMENT OF COMMON SYMPTOMS

12

Intraspinal Analgesic Therapy in Palliative Care: Evolving Perspective

STUART L. DU PEN AND ANNA R. DU PEN

In the mid-twentieth century, the hospice movement in England epitomized the "death with dignity" philosophy—the picture of the patient with a peaceful, rapturous countenance attended at home by a modern Florence Nightingale. Nowhere did the anesthesiologist in scrubs appear, with catheters, needles, and infusion pumps. Later, in the United States, the Diagnosis Related Groups atmosphere of the 1970s and 1980s gave way to a growing adversarial relationship between hospice enthusiasts, for whom no invasive (and costly) technologies were ever deemed appropriate, and the infant subspecialty of anesthesia pain management, for which the hospice represented a deplorable sisterhood of euthanasia activists. Thankfully, a more well-defined middle ground has taken shape over the last several years for intraspinal analgesia in palliative care.

The state of the art in palliative pain management today reflects a softening on both sides, reflecting the combined experiences of the last 20 years. Physicians and nurses practicing palliative care were faced with increasing numbers of patients with intractable pain syndromes, for whom nothing short of conscious sedation seemed to offer relief. The anesthesia pain specialist, initially eager to try new procedural techniques, was repeatedly exposed to overburdened family caregivers, staggering infusion therapy costs, and the dilemma of complications of technology.

The advanced cancer patients of today present an increasingly complex pain management challenge. Coyle and colleagues reported that over one-half of patients in a supportive care program required more than two routes of drug delivery during their palliative care, and one-third required three routes to manage pain effectively.[1] Advances in antitumor therapy have resulted in patients living longer with residual tumor, weakened surrounding structures, and significant treatment-related pain syndromes. Neuropathic pain syndromes, once relatively obscure, have become a common problem for palliative care specialists. Fortunately, the state of the science in oral pharmacologic management of cancer pain has also made astounding gains in the last 20 years. Clinicians have access to effective long-acting opioid agents and fast-onset opioids for relief of episodic pain. Clinical research in the area of adjuvant drug therapy for neuropathic pain syndromes is escalating.

There is broad global agreement that the goal of pain relief in the terminally ill patient is a high priority, and that invasive techniques should be reserved for those patients for whom simpler, less caregiver-intensive, and less costly alternatives have been unsuccessful. The role of intraspinal analgesic techniques in palliative medicine is small but important, and its evolution bears further review.

Reports of Experience with Intraspinal Techniques

In 1977, Joseph Wang, M.D., an assistant professor of anesthesiology at the Mayo Medical School, published a report on the analgesic effects of intrathecally administered morphine in rats. In the last paragraph, he described a clinical trial for "intractable pain of inoperable cancer" in humans, with preliminary results that were encouraging.[2] This was the first mention of the use of spinal opioids in palliative care. The discovery of selective analgesic mechanisms at the spinal cord level produced substantial interest in pain management among the anesthesia and neurosurgery disciplines.

In 1983, Coombs and others[3] reported on 10 patients with intractable pain treated with continuous intraspinal morphine for 12 weeks. Five patients had cancer, and five had pain of nonmalignant origin. The cancer patients reported a significant reduction in pain; the nonmalignant group did not. Both groups required significant dose increases, which the authors interpreted as proof of the development of tolerance. Cautious encouragement for developing spinal therapies for cancer pain patients was offered, and the use of such therapies in nonmalignant pain patients was discouraged.

In 1985, Max and colleagues[4] presented pharmacokinetic profiles of spinal opioids during administration to 17 cancer patients. The investigators measured plasma levels and cerebrospinal fluid (CSF) levels at both lumbar and cervical sites. After epidural injection, peak levels in lumbar CSF occurred within 34 min and were 50 to 1300 times higher than concentrations in plasma. Comparisons were made among morphine, methadone, and beta-endorphin. The rate of decline in CSF levels correlated with drug lipid solubility. Plasma levels were comparable to those after intragluteal injection of the same dose. The investigators followed the patients for 2 weeks, during which 3 of the 17 reported improved analgesia initially. None were improved over baseline at 2 weeks. The authors concluded that spinal opioids, particularly hydrophilic drugs like morphine, were active at spinal and supraspinal sites and that there was likely to be little advantage of spinal morphine over high-dose systemic morphine.

Yaksh and Onofrio[5] published a retrospective review of intrathecal morphine dosing in 163 patients in 1987. The subjects included 130 cancer patients, who had a median infusion duration of 13 weeks. The authors reported that 48% of patients receiving therapy for more than 3 months had less than a twofold increase in dose, despite progressive metastatic disease.

Further work published in 1990 by the same authors[6] evaluated a predictive "analgesic index" to assess the "sensitivity" of the patient to spinal opioids. Fifty three patients with metastatic cancer and a median postimplant survival time of 4 months were infused with intrathecal morphine. The analgesic index, calculated following a trial of this medication, consisted of a quality indicator of pain relief multiplied by the duration of pain relief in hours divided by the trial morphine dose in milligrams. When the authors examined the variability in dose escalation, they found that the maximum increase in dose over time was observed in patients with a low analgesic index (i.e., less efficacy at screening) and that this finding usually correlated with an unsatisfactory overall outcome. This work seemed to indicate that at least some dose escalation might be explained by disease progression, and that some cancer patients were probably less responsive to opioids and less likely to have successful outcomes with spinal opioid therapy.

In 1991, Plummer, Cherry, and their Australian colleagues[7] shared their experience with intraspinal analgesia in the cancer patient. Records of 313 cancer patients implanted with catheter-port systems and treated for a mean period of 96 days were reviewed retrospectively. No clear efficacy data were reported, but complications were described. These included pain on injection (12%), occlusion of the portal system (10.9%), infection (8.1%), and leakage of administered morphine such that it did not reach the epidural space (2.1%). The most impressive finding was the wide variability in dosing, with maximum daily doses ranging from 1 to 3072 mg, and no clear trend toward increasing doses as the period of drug administration increased. The authors concluded that considerable variability within the cancer population exists with respect to epidural opioid dosing.

In a review of "key unanswered issues" in the administration of spinal opioids, Cousins and colleagues noted that the relationship between epidural/intrathecal dosing and oral/intramuscular dosing of opioids was a pharmacodynamic mystery.[8] Cousins and Plummer introduced a "dose optimization" method of initiating epidural morphine therapy, based on previous oral morphine use, as a logical approach to spinal opioid therapy.[9] The method used a scaling factor, based on previous oral morphine use, to define the starting dose, and included parameters for dose stabilization over a period of 24 hr.

The Australian group also examined differences in drug administration technique. Gourlay and colleagues examined intermittent bolus injection versus continuous infusion in 29 cancer patients treated with epidural analgesia.[10] No differences were found in efficacy, as defined by a pain visual analogue scale (VAS), categorial ratings of patient satisfaction, or neuropsychological function. However, there was a significantly greater dose escalation in the continuous infusion group, suggesting the possibility of a more rapid onset of tolerance.

Turkish authors Erdine and Aldemir[11] reported their experience with 225 cancer patients treated with intermittent injections of epidural morphine. The mean duration of therapy was 47 days, and the mean dose of morphine was 13.4 mg/day (range, 5–80 mg/day) delivered by intermittent injection. The number of injections per day ranged from 1 to 8 (mean, 2.6), and the mean duration of action was 9.3 hr. The authors reported satisfactory analgesia in 133 patients (59.1%). Of those who achieved relief, a significant number were patients with pain "arising from the abdomen," perhaps indicating visceral or somatic pain syndromes.

One report described intermittent injections via an intrathecal device. Madrid and colleagues[12] from Spain described 100 cancer patients who were implanted with an intrathecal catheter attached to a subcutaneous port system. These patients had not been previously exposed to systemic opioids. They were given an initial dose of 0.5 mg as a screening trial, and the degree of analgesia was assessed using a VAS score. A 75% reduction in pain was considered good analgesia, and the port device was then implanted. After implantation, the patient's family was instructed on the injection technique through the port, and the patient went home. The duration of pain relief with each dose reportedly ranged from 14 to 32 hr. At 2 months, the average dose administered was 1 to 2 mg every 12 hr. By the seventh month, 16 of the surviving patients required 2 mg of morphine every 6 hr to achieve analgesia. No infections were reported. Technical complications included catheter occlusion at the port assembly in one patient and seroma development around the port in four patients. The authors felt that from a cost and technical standpoint, intermittent injections were a more practical approach than continuous infusion.

Hogan and colleagues[13] from Wisconsin reported on 16 cancer patients treated with epidural infusion combinations. These patients were treated with standard epidural catheters designed for obstetric or postsurgical use. Six patients achieved relief with epidural morphine alone. The remaining 10 patients achieved relief with the addition of bupivacaine, but only 6 maintained chronic relief. Of note was the 69% complication rate, most significantly dislodged or broken catheters.

In contrast, Samuelsson and colleagues[14] from Sweden reported experience with 146 consecutive cancer patients, who were also treated with standard epidural catheters tunneled subcutaneously. The majority of these patients (121) improved and stayed on lifelong chronic epidural opioids (mean treatment time, 92 days). The dose of epidural morphine ranged from 2 to 540 mg/day, with a mean daily dose at death of 69 mg. Only 17 of the 121 patients had local anesthetic added. Catheter-related complications occurred in nine patients. Poor responders included those with neuropathic pain, pain from cutaneous ulcerations, some visceral pain syndromes, and severe incident pain on movement.

Earlier, Samuelsson and Hedner[15] had examined the efficacy of epidural morphine in 28 cancer patients. CSF and plasma morphine concentrations at a minimum steady state were related to the degree of pain relief on a VAS. The efficacy of spinal treatment was greatest in somatic pain states, followed first by visceral pain and then by neuropathic pain; there was a significant difference when somatic pain was compared to neuropathic pain. No correlations were found between CSF or plasma morphine levels and the degree of pain relief, suggesting that not all pain impulses were being modulated in a dose-dependent manner by morphine at the spinal level.

Clinicians have also looked at the influence of spinal drug delivery on drug-related side effects. In Switzerland, Schneider and Eichner[16] evaluated 165 patients with gastrointestinal (GI) tract cancers—a group of patients that could be considered more at risk for complications of high-dose systemic opioids because of slowed gut motility. The authors attempted to compare the World Health Organization (WHO) analgesic ladder approach with implantation of epidural or intrathecal systems with portable externalized morphine pumps. A reduction in reports of nausea, vomiting, obstipation, and fatigue, as well as a decline in VAS pain scores, were reported in the spinal group compared to the systemic group. The authors advance the idea of earlier use of spinal techniques in patients with GI tumors, in whom side effects are particularly problematic.

The use of different types of catheter materials has also been explored. Du Pen and colleagues[17] in Seattle studied 55 cancer patients implanted with silicone rubber epidural catheters modeled after the Hickman catheter technology. This study examined the efficacy and safety of a two-piece permanent epidural catheter and led to the first epidural delivery system granted Food and Drug Administration (FDA) approval in the United States for long-term use. The catheter system allowed for passage of the epidural component with a stiffer guidewire segment and a tunneled segment secured with a Dacron cuff. Postmortem studies on three patients showed no signs of epidural space reaction, inflammation, or spinal cord abnormalities. Postimplant hospitalization for pain-related reasons decrease dramatically, as patients were able to remain home with epidural analgesia. Subsequently, Du Pen and colleagues[18] reported an infection rate with this catheter of 5.5% (19 of 350 patients) over a 4-year period. They distinguished local, track, and epidural space infection characteristics.

Du Pen, Kharasch, and others[19] also evaluated the plasma concentrations and toxicity profiles of cancer patients receiving opioid-bupivacaine epidural infusions. Venous plasma bupivacaine levels were determined on a weekly basis from 15 consecutive cancer patients converted to bupivacaine-containing solutions because of poor pain relief with an epidural opioid alone. Epidural bupivacaine was infused in a volume consistent with the desired blockade. Doses ranged from 150 to 1320 mg/day. No cardiovascular or central nervous system events were attributed to epidural infusions of high-dose bupivacaine. Several patients in the study routinely had plasma concentrations of 4–5 mg/ml, whereas previously the toxicity threshold was believed to exist at plasma concentrations above 1.5 mg/ml. The authors concluded that epidural bupivacaine infusions could be used safely in advanced cancer patients with intractable pain syndromes.

The Scandinavian literature is rich with experience in the use of intrathecal drug delivery systems with externalized pumps. In Sweden, Devulder and others[20] reported their experience with 33 cancer patients treated with intrathecal catheters attached to subcutaneous ports. Sixteen of these patients were categorized as having nociceptive pain and 17 patients as having either neuropathic pain or mixed pain disorders. The intrathecal port systems were accessed from outside, and drugs were administered via either an external patient-controlled analgesia (PCA) pump or a bolus injection. Morphine was administered to all patients, and more than one-half of them required less than 10 mg/day. Interestingly, concomitant spinal therapy included clonidine 150 μg/day in 10 patients, salmon calcitonin 200–500 IU/day in 4 patients, and bupivacaine 15 mg/day in 1 patient. Of the 33 patients, 25 maintained good pain relief (defined as <4 on a 10-point scale) until death. Seven patients experienced >4/10 pain only at the end of life, and pain relief was unachievable in only one patient. Twenty patients were treated with continuous intrathecal infusion plus PCA via an external system. It should be noted that an intrathecal patient-activated bolus would not be available on the FDA-approved implantable intrathecal pump systems currently available in the United States, nor has morphine been combined successfully with clonidine intrathecally in the United States because of inadequate concentrations for implanted pump delivery. Using their access to adjuvant spinal drugs and patient bolus capability, the authors were successful in managing patients with varied pain syndromes. Thirteen of 16 nociceptive pain patients (76%) achieved consistent <4/10 pain levels until death, and 12 of 17 neuropathic or mixed pain patients (70%) achieved similar responses. However, infection was a serious complication in three patients (9%) with this external intrathecal system, all of whom developed bacterial meningitis. These infections were attributed to accidental disconnection and contamination of the tubing/needle/port system. The infections were treated with intrathecal antibiotic therapy (gentamicin 2 × 4 mg daily)—a therapy the authors admit is controversial—in combination with intravenous antibiotics. This approach prevented explantation of the access port in all three cases, allowing the system to continue to be used until death.

In Belgium, Nitescu and others[21] described their experience with 142 cancer patients implanted with externalized intrathecal catheters. Their technique incorporated a tunneled, externalized intrathecal catheter attached to ambulatory infusion devices. Outcomes were described for 52 patients who received a combination of morphine and bupivacaine for a median period of 23 days. Pain on a VAS, daily opioid dose, nonopioid analgesic and sedative consumption, gait and daily activities, and amount and pattern of sleep were measured. Forty-four patients obtained continuous relief, described as VAS scores of 0–2. Thirteen patients required relatively high intrathecal bupivacaine doses (>60 mg/day), and even then, some of them did not obtain acceptable pain relief. These patients were described as having "deafferentation" pain. The intrathecal treatment was reported to decrease opioid consumption significantly and improve sleep, gait, and daily activities. Overall, the therapy was assessed as good in 23.1%, very good in 59.6%, and excellent in 13.5% of cases. Adverse drug effects, which occurred in the group receiving >60 mg/day of intrathecal bupivacaine, included paresthesias, paresis, gait impairment, urinary retention, anal sphincter disturbances, and orthostatic hypotension. Procedural difficulties while accessing the subarachnoid space were noted as follows: difficult dural puncture (18%), difficult tunneling (11%), accidental puncture of an extradural vessel (10%), bloodstained CSF (9%), difficult advancement of the catheter (6%), absence of free dripping CSF in spite of successful puncture (4%), radicular pain or paresthesia (4%), and bleeding in the tunnel track (0.7%). Meningitis occurred in only 1 of the total sample of 142 patients. In a subsequent report, Nitescu and others[22] reported on infection risks with externalized intrathecal systems. Random sampling of drug reservoirs and filters was undertaken in a sample of 89 cancer patients. Seventeen cultures taken from the spinal drug delivery systems of 13 patients were found to be colonized, without symptoms of meningeal infection, again raising the problem of contamination and the question of occult infection.

In the United States, the standard of care for intrathecal drug delivery has been the totally implanted pump system. Hassenbusch and others[23] described 69 patients who were evaluated for intrathecal morphine therapy. Forty-one patients (59.4%) achieved relief during a trial and were implanted with intrathecal implanted pump devices. VAS pain scores decreased from a mean of 8.6 before implantation to a 1-month mean score of 3.8 ($p < .001$) afterward. Over the same 1 month of treatment, the systemic morphine requirements of these patients decreased by 79.3%. No respiratory depression, epidural scarring or infection, or catheter blockage was noted. One patient developed apparent drug tolerance.

Hassenbusch and colleagues continued to be interested in long-term pain relief and in 1995 reported on 18 patients with implantable intrathecal infusions devices followed for a mean period of 2.4 years.[24] This noncancer cohort achieved 61% good or fair pain relief, with average pain scores decreased by 39% from baseline. Five patients were categorized as having lower opioid dose requirements (12–24 mg/day of intrathecal morphine), and six patients required high opioid doses (>34 mg/day). Failure to achieve long-term pain relief occurred in 39% of the patients despite good relief in trial infusions. Technical problems were reported in 33% of patients. The conclusions were that long-term infusions can be efficacious but may require higher doses, and that in many cases technical problems appear to be preventable.

In a recent restrospective multicenter survey, Paice and colleagues[25] evaluated the outcomes achieved with implantable intraspinal systems. Their sample included 35 implanting physicians and 429 patients. Physicians were asked to categorize patients as having somatic (16.8%), neuropathic (37.7%), visceral (8%), or mixed pain syndromes (37.5%). They were also asked to provide a global rating of pain relief using changes in supplemental analgesic use, pain intensity scores, and activities of daily living to determine if relief was poor (4.8%), good (42.9%), or excellent (52.4%). In addition, they were asked for permission by the study team to contact patients directly. Patients who agreed to be interviewed were contacted by telephone and asked to review their outcomes of spinal therapy. Physicians gave higher overall pain relief ratings than patients in 39.8%

of cases. In 13.3% of cases the physicians' rating was lower than the patients' rating, and in 47% of cases the outcome measures provided by physicians and patients were the same. As in other studies, patients with somatic pain tended to have greater relief than did patients with other types of pain (Mann-Whitney, $p < .0003$). Morphine doses and dose escalations up to 6 months were statistically greater in patients with malignant disease than in those with nonmalignant pain syndromes (Kruskal-Wallis test, $N = 175$–$259, p < .00005$). At 6 months, patients with neuropathic pain tended to have higher doses of intrathecal morphine than did other patients (Kruskal-Wallis test, $N = 186, p = .0073$). Physicians chose to add local anesthetics in 85 patients (19.8%), suggesting that morphine alone was not always effective. System complications occurred in 82 patients (19%) and were most often associated with catheter withdrawal or disconnection.

This literature provides a picture of clinical experience with spinal opioid therapy over the last 20+ years. The majority of published reports are related to experience with advanced cancer patients. The conclusions repeated in the literature include the efficacy of spinal opioids, the relatively reduced responsiveness to opioids in neuropathic pain states, the potential for side effects, the possibility of complications of spinal drug delivery techniques, and tolerance. The experience to date provides a backdrop for clinicians in weighing the advantages and disadvantages of the various spinal drug delivery options.

Range of Spinal Drug Delivery Techniques

There is a range of available techniques for using intraspinal analgesia. In the palliative care setting, the classic candidate is likely to have end-stage cancer or another life-threatening disease, with pain that is uncontrolled despite the use of maximized noninvasive modalities. Character of the pain, prognosis, caregiver ability, and skill and comfort level of the interventional physician will all have a significant impact on the selection of drug delivery systems.

Standard percutaneous epidural catheterization

Standard epidural catheters, designed for obstetrical and short-term postoperative pain management, have been used successfully for years in palliative care. Blind placement as a clean bedside procedure is an acceptable practice, with a lidocaine challenge test dose providing confirmation of epidural catheter placement. Some anesthesiologists involved in palliative care place these catheters in the home. The procedure involves percutaneous placement through a needle, most often in the lumbar canal, with a short subcutaneous tunnel used to create stability and avoid a direct open track to the epidural space. Some clinicians suture the catheter at the skin exit site. This method is a very simple, inexpensive way to access the epidural space. Every anesthesiologist has the stability to perform the procedure; no special training is necessary. Unfortunately, the temporary nature of the catheter may lead to frequent mechanical failure if the catheter is used long-term. The catheter may become stiff over time and break off or puncture the dura. This could result in inadvertent intrathecal drug delivery and a resultant overdose. The catheter connectors are often plastic snap-ons that may dislodge in the patient's bed. With the absence of any internal fixation, the catheter can slide out of place during normal activities such as sliding up in the bed. There are no antimicrobial features that protect the line from organism entry along the catheter track. Despite these drawbacks, standard epidural catheters should be considered for patients with a life expectancy of days to weeks for whom the advantage of ease of placement and cost efficiency outweigh the mechanical difficulties inherent in the catheter's short-term design.

Implantable epidural catheterization

Implantable epidural catheters developed with the Broviac/Hickman silastic material technology are designed to provide longer-term externalized access to the epidural space. The two-part system requires operating room placement with fluoroscopy. A small incision is made, and a guidewire-stiffened catheter is placed through a needle at the desired spinal canal level. A second, tougher subcutaneous portion of catheter is tunneled from an exit site location on the abdominal wall around to join with the epidural catheter at the lumbar insertion site. The cost of the procedure includes materials, operating room time, surgical implantation fees, radiology fees, and, in most cases, 1 day of hospitalization. Most systems have a Dacron cuff for internal stabilization, as well as a Vitacuff antimicrobial system. Exit site care is similar to that for central venous access catheters. These catheters should be considered only when patients have a life expectancy of weeks to months, so that the cost and extent of the procedure are outweighed by the durability and reliability of the system for home care.

An implantable port system is another option for access to the epidural space. This system is completely buried subcutaneously, similar to the central venous access port systems. Although some clinicians prefer port systems to externalized catheters, access for pain management is generally required continuously, making the advantage of the port systems less clear. Port devices also add expense. As longer-acting injectable drugs for epidural delivery are developed, clearer indications for port systems may develop in patients with weeks to months of life.

Epidural drug delivery

Morphine is often the first-line opioid for epidural analgesia due to its long duration of action, excellent analgesia, accessibility, and relatively low cost. The hydrophilic properties of this drug may result in side effects associated with rostral spread. The duration of action of chronically administered epidural morphine is generally 6–10 hr in the opioid-tolerant cancer population. Morphine, being widely available, is easily accessible even in rural communities. Because of its long duration of action, it can be administered on an intermittent injection basis in outpatients. Individual bolus injections of morphine are less costly than an epidural infusion system in the vast majority of cases and are less burdensome for the caregiver in the home situation, a very important factor that is often overlooked by interventionists. Thus, patients with opioid-responsive pain may be candidates for a simple regimen of scheduled epidural bolus injections.

Hydromorphone and fentanyl are most often considered second-line drugs. If bolus injection is desirable, hydromorphone may be a particularly good choice in patients for whom morphine previously had been efficacious without side effects, but side effects may occur with escalating doses. A smaller amount of hydromorphone may re-establish efficacy with a better side effect profile.

If the patient seemed to be very sensitive to epidurally administered morphine from the start of therapy, a more lipid-soluble drug, such as fentanyl, may be a better choice. Lipid-soluble drugs have been promoted as the answer to the central nervous system side effects encountered with epidural morphine. However, lipid-soluble drugs are also reabsorbed more rapidly from spinal cord and CSF into the plasma. This pharmacokinetic phenomenon could translate into side effects from high plasma levels, which may offset the benefit of local segmental effect.

The titration of epidural opioids follows the same general principles of systemic opioid titration. There is no ceiling dose for epidurally administered opioids. Anecdotally, our highest dose of epidural morphine has been 75 mg/hr by continuous infusion. The first 24 hr of epidural opioid therapy require frequent pain assessment and continuous evaluation of efficacy and toxicity. Pain and sedation levels are generally assessed every 4–8 hr, with dosage adjustments being made accordingly. Patients must be weaned from systemic opioids as epidural opioid therapy begins. They will need to remain on 50% of their systemic opioid dose the first day, cutting the dose by an additional 30–50% each subsequent day to avoid symptoms of withdrawal. Initial dosing and titration may require significant drug manipulation. Stabilization is achieved within 1–3 days, during which time patients are taught about catheter care and maintenance to provide for better home care outcomes. A flexible "titration range" can be ordered for the patient. This becomes particularly important for home care nurses working with patients experiencing escalating pain at the end of life. A typical example would be "epidural morphine 10–15 mg in 8 ml every 8 hr" or "epidural MS 0.5 mg/ml at 5 ml/hr—may increase to 10 ml/hr prn." A general "standing order" for 20% titration of the current dose within any 24-hr period can be very helpful in facilitating home care.

The addition of local anesthetics such as bupivacaine can be done when the epidural opioid alone fails to provide analgesia. Bupivacaine provides volume/concentration-dependent sensory blockade. The location of the catheter tip becomes critical for anesthetic blockade, as the infusate literally must bathe the targeted nerve roots. Low-dose bupivacaine in the range of 0.08–0.125% infusing at a rate of 5–10 ml/hr can achieve nociceptive blockade with minimal sensory blockade, whereas epidural bupivacaine at 0.125–0.25% will create more dramatic nociceptive blockade and may result in sensorimotor blockade. Clinicians must take safety precautions when initiating therapy because of the initial orthostatic hypotension associated with sympathetic blockade. Intravenous fluid may be required, but hypotension is rarely more than a transient effect. PCA bolus functions can be very effective with opioid/bupivacaine combinations, particularly with severe incident-type pain. Experienced clinicians can manipulate doses of opioid and bupivacaine to balance their effects and achieve efficacy with minimal side effects. Even in experienced hands, however, epidural therapy is not always successful.

Intrathecal drug delivery

Direct drug access to the intrathecal space is another option. Clinicians who favor intrathecal drug delivery argue that the intrathecal space has many significant advantages over the epidural space, all related to the complex diffusion pathways of epidurally administered drugs. Opioid administered into the epidural space crosses the dura and enters the CSF, where it is available for diffusion into the tissues of the spinal cord. However, there are at least three other possible endpoints for an epidurally administered opioid. It is well known that drug in the epidural space is absorbed into the significant vascular bed that lies within the epidural space. Studies show that the plasma level following a single epidural injection of opioid closely approximates that of an intramuscular injection. Thus, a fair amount of systemic opioid is always present with epidural administration. A second fraction of opioid is mixed with the passive circulation of CSF that flows through dural root sleeves and via arachnoid villi. A third fraction of opioid enters the fatty depot of the epidural space, where it is available for either reabsorption into the vascular route or transdural spread into the CSF.

Direct intrathecal administration ensures delivery of drug directly into the CSF. Intrathecal morphine is roughly 10 times as potent as epidural morphine, providing a presumed advantage in dosing for the morphine-tolerant cancer patient. As with the epidural route, a variety of other opioids and adjuvant drugs can be administered intrathecally, using an approach tailored to the specific pain syndrome.

The European reports suggest a role for externalized intrathecal catheters. The same catheters used epidurally can be placed intrathecally, both the standard percutaneous type and the implantable silastic catheters tunneled externally. The external infusion pumps can then deliver any concentration of opioid, local anesthetic, alpha-2 agonist, or another agent to the intrathecal space, with the goal of achieving a balance between pain relief and side effects. This flexibility with the externalized systems contrasts to the relative inflexibility of the implantable infusion pumps used for cancer and nonmalignant pain syndromes. The smaller reservoir volumes of the internalized devices are fixed, and the lack of high-concentration drug availability limits the clinician's ability to tailor the therapy. Implantable pumps are costly and inappropriate for patients with a prognosis of less than 3 months.

The major disadvantage of externalized intrathecal drug delivery is the risk of meningitis. The dura-arachnoid membrane provides a natural barrier to infection for epidural drug delivery that is lost when direct intrathecal access is chosen. Meningitis in the setting of palliative care may be a terminal event and would require a preplacement discussion to consider the ultimate course of action should infection occur. However, if comfort is the only goal, and pain is severe and unrelenting, the bedside placement of a standard catheter in the intrathecal space may be effective.

Alternatives to Spinal Drug Delivery Techniques

Oral, subcutaneous, intravenous, and other noninvasive routes for opioids and adjuvant therapy should be considered before spinal delivery techniques.[26] These therapies should be maximized until side effects dictate either sequential opioid trials or a change in analgesic technique. A number of physicians still believe that there is a ceiling dose for opioids above which additional drug will lead to overdosage. This treatment restriction may lead to the unnecessary early use of interventional procedures. The aggressive and artful use of systemic analgesics is successful in the management of 80–90% of patients with intractable pain.[9] To achieve this goal, one must titrate the analgesic dosage to the effect or the side effects.

Patient selection for invasive procedures, including both regional anesthesia techniques and neurosurgical intervention, should be based on pain assessment, pain character, life expectancy, and response to previous therapeutic endeavors.[27] Pain assessment during activity should measure the worst, least, and average pain to give a temporal quality and intensity description of pain. The pain character (neuropathic, visceral, or somatic) relates the pain experience to its presumed origin. Neuropathic pain states from malignant (tumor or treatment-related) or non malignant sources are considered most intractable, whereas visceral pain is most often opioid responsive.[28] Samuelsson et al. state that certain types of visceral pain, movement-related somatic pain, and cutaneous ulceration pain may be as difficult to treat as neuropathic pain.[14] Therefore, the character of the pain alone only gives the clinician an indication of treatment responsiveness and should be used only as a therapeutic guide. Serial trials of therapeutic interventions starting with systemic opioids and moving to interventional techniques is a time-proven algorithmic approach to achieve the best possible outcome.[29]

There are no guidelines on the steps to be taken in the interventional decision-making process. The guidelines on cancer pain management issued by the U.S. Agency for Health Care Policy and Research list the possible interventional techniques individually, with benefits and complications, but do not establish an algorithm for application of these techniques.[30] Krames published his concept of how intraspinal opioid infusions and spinal cord stimulation fit into the therapeutic continuum for nonmalignant pain management.[31,32] The literature contains a number of individual and small series case reports with conclusions on how these techniques should be used clinically. The variables of nociceptive and neuropathic pain character, pain intensity, life expectancy, economic impact, and psychosocial makeup of the patient/family make it difficult to establish a standard algorithm for interventional pain management. The clinician is left alone in a sea of individual reports to determine the best technique for the patient at any specific point in the pain continuum. However, these techniques can be presented in a logical order of consideration based on the many variables encountered in treating the cancer patient with intractable pain.

Whenever clinically possible, these interventional techniques should be tested before clinical application. This is not possible for some neurosurgical procedures, but neuroablative procedures and infusion devices may be tested with individual local anesthetic blocks or with temporary infusions or injections. Table 12.1 lists some of the chemical and surgical neurolytic procedures that have been incorporated into a cancer pain treatment continuum after systemic pain management has been unsuccessful.

Peripheral neurolytic blocks are ideal when the pain source is innervated by three or fewer single nerve roots. Alcohol and phenol are effective neurodestructive agents, but their effect is limited (2–3 months).[33] Cryoneurolysis is also a time-limited technique that results in neurodestruction after freezing the nerve with a $-196°C$ liquid nitrogen–filled needle probe tip.[34] These procedures are effective on small peripheral nerves but not on larger, protected nerve trunks (brachial or lumbar plexus). Care must be taken not to destroy critical motor branches, which may result in unacceptable secondary effects. Diagnostic local anesthetic blocks are a good predictor of the outcome of the neurodestructive procedure.[35] When these blocks are effective, there will be a dramatic impact on the patient's overall functional outcome and the requirement for opioid use. Intercostal blockade for invasive chest wall involvement is the most frequent application of this technique.[35]

Table 12.1. Examples of chemical and surgical neurolytic procedures for management of cancer pain

1. Neurolytic peripheral blocks (intercostal and other peripheral nerves, nerve root blocks)
2. Neurolytic sympathetic blocks (celiac plexus, stellate ganglion, superior hypogastric plexus)
3. Neurolytic intraspinal blocks (phenol and alcohol subarachnoid blocks, epidural phenol and alcohol blocks)
4. Neuroablative procedures (peripheral destruction)—radiofrequency neurodestructive procedures, including ganglionic and nerve root destruction
5. Neuroablative procedures (central destruction)—cordotomy, dorsal root entry zone (DREZ) lesioning, alcohol destruction of the pituitary gland, thalamotomy, cingulotomy
6. Other neurosurgical interventions including deep brain stimulation and gamma-knife procedures

Blockade of sympathetic ganglia is an effective means of interrupting sympathetically maintained pain. An understanding of neuroanatomy is essential in determining when this approach is indicated. The sympathetic ganglia accessible to blockade are the stellate ganglion, celiac ganglion, lumbar sympathetic plexus, and superior hypogastric plexus. The celiac plexus also includes afferent fibers that mediate nociceptive sensation from the lower esophagus, stomach, liver, pancreas, and upper small intestine. Blockade of this ganglion may lead to dramatic visceral pain relief from pancreatic cancer and should be considered before spinal drug delivery.[36] The use of a diagnostic celiac plexus block allows the clinician to determine the efficacy of the technique before the neurodestructive procedure is performed. Stellate ganglion blockade relieves sympathetically maintained pain in the upper extremity, whereas superior hypogastric plexus blockade relieves visceral pain from the pelvis.[37] The opioid responsiveness of visceral pain often results in effective treatment with oral opioids until the tumor stimulates pain beyond the coverage of the affected plexus. At this point, blockade becomes ineffective.[38,39] Similarly, early analgesic loss may occur after successful celiac blockade when tumor growth involves additional pain sources.

Neurolytic intraspinal procedures have been proposed for the control of both nociceptive and neuropathic pain sources.[33] Alcohol and phenol are effective for this purpose, and butamben is being investigated.[35,40] The epidural instillation of both alcohol and phenol has a bilateral effect with difficult-to-predict spread.[33] Subarachnoid alcohol and phenol are much more controllable due to the hypobaric nature of alcohol and the hyperbaric composition of phenol, but the risk of neurological deficit is greater with subarachnoid instillation.[33] Most oncology patients elect to avoid procedures that may result in an irreversible neurological deficit. Neurosurgical consultation in cases that may require extensive neurodestruction should focus on risk versus benefit.

Neurosurgical peripheral interventions include both nerve root transection and radiofrequency ablation. Radiofrequency peripheral nerve or ganglion ablation may be used for the control of pain associated with the trigeminal nerve or individual spinal nerve roots.[41] The application of this technique requires that the pain source be limited to two or three peripheral nerves. This technique is rarely used, but it is effective if the circumstances warrant it.

More aggressive neurosurgical procedures, such as cordotomy and dorsal root entry zone (DREZ) lesions, may be used when pain is somatic or neuropathic in origin and has a unilateral distribution.[42] Cordotomy can be useful in a patient with severe unilateral pain syndrome. The risks of loss of bladder or bowel control and motor loss must be weighed against the benefits of the procedure. The DREZ lesion, which is a form of selective posterior rhizotomy, may be an effective means of controlling pain associated with the brachial or lumbar plexus, with less risk to motor function than rhizotomy.[42] Anesthesia risk and postoperative recovery may be determining factors, depending on the life expectancy of the patient.

Procedures such as alcohol ablation of the pituitary, thalamotomy, and cingulotomy have been used by surgeons experienced with these procedures, but the risk–benefit ratio is difficult to determine, as there are so few cases in the literature. These aggressive surgical techniques are available in extremely rare cases when no other alternative has been successful.

Deep brain stimulation is considered the leading edge of neurosurgical interventions that may be used to control pain.[43,44] The mechanism of action may be dopaminergic.[43] The gamma-knife is another innovative procedure that focuses 201 hemispherically arrayed cobalt-60 sources to deliver a high dose of radiation to a small, focused deep brain target.[45] Both of these procedures may hold promise in the future, but they are being used clinically in only a small number of institutions.

In summary, there are a number of chemical and surgical techniques for ameliorating pain in the rare cases where traditional systemic pharmacotherapy fails to provide relief in the patient with life-threatening disease. Spinal drug delivery provides a reversible pharmacological approach that generally falls between oral therapy and neurolytic or neuroablative techniques. These techniques may meet the changing pain management needs of end-stage patients and will likely continue to have a role in the treatment of intractable pain.

What the Future Holds

The future of intraspinal analgesia is exciting. New technological advances in delivery devices for epidural and subarachnoid space access will make the procedures more accessible and safer for more cancer patients. A better understanding of the infection risk, system contamination, and system design will allow externalized access to the subarachnoid space for long-term infusion techniques. New long-acting local anesthetic agents and long-acting, intraspinally administered opioids will allow the use of implantable port systems to deliver intermittent drug therapy with a reduced risk of infection.

Alpha-2-agonists like clonidine will become more commonly used spinal drug adjuvants. Coombs et al. reported the efficacy of clonidine in conjunction with opioids in a case of intractable invasive cervical cancer in the early 1980s.[46] Yaksh et al. demonstrated dose-dependent analgesia with spinal clonidine, without signs of systemic or spinal cord toxicity, in their long-term dog model.[47] Eisenach et al. demonstrated the safety and efficacy of epidural clonidine with morphine in relieving neuropathic pain in a multicenter study involving 85 cancer patients.[48] The future development of new alpha-2 agonists, perhaps with a decreased incidence of hypotension, may allow more widespread use of the technique.

N-Methyl-D-Aspartate (NMDA) receptor antagonists administered intraspinally, subcutaneously, and intravenously all have a dose-dependent antinociceptive effect.[49] Of particular interest is the role these drugs may play in opioid tolerance. Studies in mice suggest that mu-opioid tolerance but not kappa tolerance involves mediation by NMDA receptors.[50] As more data become available, we may have a new tool to use in avoiding opioid tolerance while increasing analgesia. These agents may play a role in the delivery of analgesia to patients with a previous history of drug abuse and tolerance.

Butamben, a highly lipid-soluble local anesthetic, has stirred great interest. In 1990, Shulman et al. demonstrated in dogs that the use of subarachnoid 10% butamben resulted in adhesive arachnoiditis, but when injected into the epidural space, the drug produced analgesia with no demonstrable pathology.[51] Korsten et al. examined 12 cancer patients who failed to achieve acceptable analgesia with epidural opioid with local anesthetics but had prolonged analgesia from butamben.[40] Five of these patients required no further use of opioids. Korsten et al. further postulate that this drug may replace the need for cordotomy.

Manipulation of the lipid solubility of opioids in the spinal canal has generated some future possibilities. Drug vehicles such as 2-hydroxypropyl-betacyclodextrin may help reduce the rate of clearance from spinal cord to the vascular tree, thereby retaining the properties of lipophilic drugs that enhance efficacy but eliminating the systemic reabsorption problem that increases the risk of side effects.[52] Adjustments of the lipid solubility of opioids may prolong the duration of efficacy of our well-tested and effective drugs.

The future of pain management is truly exciting, with many new avenues of drug investigation and device development. Our goal will be to create better spinally administered pharmacologic regimens, with safer and easier delivery systems, to meet the goal of pain relief in palliative care.

References

1. Coyle N, Adelhart J, Foley KM, et al. Character of terminal illness in the advanced cancer patient: pain and other symptoms during the last four weeks of life. *J Pain Symptom Manage* 1990; 5:83–93.
2. Wang JK. Analgesic effect of intrathecally-administered morphine. *Regional Anesth* 1977; 2:3–4.
3. Coombs DW, Saunders RL, Gaylor MS, et al. Relief of continuous chronic pain by intraspinal narcotics infusion via an implanted reservoir. *JAMA* 1983; 250:2336–2339.
4. Max MB, Inturrisi CE, Kaiko RF, et al. Epidural and intrathecal opiates: cerebrospinal fluid and plasma profiles in patients with chronic cancer pain. *Clin Pharm Ther* 1985; 38:631–641.
5. Yaksh TL, Onofrio BM. Retrospective consideration of the doses of morphine given intrathecally by chronic infusion in 163 patients by 19 physicians. *Pain* 1987; 31:211–223.
6. Onofrio BM, Yaksh TL. Long-term pain relief produced by intrathecal morphine infusion in 53 patients. *J Neurosurg* 1990; 72:200–209.
7. Plummer JL, Cherry DA, Cousins MJ, et al. Long-term spinal administration of morphine in cancer and noncancer pain: a retrospective study. *Pain* 1991; 44:215–220.
8. Cousins MJ, Cherry DA, Gourlay GK. Acute and chronic pain: use of spinal opioids.

In: Cousins MJ, Bridenbaugh PO, eds. *Neural Blockade in Clinical Anesthesia and Pain Management.* 2nd ed. Philadelphia: J.B. Lippincott Co., 1988:955–1029.

9. Cousins MJ, Plummer JL. Spinal opioids in acute and chronic pain. In: Max M, Portenoy RK, Laska E, eds. *Advances in Pain Research and Therapy.* New York: Raven Press, 1991:457–473.

10. Gourlay G, Plummer J, Cherry D, et al. Comparison of intermittent bolus with continuous infusion of epidural morphine in the treatment of severe cancer pain. *Pain* 1991; 37(2):135–140.

11. Erdine S, Aldemir F. Long-term results of peridural morphine in 225 patients. *Pain* 1991; 45:155–159.

12. Madrid JL, Fatela LV, Guillen AF, et al. Intermittent intrathecal morphine by means of an implantable reservoir: a survey of 100 cases. *J Pain Symptom Manage* 1988; 3:67–71.

13. Hogan Q, Haddox JD, Abram S, et al. Epidural opiates and local anesthetics for the management of cancer pain. *Pain* 1991; 46:271–279.

14. Samuelsson H, Malmberg F, Erikson M, et al. Outcomes of epidural morphine treatment in cancer pain: nine years of clinical experience. *J Pain Symptom Manage* 1995; 10:105–112.

15. Samuelsson H, Hedner T. Pain characterization in cancer patients and the analgetic response to epidural morphine. *Pain* 1991; 46:3–8.

16. Schneider M, Eichner C. Pain therapy of tumor patients with special reference to tumors of the gastrointestinal tract: WHO staged schedule versus para-spinal analgesia techniques. *Chirurgie* 1994; 56:551–555.

17. Du Pen SL, Peterson DG, Bogosian AC, et al. A new permanent externalized epidural catheter for narcotic self-administration to control cancer pain. *Cancer* 1987; 59: 986–993.

18. Du Pen SL, Peterson DG, Williams AR, et al. Infection during chronic epidural catheterization: diagnosis and treatment. *Anesthesiology* 1990; 73:905–909.

19. Du Pen SL, Kharasch ED, Williams AR, et al. Chronic epidural bupivacaine-opioid infusion in intractable cancer pain. *Pain* 1992; 49:293–300.

20. Devulder J, Ghys L, Dhondt W, et al. Spinal analgesia in terminal care: risk versus benefit. *J Pain Symptom Manage* 1994; 9:75–81.

21. Nitescu P, Appelgren L, Hultman E, et al. Long-term open catheterization of the spinal subarachnoid space for continuous infusion of narcotic and bupivacaine in patients with refractory cancer pain. A technique of catheterization and its problems and complications. *Clin J Pain* 1991; 7:143–161.

22. Nitescu P, Hultman E, Allepgren L, et al. Bacteriology, drug stability and exchange of percutaneous delivery systems and antibacterial filters in long-term intrathecal infusion of opioid drugs and bupivacaine in refractory pain. *Clin J Pain* 1992; 8:324–337.

23. Hassenbusch SJ, Pillay PK, Magdinec M, et al. Constant infusion of morphine for intractable cancer pain using an implanted pump. *J Neurosurg* 1990; 73:405–409.

24. Hassenbusch SJ, Stanton-Hicks M, Covington EC, et al., Long-term intraspinal infusions of opioids in the treatment of neuropathic pain. *J Pain Symptom Manage* 1995; 10:527–543.

25. Paice JA, Penn RD, Shott S. Intraspinal morphine for chronic pain: a retrospective multicenter study. *J Pain Symptom Manage* 1996; 11:71–80.

26. Foley KM, Inturrisi CE. Analgesic drug therapy in cancer pain: principles and practice. *Med Clin North Am* 1987; 71(2):207–232.

27. Du Pen SL, Du Pen AR. Spinal analgesia. In: Ashburn MA, Rice LJ, eds. *The Management of Pain.* New York: Churchill Livingstone, 1998.

28. Cousins MJ, Bromage PR. Epidural neural blockade In: Cousins MJ, Bridenbaugh PO, eds. *Neural Blockade in Clinical Anesthesia and Management of Pain,* 2nd ed. Philadelphia: J.B. Lippincott Co., 1988:253–360.

29. Portenoy R, Foley K, Inturrisi C. The nature of opioid responsiveness and its implications for neuropathic pain: new hypotheses derived from studies of opioid infusions. *Pain* 1990; 43(3):372–286.

30. Agency for Health Care Policy and Research. *Clinical Guideline: Cancer Pain Management.* Bethesda, MD: Public Health Service, 1993.

31. Krames E. Intraspinal opioid therapy for chronic nonmalignant pain: current practice and clinical guidelines. *J Pain Symptom Manage* 1996; 11(6):333–352.

32. Krames E. The role of implantable pain management technologies: an algorithm for decision-making. In: Waldman S, Winnie A, eds. *Interventional Pain Management.* Philadelphia: W.B. Saunders Co., 1996:501–510.

33. Myers RR, Katz J. Neural pathology of neurolytic and semidestructive agents. In: Cousins MJ, Bridenbaugh PO, eds. *Neural Blockade in Clinical Anesthesia and Management of Pain,* 2nd ed. Philadelphia: JB Lippincott, 1988:1031–1051.

34. Saberski LR. Cryoneurolysis in clinical practice. In: Waldman S, Winnie A, eds. *Interventional Pain Management.* Philadelphia: W.B. Saunders Co., 1996:172–184.

35. Jain S, Gupta R. Neurolytic agents in clinical practice. In: Waldman S, Winnie A, eds. *Interventional Pain Management.* Philadelphia: W.B. Saunders Co., 1996:167–171.

36. Waldman S, Patt R. Celiac plexus and splanchnic nerve block. In: Waldman S, Winnie A, eds. *Interventional Pain Management.* Philadelphia: W.B. Saunders Co., 1996: 360–374.

37. Patt R, Plancarte R. Superior hypogastric plexus block: a new therapeutic approach for pelvic pain. In: Waldman S, Winnie A, eds. *Interventional Pain Management.* Philadelphia: W.B. Saunders Co., 1996:384–391.

38. Bonica JJ. Autonomic innervation of the viscera in relation to nerve block. *Anesthesiology* 1968; 29:793.

39. Patt RB. Neurolytic blocks of the sympathetic axis. In: Patt RB, ed. *Cancer Pain.* Philadelphia: J.B. Lippincott Co., 1993:393–411.

40. Korsten HH, Ackerman EW, Grouls RJ, et al. Long-lasting epidural sensory blockade by *n*-butyl-*p*-aminobenzoate in the terminally ill intractable cancer pain patient. *Anesthesiology* 1991; 75(6):950–960.

41. Arbit E, Krol G. Percutaneous radiofrequency neurolysis guided by computer tomography for the treatment of pain. *Neurosurgery* 1991; 29:580–582.

42. Augustinsson LE. The role of neurosurgery in the management of intractable pain. In: Waldman S, Winnie A, eds. *Interventional Pain Management.* Philadelphia: W.B. Saunders Co., 1996:511–518.

43. Kumar K, Wyant GM, Nath R. Deep brain stimulation for control of intractable pain in human, present and future: a ten-year follow-up. *Neurosurgery* 1990; 26(5):774–781.

44. Gybles J, Kupers R. Deep brain stimulation in the treatment of chronic pain in man: where and why? *Neurophysiol Clin* 1990; 20(5):389–398.

45. Blond S, Coche-Dequeant B. Stereotactically-guided radiosurgery using the linear accelerator. *Acta Neurochir Wien* 1993; 124(1):40–44.
46. Coombs DW, Saunders RL, Fratkin JD, et al. Continuous intrathecal hydromorphone and clonidine for intractable cancer pain. *J Neurosurg* 1986; 64(6):890–894.
47. Yaksh TL, Rathbun M, Jage J, Mirzai T, Grafe M, Hiles RA. Pharmacology and toxicology of chronically infused epidural clonidine HCl in dogs. *Fundament Appl Toxicol* 1994; 23(3):319–335.
48. Eisenach JC, Du Pen S, Debois M, et al. Epidural clonidine analgesia for intractable cancer pain. The epidural clonidine study group. *Pain* 1995; 61(3):391–399.
49. Sosnowski M. Pain management: physiopathology, future research and endpoints. *Supportive Care in Cancer* 1993; (2):79–88.
50. Elliott K, Minami N, Kolesnikov YA, et al. The NMDA receptor antagonists, LY274614 and MK-801, and the nitric oxide synthase inhibitor, NG-nitro-L-argine, attenuate analgesic tolerance to the mu-opioid morphine but not to kappa opioids. *Pain* 1994; 56(1):69–75.
51. Shulman M, Joseph NJ, Haller CA. Effect of epidural and subarachnoid injections of a 10% butamben suspension. *Regional Anesth* 1990; 15(3):142–146.
52. Jang J, Yaksh T, Hill H. Use of 2-hydroxypropyl-beta-cyclodextrin as an intrathecal drug vehicle with opioids. *J Pharmacol Exp Ther* 1992; 261(2):592–600.

13

Pathophysiology and Assessment of Dyspnea in the Patient with Cancer

DEBORAH J. DUDGEON AND SUSAN ROSENTHAL

Dyspnea, an uncomfortable awareness of breathing, can seriously affect the quality of life of cancer patients. Management of this symptom in these patients requires an understanding of the multidimensional nature of dyspnea,[1] the neural pathways and receptors that may be involved, the pathophysiological mechanisms that may underline the problem, the methods of evaluation and assessment of dyspnea, and the clinical syndromes that are common in cancer. Relief of breathlessness should be the goal of treatment at all stages of cancer. Good control of this symptom will improve function and quality of life.

Dyspnea, like pain, is a subjective experience involving many factors that modulate both the quality and the intensity of its perception. Dyspnea incorporates not only physical neuroanatomical elements but also affective components, which are shaped by previous experience.[2,3] Individuals with comparable degrees of functional lung impairment may experience considerable differences in the intensity of dyspnea they perceive.[2] Furthermore, objective signs often do not match the patient's perception of dyspnea,[4] and dyspnea cannot be predicted by an isolated pulmonary function test.[5] This lack of correlation and predictability may be due to any one or a combination of factors including adaptation, differing physical characteristics, and psychological conditions.[2] Variations in the pattern of breathing, changes in respiratory impedance and respiratory muscle operating characteristics, and changes in circulatory function during a given physical activity may account for differences in clinical ratings of dyspnea among patients with comparable degrees of lung impairment.[2,6,7] A psychological explanation may also underline, at least in part, differences in perception of the intensity of breathlessness.

Neuroanatomical Elements Involved in Breathing

Breathing is usually an automatic function controlled by centers in the medulla and the pons. Afferent information from various receptors travels to the brainstem and influences the frequency and depth of ventilation (Fig. 13.1). Voluntary control by the cerebral cortex can override the activity of the respiratory centers during speech and other activities.[3] Spinal cord reflexes, in response to local sensory input, also can override the automatic function of the respiratory centers.[8]

The neural pathways responsible for the sensation of dyspnea are poorly understood,[9] and no simple physiological mechanism or unique peripheral site can explain the varied circumstances that lead to the perception of breathlessness.[2,10] Stimulation of a number of different receptors and the conscious perception this invokes can alter ventilation and result in the sensation of breathlessness. Dyspnea in patients with cancer and other diseases is probably caused by the interaction of many stimuli. The stimuli that influence the level and pattern of breathing fall into four categories: mechanical, biochemical, vascular, and psychogenic.[11]

Mechanical stimuli

A variety of receptors in the chest wall, diaphragm, airways, oral mucosa, and lung parenchyma respond to mechanical stimuli, and this afferent information modi-

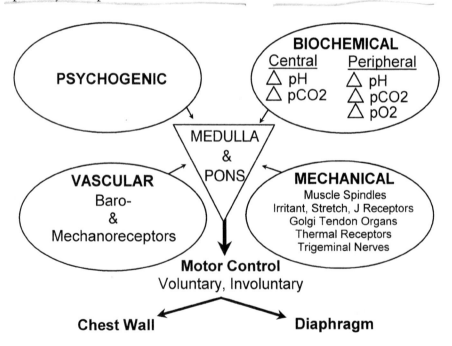

Figure 13.1. Schematic diagram of the neuroanatomical elements involved in the control of ventilation.

fies the intensity of dyspnea. Muscle spindle receptors in the intercostal muscles and the Golgi tendon organ receptors of the diaphragm mediate the sense of muscle length tension "inappropriateness" or variation from normal. Stretch receptors located in bronchial smooth muscle respond to inflation pressures. Physical distortion of the lung interstitium resulting from congestion, embolism, tumor, or infection, as well as the action of a number of chemical substances, can stimulate the juxtapulmonary or J receptors. The vagus nerve transmits the afferent neural messages from stimulation of the J receptors to the central nervous system. Receptors in the nasopharynx and in the distribution of the trigeminal nerve respond to air cooling and air flow, decreasing the perceived intensity of breathlessness.[12,13] A rise in deep body temperature increases ventilation by stimulating thermal receptors in the hypothalamus. A change in the level of stimulation of any of these receptors alters the afferent information transmitted from the respiratory system to the central nervous system, modulating ventilation and thereby the sensation of breathlessness.

Biochemical stimuli

Receptors in the medulla, the aortic arch, and the carotid bodies respond to biochemical changes, producing changes in ventilation. Carotid body receptors perceive hypoxemia, hypercapnia, and acidosis and stimulate ventilation in response. Acidosis and hypercapnia also stimulate central chemoreceptors.[11] Ventilation increases when the partial pressure of oxygen drops below 60 mm Hg, but the response to hypercapnia is even more sensitive: increases in the partial pressure of carbon dioxide as small as 2–3 mm Hg produce increases in ventilation. Some evidence suggests that chemoreceptor stimulation produced by hypercapnia or hypoxemia causes a sensation of distress and breathlessness even without any change in ventilation.[2,14,15]

Vascular stimuli

Mechanoreceptors in the atria and right ventricle respond to increased vascular pressures and cause an increase in ventilation. Baroreceptors in the pulmonary artery respond to abnormal pressures and increase ventilation as well.[11] Reduced carotid sinus pressures also stimulate ventilation.[11] Alterations in the afferent information from these receptors may produce the perception of breathlessness.

Psychogenic stimuli

Perception of the intensity and quality of dyspnea requires cognitive interpretation, which can be influenced by past experience, emotional state, response style, and behavioral characteristics.[16] Dyspnea may also develop in some patients who have a psychiatric disorder and no underlying lung pathology.[11,17,18]

Pathophysiology of Dyspnea

The causes of breathlessness derive from impairment of the respiratory, cardio-vascular, hematological, musculoskeletal, and psychological systems.

Respiratory impairment

Respiratory impairment is assessed by means of pulmonary function tests, the results of which help to determine the etiology of dyspnea and guide therapy. The broad categories of respiratory impairment are obstructive, restrictive, decreased diffusion, and mixed obstructive and restrictive.

Obstructive impairment

Obstructive impairment refers to impedance to the flow of air, Progressive nar-rowing of the airways can result from both structural and functional changes. Extramural compression or endomural obstruction of the lumen of the airway results from tumor, mucus, inflammation, or edema. Increased bronchomotor tone due to release of histamine, leukotrienes, and other mediators produces bronchoconstriction. Loss of radial traction on intrapulmonary airways is the major cause of airflow obstruction in emphysema, which is associated with large lung volumes. Less commonly, loss of radial traction on intrapulmonary airways occurs in the setting of small lung volumes and in the elderly.[8] A reduced forced expiratory volume in 1 min as a fraction of vital capacity (FEV_1/FVC) and an increase in total lung capacity (TLC), residual volume (RV), and functional resid-ual capacity (FRC) are the usual hallmarks of an obstructive ventilatory defect.

Restrictive impairment

The principal diagnostic features of a restrictive ventilatory defect are a concur-rent reduction in both FEV_1 and FVC, decreased TLC and RV, and often decreased diffusing capacity as well. A restrictive ventilatory defect results from decreased distensibility of the lung parenchyma, pleura, or chest wall or from a reduction in the maximum force exerted by the respiratory muscles. Interstitial infiltration, pneumonitis, fibrosis, or edema; fibrosis or infiltration of the pleura or subpleural tissue; a space-occupying lesion of the parenchyma; pleural effu-sion; muscle weakness; obesity; and ascites can limit lung expansion and result in a restrictive ventilatory defect.[8]

Decreased diffusion

A low diffusing capacity usually results from the loss of functioning alveolocapil-lary surface area, with the obliteration of the pulmonary vascular bed, and seldom from thickening of alveolar walls.[19] Interstitial lung disease (from tumor, pneu-monitis, or fibrosis), emphysema, and pulmonary vascular disease can cause the defective transfer of oxygen and, to a lesser extent, carbon dioxide.[8]

Mixed obstructive and restrictive impairments

This category is a combination of obstructive and restrictive impairments as outlined above.

Cardiovascular impairment

Cardiovascular causes of dyspnea are related to the development of congestive heart failure, with decreased cardiac output and increased pulmonary venous pressure. Cardiomyopathies, valvular or pericardial disease, and congenital abnormalities can cause a decrease in cardiac output, with a resultant decrease in delivery of oxygen to the tissues. Diastolic dysfunction, mitral stenosis, pulmonary venous occlusive disease, hypercapnia, acidosis, chronic hypoxia, thromboemboli or tumor emboli,[20] and right-to-left shunts cause elevation of the pulmonary venous pressure with pulmonary congestion and a decrease in the diffusion of oxygen.[8]

Hematological impairment

Oxygen is transported to the tissues and lungs bound to intracorpuscular hemoglobin. Maximum oxygen uptake is reduced when the hemoglobin concentration is less than 80% of normal.[8] Anemia from a variety of causes results in decreased oxygen delivery to the tissues.

Musculoskeletal impairment

The respiratory muscles consist of two functional groups: the inspiratory muscles, which include the diaphragm, sternocleidomastoids, scalenes, and external intercostals, and the expiratory muscles, which include the internal intercostals and abdominal muscles. Breathing is the main function of the respiratory muscles and is performed largely by the muscles of inspiration (mostly the diaphram). Respiratory muscle weakness and dysfunction can cause acute and chronic respiratory failure and lead to dyspnea and even death on occasion. If respiratory muscle strength is reduced to less than 30% of the predicted level, respiratory failure may occur.[21] Causes of respiratory muscle dysfunction include neuromuscular diseases; malnutrition; deficiencies of potassium, magnesium, and inorganic phosphate[22]; poor oxygenation; neurohormonal changes in levels of cortisol, catecholamines, and tissue necrosis factor; and muscle fatigue.[23] Respiratory muscle strength is measured by maximum inspiratory and maximum expiratory pressures.

Psychological impairment

Psychological variables influence the perception of breathlessness. Anxious, obsessive, depressed, and dependent persons appear to experience dyspnea that is disproportionately severe relative to the extent of pulmonary disease.[2] Burns and Howell found that patients with airway disease who had disproportionately severe breathlessness were more likely to have obvious psychogenic stress factors, a previous personal or family history of psychiatric illness, or an obsessional type of premorbid personality than patients with an appropriate degree of breathlessness for the degree of airway disease.[18] They also found that patients with disproportionate breathlessness manifested symptoms of a psychiatric disorder (most commonly depression) more frequently, and that their breathlessness resolved with resolution of the psychiatric disorder. Others have found that anxiety and depression seem to perpetuate episodes of disproportionate breathlessness.[24]

Epidemiology of Dyspnea

In a recent study by Dudgeon and colleagues, 46% of a general cancer population reported breathlessness, and 15% described symptoms in the moderate to severe range.[25] Muers and Round noted that breathlessness was a complaint at presentation in 60% of 289 patients with non-small cell lung cancer.[26] One-half of this group described their shortness of breath as moderate or severe. Just prior to death, nearly 90% of this patient group experienced dyspnea. Among 1500 cancer patients studied by Reuben and Mor, 70% suffered from dyspnea during the last 6 weeks of life.[27] In Reuben and Mor's study, dyspnea was moderate to severe in more than 28% of terminally ill cancer patients who were able to grade their shortness of breath. Others[28,29] have found that 45–50% of hospitalized, terminally ill cancer patients complain of dyspnea. One study noted that dyspnea was the main symptom in 21% of 86 terminal cancer patients cared for at home.[30]

Dudgeon and colleagues[25] found that shortness of breath was significantly more common among patients with mediastinal, hilar, lung parenchymal, or rib metastases; previous thoracic surgery or lung irradiation; environmental exposures to asbestos, chemicals, sprays, coal and grain dust, and moldy hay; current use of respiratory medications; and a history of cigarette smoking or nonmalignant pulmonary disease. In Reuben and Mor's National Hospice Study, the best predictor of dyspnea in terminally ill patients was the presence of lung or pleural involvement with cancer.[27]

Causes of Dyspnea in Cancer Patients

The optimal therapy for breathlessness is correction of the cause. This remedy is possible only if the cause of dyspnea is reversible. Reuben and Mor retrospectively examined the results of the National Hospice Study to determine the prevalence and etiology of dyspnea in this group of patients with terminal cancer.[27] They found that patients with lung or pleural involvement constituted only 39% of the terminally ill patients reporting dyspnea. Thirty-four percent of the patients in the National Hospice Study had a history of cardiac disease, and 24.3% had a history of respiratory disease. No etiology for dyspnea could be determined in 23.9% of

Table 13.1. Radiological findings in 100 cancer patients with dyspnea

Radiological abnormality	Percent of patients°
Parenchymal abnormality	54
Hilar/mediastinal adenopathy	30
Pleural effusion(s)	36
Pleural involvement	16
Pneumonia	11
Lymphangitic carcinomatosis	8
Pneumothorax	2
Pulmonary edema	1
Normal	9
Unavailable	3

°Many patients had more than one radiological abnormality.

dyspneic terminal cancer patients in the National Hospice Study; in these patients, dyspnea was attributed to the general debility caused by terminal cancer.

In a prospective study of 100 dyspneic patients with advanced cancer, Dudgeon and Lertzman found that 91% had an abnormal chest radiograph[31] (Table 13.1). Spirometry test results were abnormal in 93% of patients; 87% had a restrictive component, and 52% had an obstructive component. The median maximum inspiratory pressure was only 16 cm H_2O, indicating severe respiratory muscle impairment. Hypoxia (O_2 saturation <90%) was implicated as the cause of dyspnea in only 40% of the patients. These investigators also found that anxiety and shortness of breath, as measured by visual analogue scales, had a low correlation ($r = .29$). Anxiety was implicated as the cause of dyspnea in only one patient.

In a clinical classification, the causes of dyspnea in cancer patients[4,32–35] fall into four categories: direct tumor effects, indirect tumor effects, treatment-related causes, and problems unrelated to the cancer (Table 13.2).

Dyspnea due directly to cancer

The causes of dyspnea due directly to cancer include parenchymal involvement by tumor (primary or secondary), lymphangitic carcinomatosis, extrinsic or intrinsic obstruction of airways by tumor, pleural tumor (particularly mesothelioma), pleural effusion, pericardial effusion, ascites, hepatomegaly, phrenic nerve involvement, superior vena cava obstruction, multiple tumor microemboli, and pulmonary leukostasis.

Pleural effusion
Pleural effusion may be the initial symptom of cancer, or it may accompany progressive advanced disease. Patients with pleural effusions usually complain of

Table 13.2. Causes of dyspnea in cancer patients

Dyspnea Due Directly to Cancer	Dyspnea Due to Cancer Treatment
Pulmonary parenchymal involvement (primary or metastatic)	Surgery
Lymphangitic carcinomatosis	Radiation pneumonitis/fibrosis
Intrinsic or extrinsic airway obstruction by tumor	Chemotherapy-induced pulmonary disease
Pleural tumor	Chemotherapy-induced cardiomyopathy
Pleural effusion	Radiation-induced pericardial disease
Pericardial effusion	
Ascites	**Dyspnea Unrelated to Cancer**
Hepatomegaly	Chronic obstructive pulmonary disease
Phrenic nerve paralysis	Asthma
Multiple tumor microemboli	Congestive heart failure
Pulmonary leukostasis	Interstitial lung disease
Superior vena cava syndrome	Pneumothorax
	Anxiety
Dyspnea Due Indirectly to Cancer	Chest wall deformity
Cachexia	Obesity
Electrolyte abnormalities	Neuromuscular disorders
Anemia	Pulmonary vascular disease
Pneumonia	
Pulmonary aspiration	
Pulmonary emboli	
Neurological paraneoplastic syndromes	

Source: Dudgeon D, Rosenthal S. Management of dyspnea and cough in patients with cancer. In: Cherny NI, Foley KM, eds. *Hematology/Oncology Clinics of North America: Pain and Palliative Care,* Vol. 10. Philadelphia: W.B. Saunders Co., 1996; 1:151–171.

dyspnea, cough, or, less often, chest pain that is often pleuritic. Physical examination reveals the classic findings of dullness to percussion, decreased breath sounds, decreased tactile fremitus, and egophony. A chest radiograph confirms the diagnosis.

About one-half of all pleural effusions are due to cancer.[36] Virtually any type of cancer can cause pleural effusion, but nearly two-thirds of all malignant pleural effusions are due to only three tumor types: lung cancer, breast cancer, and lymphoma. Although a pleural effusion in an individual with a known malignancy is probably caused by the cancer, other possibilities, including congestive heart failure, pneumonia, pulmonary embolus with infarction, postradiation changes, tuberculosis, and vasculitis, should be considered.

Diagnostic thoracentesis is the first step in the evaluation of patients with effusions. Although most malignant effusions are exudates (pleural fluid to serum lactate dehydrogenase [LDH] ratio of >.6, a fluid to serum protein ratio of >.5, or a pleural LDH value of >200 U),[36] 5–15% are transudates.[37] Therefore, the definitive diagnosis of malignant pleural effusion requires the demonstration of malignant cells in a fluid specimen. Pleural fluid cytology is positive after a single thoracentesis in about 60–90% of cases; additional samples often lead to conclusive diagnoses in the remainder.[38] Closed pleural biopsy is less valuable in the evaluation of suspected malignant pleural effusion but should be performed if repeated tests of cytology specimens are negative.[39,40] Thoracoscopy has become the procedure of choice when the diagnosis remains elusive.[41] Thoracoscopy with pleural biopsy yields a diagnosis in essentially 100% of patients with malignant pleural effusions. The use of panels of monoclonal antibodies against a variety of tumor antigens has shown promise in small series, but flow cytometry and oncogene analysis have yet to prove their worth in this setting.

Pericardial effusion
Metastatic disease involving the heart is discovered in up to 20% of autopsied cancer patients, but clinically significant cardiac involvement is much less common. Pericardial involvement is most frequently encountered in patients with cancers of the lung, breast, gastrointestinal tract, melanoma, lymphoma, and leukemia. Malignancy is the most common cause of pericardial tamponade (16–41%),[42] but radiation, drugs, infection, hypothyroidism, autoimmune disorders, and other nonmalignant etiologies underlie 50% of symptomatic pericardial disease in patients with cancer.[43] Benign etiologies are most likely, in patients free of known metastatic disease at the time the pericardial effusion is detected.[44] The clinical significance of a pericardial effusion is determined by the rate of fluid accumulation, the compliance of the pericardium, the mass of the myocardium, and the total blood volume.[41] Malignant effusions tend to accumulate rapidly, causing orthopnea, chest pain, and exertional dyspnea. Physical findings may include edema, hypotension, soft heart sounds, significant pulsus paradoxus, elevated jugular venous pressure, and pericardial friction rub.

Characteristics electrocardiographic findings (low QRS voltage, T-wave changes, and electrical alternans) and an enlarged cardiac silhouette on a chest radiograph should raise the suspicion of pericardial effusion. Echocardiography is the most useful diagnostic test to detect the presence of pericardial fluid and the degree of myocardial dysfunction. Computed tomography (CT) provides further information if echocardiographic results are inconclusive. Cytological tests of pericardial fluid are positive in 65–85% of malignant effusions,[45] and pericardial biopsy is positive in 55%.[42] often, the histological diagnosis is made at the time of emergency surgery (pericardial window formation) performed to relieve pericardial tamponade.

Superior vena cava syndrome
Malignancies cause 85–90% of cases of superior vena cava syndrome (SVCS) in adults.[46] The obstruction may result from invasion of the venous wall by tumor or

from occlusion due to extrinsic compression or intraluminal thrombosis.[47] The tumors most frequently associated with the SVCS are lung cancers, lymphomas, and other tumors metastatic to the mediastinum.[48] The diagnosis of SVCS is essentially clinical, based on characteristic physical signs and symptoms. Patients may note dyspnea worsened by recumbency, a sensation of fullness in the head, and cough. The neck and thoracic veins are distended, and the face and neck are edematous and cyanotic. The voice is often hoarse. An infused CT scan of the chest is the diagnostic imaging technique of choice; it helps confirm the diagnosis, determine the extent of the tumor, and visualize the actual occlusion.

Dyspnea due indirectly to cancer

Cancer causes dyspnea indirectly as a consequence of malnutrition or cachexia, mineral and electrolyte deficiencies, infections due to obstruction or immuno-compromise; anemia due to bone marrow replacement, gastrointestinal blood loss, or chronic disease; pulmonary embolism, neurological paraneoplastic syndromes, and pulmonary aspiration.

Cachexia and electrolyte deficiencies
Respiratory muscle weakness can result from impaired nutritional status. Diaphragmatic mass is reduced in undernourished individuals, and contractile force per unit of muscle cross-sectional area is diminished as well.[22] Hypocalcemia, hypokalemia, hypomagnesemia, and severe hypophosphatemia can impair the function of the respiratory muscles.[21] Phrenic nerve paralysis and muscle atrophy due to disuse may also contribute to respiratory muscle weakness.[32,49]

Immunocompromise
Patients with cancer are at increased risk of pneumonia due to immunosuppression caused by the disease or its treatment, and also as a consequence of local phenomena such as mucosal erosion and mass effect producing abscess, fistula, or obstruction. Granulocytopenia due to bone marrow involvement with malignancy or due to cytotoxic treatment, and impaired granulocyte function as a consequence of an underlying myeloproliferative disorder or treatment with cytotoxic agents, radiation, or steroids increase the risk of bacterial and fungal infections. Impaired cell-mediated immunity as a consequence of malignancy and its treatment predisposes to infections with intracellular pathogens and viruses. Defective humoral immunity due to multiple myeloma, acute and chronic leukemias, asplenia, and cytotoxic treatments results in a predisposition to infections with encapsulated organisms.

Pulmonary emboli
The association of cancer with venous thrombosis and pulmonary embolism (Trousseau's syndrome) has been recognized for well over a century.[50,51] Numerous studies document this relationship, especially in patients with mucinous

adenocarcinomas of the upper gastrointestinal tract, pancreas, and lung.[52] The mechanisms by which cancers predispose to thromboembolism include stasis and immobility, venous compression or direct invasion by tumor, and a variety of interactions between tumor cells and the coagulation system, the fibrinolytic system, platelets, and the endothelium.[51] Cancer chemotherapy in some settings also appears to increase the risk of thromboembolic phenomena.[53] In one study, patients over the age of 50 receiving adjuvant chemotherapy for Stage II breast cancer had a 10% incidence of venous thrombosis during treatment.[54]

Patients with acute pulmonary embolic disease due to large blood clots arising in the legs or the heart typically describe a single episode or multiple episodes of acute shortness of breath. Less commonly, multiple small emboli produce pulmonary hypertension with no history of acute episodes.[55] Rarely, sudden severe dyspnea results from multiple tumor embolization. Autopsy studies of patients with solid tumors reveal massive pulmonary embolic carcinomatosis in 2.4% of cases.[56] Cancers of the breast, stomach, prostate, and liver, as well as germ cell tumors, most often produce this syndrome, which is usually rapidly fatal. Treatment other than supportive measures is rarely of any value.

Neurological paraneoplastic syndromes

Neurological paraneoplastic syndromes can contribute to the development of dyspnea in cancer patients. Thirty percent of patients with malignant thymoma have myasthenia gravis, which can weaken respiratory muscles and cause respiratory failure.[57,58] The diagnosis is confirmed by the edrophonium test; by electromyography, which reveals a decreasing motor response with repetitive nerve stimulation; or by radioimmunoassay for antibody to the acetylcholine receptor.[58] A few patients with polymyositis develop cardiac conduction abnormalities and interstitial lung disease.[58] Eaton-Lambert syndrome associated with lung, rectal, kidney, breast, stomach, skin, and thymic cancers can also produce respiratory muscle weakness, resulting in dyspnea.[59,60] Neurophysiological studies demonstrating that the amplitude of the action potential of muscle evoked by nerve stimulation increases by more than 200% after the muscle has exercised for 10 to 15 sec help to confirm the latter diagnosis.[58] Dyspnea in patients with neuromuscular disease probably results from a perception of increased respiratory muscle effort because of the increased neural drive required to activate weakened respiratory muscles.[9]

Dyspnea due to cancer treatment

Treatment-related causes of dyspnea include surgery, radiation pneumonitis or fibrosis, chemotherapy-induced pulmonary and cardiac damage, and infection.

Surgery

Pneumonectomy or even lobectomy can result in shortness of breath in patients with pre-existing impairment of pulmonary function.

Table 13.3. Chemotherapeutic agents that produce dyspnea

Hypersensitivity Lung Disease

Bleomycin

Methotrexate

Procarbazine

Mitomycin

Noncardiogenic Pulmonary Edema

Cytosine arabinoside

Methotrexate

Teniposide

Ifosfamide

Cyclophosphamide

Chronic Pneumonitis/Pulmonary Fibrosis

Bleomycin

Methotrexate

Busulfan

Cyclophosphamide

Carmustine (BCNU)

Mitomycin

Ifosfamide

Fludarabine

Congestive Heart Failure

Doxorubicin

Daunorubicin

Mitoxantrone

Amsacrine

Estrogens

Progestins

Androgens

Corticosteroids

Source: Dudgeon D, Rosenthal S. Management of dyspnea and cough in patients with cancer. In: Cherny, NI, Foley KM. *Hematology/Oncology Clinics of North America: Pain and Palliative Care,* vol. 100 Philadelphia: W.B. Saunders Co., 1996; 1:157–171.

Radiation therapy

Thoracic irradiation can induce two clinical syndromes: radiation pneumonitis occurring 6–12 weeks following treatment and radiation fibrosis 6–12 months later.[61] Clinically significant radiation effects on the lung occur in up to 10% of treated patients. The degree of lung damage is determined by the radiation dose and the volume of lung irradiated. Concomitant chemotherapy with certain agents and steroid withdrawal may exacerbate the process.[61,62]

Symptomatic radiation pneumonitis ranges in severity from a mild cough with fever and dyspnea to severe respiratory distress and death.[63] Chest radiography usually reveals an infiltrate with well-defined borders that correspond to the radiation field. Radiation fibrosis develops in areas of previous pneumonitis but is usually asymptomatic except in patients with underlying pulmonary functional impairment or severe radiation pneumonitis.[61] Thoracic irradiation is also associated with pleural effusions, spontaneous pneumothoraces, pericardial effusions, and acute airway obstruction.[61]

Systemic therapy

Numerous pharmacological agents used to treat cancer can cause pulmonary damage (Table 13.3). Three patterns of pulmonary injury can be recognized: chronic pneumonitis/fibrosis, acute hypersensitivity lung disease, and noncardiogenic pulmonary edema. Chronic pneumonitis/fibrosis is the most frequent pattern and is associated with most cytotoxic agents that cause pulmonary damage. Bleomycin, methotrexate, and procarbazine can each cause hypersensitivity lung disease. Cytosine arabinoside, VM-26 (teniposide), methotrexate, and cyclophosphamide have each been associated with noncardiogenic pulmonary edema. Risk factors for development of pulmonary toxicity include cumulative dose (bleomycin, busulfan, carmustine), age (bleomycin), previous or subsequent thoracic radiotherapy (bleomycin, busulfan, mitomycin), high concentrations of inspired oxygen (bleomycin, cyclophosphamide, mitomycin), concomitant or subsequent use of other chemotherapeutic agents (carmustine, mitomycin, cyclophosphamide, bleomycin, methotrexate), steroid withdrawal,[62] and pre-existing pulmonary disease (carmustine).[64]

Dyspnea unrelated to the cancer

Risk factors for dyspnea unrelated to cancer include pre-existing chronic obstructive pulmonary disease, cardiovascular insufficiency, asthma, interstitial lung disease, pneumothorax, anxiety, chest wall deformity, obesity, neuromuscular disorders, and pulmonary vascular disease (Table 13.2).

Evaluation of Cancer Patients with Dyspnea

Dyspnea, like pain, is a subjective experience that may not be evident to an observer. Tachypnea, a rapid respiratory rate, is not dyspnea. Just as pain is not necessarily apparent to the examiner or reflected in laboratory values or on imaging studies, dyspnea is a perception that often occurs without measurable physical correlates. Medical personnel must learn to accept patients' assessments when they say they are short of breath, in the same way that they have learned to believe patients when they say they are in pain.

Dyspnea is also not a single sensation. Recent work suggests that the sensation of breathlessness encompasses several qualities.[10,14] Just as the description of "burning" or "numb" features points to neuropathic pain, phrases such as "chest tightness," "exhalation," and "deep" were among clusters of terms associated with asthma in a study conducted by Simon et al.[10] It is possible that dyspnea mediated by similar receptors evokes common word descriptors. Simon et al. found that patients with dyspnea caused by pulmonary vascular disease and congestive heart failure—which are postulated to cause dyspnea through stimulation of J receptors—used the word *rapid* to describe their breathlessness.[10] Different disease states seem to produce different sensations of the quality of breathlessness, and these descriptions may help identify the underlying pathophysiological processes and thus point to the appropriate remedies.[65]

Clinical assessment of dyspnea should include a complete history of the symptom, including its temporal onset (acute or chronic), qualities, associated symptoms, precipitating and relieving events or activities, and response to medications. A past history of smoking, underlying lung or cardiac disease, concurrent medical conditions, and details of previous cancer therapies should be elicited as well. A careful physical examination focused on possible underlying causes of dyspnea should be performed. Particular attention should be directed at signs associated with certain clinical syndromes, such as chronic obstructive pulmonary disease (COPD), congestive heart failure, pleural and pericardial effusions, or SVCS, that are more common causes of dyspnea in cancer patients.

To evaluate the role of various interventions in relieving dyspnea, assessment tools are required. McCord and Cronin-Stubbs have critically appraised the reliability and validity of the tools currently used to evaluate dyspnea.[17] Dyspnea correlates moderately (at best) with functional (6- or 12-minute walk) and physiological (pulmonary function tests) parameters.[66] Most studies have been conducted in patients with COPD, but two studies describe the reliability and validity of a measure of breathlessness in patients with cancer.[25,67]

The visual analogue scale (VAS) is one of the most popular techniques for assessing breathlessness. This scale is usually a 100-mm vertical or horizontal line, anchored at either end by phrases such as "not at all breathless" and "very breathless," although there are no standards for anchoring the ends of the scale.[66] Brown et al. established the test-retest reliability of the VAS as a measure of dyspnea in 30 adults with lung cancer.[67] Their study demonstrated concurrent validity of the VAS and the American Thoracic Society Respiratory Disease Questionnaire at time 1 (worst dyspnea: $r = .72, p = .001$; usual dyspnea, $r = .70, p = .001$) and at time 2 (worst dyspnea, $r = .56, p = .002$; usual dyspnea, $r = .57, p = .002$). Concurrent validity was also shown by VAS and the Karnofsky Performance Scale correlations at time 1 ($r = .59, p = .001$) and time 2 ($r = .56, p = .002$). Dudgeon et al. established concurrent validity of the VAS with a verbal rating scale ("none", "mild", "moderate", "severe", "horrible") in 923 patients with cancer. The correlation between the VAS and verbal rating scale (VRS) was $r = .82$ ($p = .0001$).[25] Construct validity was also supported by this study; shortness of breath as measured by the VAS was significantly related to smoking history, thoracic surgery, history of lung disease, and other appropriate variables.

The VAS measures the perception of the intensity of dyspnea; it does not address the multidimensional nature of the symptom, and, therefore, its usefulness is limited. The reliability and validity of other established dyspnea assessment tools have not been evaluated in patients with cancer. Clearly, further research in this area will require the development and psychometric testing of multidimensional tools for the assessment of dyspnea in cancer patients.

Diagnostic tests helpful in determining the etiology of dyspnea include chest radiography; pulmonary function tests; arterial blood gases; complete blood count; serum potassium, magnesium, and phosphate levels; oxygen saturation with exercise; and tests specific for suspected underlying pathologies (e.g., echocardiogram for suspected pericardial effusion). The choice of appropriate diagnostic tests and therapies should be guided by the stage of the cancer, its prognosis, the goals of therapy (palliative or curative), and the risk–benefit ratios of any proposed interventions.

Summary

The understanding of dyspnea in patients with cancer in the 1990s is at the same level as the knowledge of cancer pain 15 or 20 years ago. Studies have shown that dyspnea is very common in patients with cancer, but little research has been done to determine the underlying pathophysiological mechanisms of this symptom.

Relief of breathlessness should be the goal of treatment in all stages of cancer. Accurate assessment and a better understanding of the mechanisms leading to dyspnea will ensure better control of this symptom and improve the function and quality of life of many patients.

Acknowledgments

We wish to thank Aleta Foreman, Joan Honer, Dr. Michael Harlos, and Dr. Morley Lertzman for their help in the preparation of this manuscript.

References

1. Rice KL. Treatment of dyspnea with psychotropic agents. *Chest* 1986; 90 (6):789–790.
2. Cherniack NS, Altose MD. Mechanisms of dyspnea. *Clin Chest Med* 1987; 8 (2):207–214.

3. Tobin MJ. Dyspnea: pathophysiologic basis, clinical presentation, and management. *Arch Intern Med* 1990; 150:1604–1613.

4. Mahler DA, Rosiello RA, Harver A, et al. Comparison of clinical dyspnea ratings and psychophysical measurements of respiratory sensation in obstructive airway disease. *Am Rev Respir Dis* 1987; 135:1229–1233.

5. Carrieri VK, Janson-Bjerklie S. The sensation of dyspnea: a review. *Clin Rev Crit Care* 1984; 13 (4):436–447.

6. Altose MD. Psychophysics—an approach to the study of respiratory sensation and the assessment of dyspnea. *Am Rev Respir Dis* 1987; 135:1227–1228.

7. Altose MD. Assessment and management of breathlessness. *Chest* 1985; 88(2 Suppl): 77S–83S.

8. Cotes JE. Lung function in disease. In: Leathart GL, ed. *Lung Function Assessment and Application in Medicine*, 5th ed. Oxford: Blackwell Scientific, 1993: 518–519.

9. Manning HL, Schwartzstein RM. Pathophysiology of dyspnea. *N Engl J Med* 1995; 333(23):1547–1553.

10. Simon PM, Schwartzstein RM, Weiss JW, et al. Distinguishable types of dyspnea in patients with shortness of breath. *Am Rev Respir Dis* 1990; 142:1009–1014.

11. Wasserman K, Casaburi R. Dyspnea: physiological and pathophysiological mechanisms. *Annu Rev Med* 1988; 39:503–515.

12. Burgess KR, Whitelaw WA. Effects of nasal cold receptors on pattern of breathing. *J Appl Physiol* 1988; 64 (1):371–376.

13. Schwartzstein RM, Lahive K, Pope A, et al. Cold facial stimulation reduces breathlessness induced in normal subjects. *Am Rev Respir Dis* 1987; 136:58–61.

14. Schwartzstein RM, Manning HL, Weiss JW, et al. Dyspnea: a sensory experience. *Lung* 1990; 168:185–199.

15. Freedman S. Chemoreflexes and breathlessness. In: McMaster University, ed. *"Breathlessness." Proceedings of the Campbell Symposium, May 16–19, 1991*. Hamilton, Canada: Boehringer Ingelheim, 1992:117–123.

16. Steele B, Shaver J. The dyspnea experience: nociceptive properties and a model for research and practice. *Adv Nurs Sci* 1992; 15 (1):64–76.

17. McCord M, Cronin-Stubbs D. Operationalizing dyspnea: focus on measurement. *Heart Lung* 1992; 21:167–179.

18. Burns BH, Howell JBL. Disproportionately severe breathlessness in chronic bronchitis. *Q J Med* 1969; 38 (151):277–294.

19. Terry PB, Ball WCJ, Peters SP. An introduction to respiratory diseases. In: Harvey AM, Johns RJ, McKusick VA, et al, eds. *The Principles and Practice of Medicine*, 22nd ed. East Norwalk, Conn.: Appleton & Lange, 1988:161.

20. Goldberg HS. Pulmonary vascular disease. In: Kryger MH, ed. *Pathophysiology of Respiration*. Toronto: Wiley, 1981:79–80.

21. Lewis MI, Belman MJ. Nutrition and the respiratory muscles. *Clin Chest Med* 1988; 9 (2):337–347.

22. Rochester DF, Arora NS. Respiratory muscle failure. *Med Clin North Am* 1983; 67 (3):573–597.

23. Mancini DM. LaManca J, Henson D. The relation of respiratory muscle function to dyspnea in patients with heart failure. *Heart Fail* 1992; 8:183–189.

24. Howell J. Behavioral breathlessness. In: McMaster University, ed. *"Breathlessness."*

Proceedings of the Campbell Symposium, May 16–19, 1991. Hamilton, Canada: Boehringer Ingelheim, 1992:149–155.

25. Dudgeon D, Kristjanson L, Sloan JA, et al. Dyspnea in cancer patients: prevalence and associated factors. Submitted to *J Pain Symptom Manage.*

26. Muers MF, Round CE. Palliation of symptoms in non-small cell lung cancer: a study by the Yorkshire Regional Cancer Organisation Thoracic Group. *Thorax* 1993; 48:339–343.

27. Reuben DB, Mor V. Dyspnea in terminally ill cancer patients. *Chest* 1986; 89:234–236.

28. Fainsinger R, MacEachern T, Hanson J, et al. Symptom control during the last week of life on a palliative care unit. *J Palliat Care* 1991; 7 (1):5–11.

29. Twycross RG, Lack SA. Respiratory symptoms. In: Twycross RG, Lack SA, eds. *Therapeutics in Terminal Cancer,* 2nd ed. London: Churchill Livinstone, 1990:123–136.

30. Higginson I, McCarthy M. Measuring symptoms in terminal cancer: are pain and dyspnoea controlled? *J R Soc Med* 1989; 82:264–267.

31. Dudgeon D, Lertzman M. Dyspnea in the advanced cancer patient. *J Pain Symptom Manage* 1998; 16:212–219.

32. Fishbein D, Kearon C, Killian KJ. An approach to dyspnea in cancer patients. *J Pain Symptom Manage* 1989; 4 (2):76–81.

33. Enck RE. The management of dyspnea. *Am J Hosp Care* 1989; 6:11–12.

34. Ajemian I. Palliative management of dyspnea. *J Palliat Care* 1991; 7:3:44–45.

35. Cowcher K, Hanks GW. Long-term management of respiratory symptoms in advanced cancer. *J Pain Symptom Manage* 1990; 5 (5):320–330.

36. Hausheer FH, Yarbro JW. Diagnosis and treatment of malignant pleural effusion. *Semin Oncol* 1985; 12 (1):54–75.

37. Sahn SA. Pleural effusion in lung cancer. *Clin Chest Med* 1993; 14 (1):189–200.

38. Johnston WW. The malignant pleural effusion: a review of cytopathologic diagnoses of 584 specimens from 472 consecutive patients. *Cancer* 1985; 56:905–909.

39. Prakash UBS, Reiman HM. Comparison of needle biopsy with cytologic analysis for the evaluation of pleural effusion: analysis of 414 cases. *Mayo Clin Proc* 1985; 60:158–164.

40. Fentiman IS. Diagnosis and treatment of malignant pleural effusions. *Cancer Treat Rev* 1987; 14:107–118.

41. Miles DW, Knight RK. Diagnosis and management of malignant pleural effusion. *Cancer Treat Rev* 1993; 19:151–168.

42. Press OW, Livingston R. Management of malignant pericardial effusion and tamponade. *JAMA* 1987; 257 (8):1088–1092.

43. Missri J, Schechter D. When pericardial effusion complicates cancer. *Hosp Pract* 1988; 23 (4):277–286.

44. Buck M, Ingle JN, Giuliani ER, et al. Pericardial effusion in women with breast cancer. *Cancer* 1987; 60:263–269.

45. Vaitkus PT, Hermann HC, LeWinter MM. Treatment of malignant pericardial effusion. *JAMA* 1994; 272 (1):59–64.

46. Yellin A, Rosen A, Reichert N, et al. Superior vena cava syndrome: the myth—the facts. *Am Rev Respir Dis* 1990; 141:1114–1118.

47. Jones LA. Superior vena cava syndrome: an oncologic complication. *Semin Oncol Nurs* 1987; 3 (3):211–215.

48. Sculier JP, Feld R. Superior vena cava obstruction syndrome: recommendations for management. *Cancer Treat Rev* 1985; 12:209–218.
49. Mier A. Respiratory muscle weakness. *Respir Med* 1990; 84:351–359.
50. Prandoni P, Lensing AWA, Buller HR, et al. Deep-vein thrombosis and the incidence of subsequent symptomatic cancer. *N Engl J Med* 1992; 327 (16):1128–1133.
51. Silverstein RL, Nachman RL. Cancer and clotting—Trousseau's warning. *N Engl J Med* 1992; 327 (16):1163–1164.
52. Rickles FR, Edwards RL. Activation of blood coagulation in cancer: Trousseau's syndrome revisited. *Blood* 1983; 62 (1):14–31.
53. Doll DC, Ringenberg QS, Yarboro JW. Vascular toxicity associated with antineoplastic agents. *J Clin Oncol* 1986; 4 (9):1405–1417.
54. Levine MN, Gent M, Hirsch J, et al. The thrombogenic effect of anticancer drug therapy in women with stage II breast cancer. *N Engl J Med* 1988; 318 (7):404–407.
55. Scully RE, Mark EJ, McNeely WF, et al. Case record of the Massachusetts General Hospital (Case 30-1987). *N Engl J Med* 1987; 317 (4):225–235.
56. Kane RD, Hawkins HK, Miller JA, et al. Microscopic pulmonary tumor emboli associated with dyspnea. *Cancer* 1975; 36:1473–1482.
57. Chad DA, Recht LD. Neurological paraneoplastic syndromes. *Cancer Invest* 1988; 6 (1):67–82.
58. Palma G. Paraneoplastic syndromes of the nervous system. *West J Med* 1985; 142: 787–796.
59. Laroche CM, Mier AK, Spiro SG, et al. Respiratory muscle weakness in the Lambert-Eaton myasthenic syndrome. *Thorax* 1989; 44:913–918.
60. Wilcox PG, Morrison NJ, Anzarut ARA, et al. Lambert-Eaton myasthenic syndrome involving the diaphragm. *Chest* 1988; 93:604–605.
61. Gross NJ. Pulmonary effects of radiation therapy. *Ann Intern Med* 1977; 86 (1):81–92.
62. Castellino RA, Glatstein E, Turbow MM, et al. Latent radiation injury of lungs or heart activated by steroid withdrawal. *Ann Intern Med* 1974; 80 (5):593–599.
63. Gibson PG, Bryant DH, Morgan GW, et al. Radiation-induced lung injury: a hypersensitivity pneumonitis? *Ann Intern Med* 1988; 109:288–291.
64. Cooper JAD, Jr, White DA, Matthay RA. Drug-induced pulmonary disease. *Am Rev Respir Dis* 1986; 133:321–340.
65. Elliott MW, Adams L, Cockcroft A, et al. The language of breathlessness: Use of verbal descriptions by patients with cardiopulmonary disease. *Am Rev Respir Dis* 1991; 144:826–832.
66. Eakin EG, Kaplan RM, Ries AL. Measurement of dypsnoea in chronic obstructive pulmonary disease. *Qual Life Res* 1993; 2:181–191.
67. Brown ML, Carrieri V, Janson-Bjerklie S, et al. Lung cancer and dyspnea: the patient's perception. *Oncol Nurs Forum* 1986; 13 (5):19–24.

14

The Role of Oxygen in Cancer-Related Dyspnea

SHARON WATANABE

Dyspnea is a prevalent and often distressing symptom in cancer patients. The role of oxygen in alleviating this symptom is controversial. Most studies examining the symptomatic benefit of oxygen have been conducted in the context of nonmalignant disease, with conflicting results. The mechanisms by which oxygen may improve dyspnea are also uncertain. This chapter will review the evidence in favor of a therapeutic effect from oxygen, explore possible mechanisms, and suggest clinical guideliness for use.

Chronic Lung Disease

Supplemental oxygen has been shown to improve exercise capacity and reduce subjective dyspnea in patients with chronic obstructive lung disease. Woodcock et al.[1] compared oxygen and room air administered at a rate of 4 l/min in a randomized, double-blind, crossover study involving 10 patients. Oxygen use resulted in increased 6-min walking distance, increased endurance walking distance, and decreased visual analogue scores for dyspnea. Outcomes were not significantly different if the oxygen cylinder was carried by the patient or an assistant. The effect of pre-dosing with oxygen for 5 min was found to be comparable to that achieved by wearing oxygen continuously.

In a study by Davidson et al.,[2] 17 patients were administered oxygen at a rate of 0, 2, 4 and 6 l/min in random sequence during bicycle exercise. Blinding was achieved by adding air to maintain the total flow rate at 6 l/min. Oxygen use increased endurance and reduced visual analogue scores for dyspnea in a dose-dependent fashion. A randomized, double-blind, crossover comparison of oxygen versus air administered at a rate of 4 l/min showed that oxygen improved endurance distance by 59% and 6-min distance by 17%.[2] The latter finding suggests that oxygen enables patients to walk longer rather than faster.

Dean et al.[3] conducted a randomized, double-blind, crossover trial comparing 40% oxygen with air in 12 patients during bicycle exercise. Again, endurance increased and visual analogue scores for dyspnea decreased with oxygen. Notably, improvement was seen even in the absence of significant desaturation during exercise with air.

The effect of oxygen on resting dyspnea in chronic obstructive lung disease is more controversial. Using a nasal cannula, Liss and Grant[4] subjected eight patients to no flow, air at 2 and 4 l/min, and oxygen at 2 and 4 l/min. Flows were administered in random order in a single-blind manner. Oxygen use did not reduce visual analogue scores for dyspnea. When the procedure was repeated after anesthetizing the nasal mucosa, dyspnea increased with each flow. The authors concluded that perceived reduction in breathlessness with the use of nasal oxygen is attributable to stimulation of nasal receptors by the cannula rather than to any effect of the gas itself.

Swinburn et al.[5] reached a different conclusion in a study involving 12 patients with obstructive lung disease and 10 patients with interstitial lung disease. Twenty-eight percent oxygen and air were administered twice each in randomized, double-blind, crossover fashion. In both groups, oxygen use reduced visual analogue scores for dyspnea, and patients blindly chose oxygen as being more helpful with greater frequency and consistency. Patients in this study were more hypoxemic than those in the study of Liss and Grant[4] (mean arterial PO_2 48 mm Hg and 50.3 mm Hg for obstructive and interstitial lung disease, respectively, versus 67 mm Hg), which may explain the discrepancy in results.

Congestive Heart Failure

Two controlled studies of the effects of supplemental oxygen on exercise capacity and dyspnea in congestive heart failure have yielded conflicting results. In a randomized, double-blind, crossover trial, Moore et al.[6] administered air, 30% oxygen, and 50% oxygen to 12 patients during bicycle exercise. Oxygen use led to a dose-dependent increase in endurance and a decrease in visual analogue scores for dyspnea and Borg scores for perceived exertion.

In a trial by Restrick et al.,[7] 12 patients received air and oxygen at a rate of 2 l/min in randomized, double-blind fashion while performing 6-min walks. They also undertook endurance walks on air administered at a rate of 2 l/min and oxygen administered at rates of 2 and 4 l/min. In neither test did oxygen use result in improved walking distances, visual analogue scores for dyspnea, or Borg scores. The discordant findings may be attributable to differences in the severity of heart failure, degree of oxygen desaturation with exercise, amount of oxygen administered, and type of exercise.

Cancer

The extent to which the aforementioned findings may be extrapolated to cancer patients may be limited, since dyspnea in this setting is often due to restrictive lung dysfunction.[8] Currently there are only two published trials addressing the role of oxygen in cancer-related dyspnea. Bruera et al.[9] studied 14 cancer patients with resting dyspnea and hypoxemia due to lung or pleural involvement. Air and oxygen at 5 l/min were administered twice each in a randomized, double-blind, crossover design. Visual analogue scores for dyspnea improved with oxygen but not with air. Patients and investigator also consistently expressed a preference for oxygen over air.

Booth et al.[10] conducted a randomized, single-blind, crossover trial in 38 cancer patients comparing air and oxygen administered at a rate of 4 l/min. Visual analogue and Borg scores for dyspnea improved with both treatments. No significant difference between treatments was observed, although the improvement with oxygen was quantitatively greater and its effect appeared to carry over into the air phase. Unlike the Bruera et al. study, in which all patients had an oxygen saturation below 90%, only six patients were similarly hypoxemic.

Possible Mechanisms of Oxygen Benefit

The mechanisms by which oxygen relieves dyspnea are incompletely understood, in part because the pathophysiology of dyspnea is itself complex. Arterial hypoxemia results in an increased rate of firing of chemoreceptors located in the carotid and aortic bodies. The impulses are transmitted via the glossopharyngeal and vagus nerves to the respiratory center in the medulla, leading to reflex activation of respiratory neurons, which in turn stimulate the anterior horn cells innervating respiratory muscles.

The sensation of dyspnea depends on cortical perception of the above process, which could occur at the level of chemoreceptor firing, activation of respiratory neurons in the medulla, excitation of anterior horn cells, or stimulation of mechanoreceptors in the lungs or chest wall. Hypoxemia does not appear to be directly perceived by the sensory cortex. This conclusion is based on the anecdotal observation that removal of the carotid bodies in chronic obstructive lung disease patients results in relief of dyspnea despite worsening hypoxemia.[11]

Adams et al.[12] further examined this issue in a study involving eight normal volunteers and six respiratory patients. Subjects were blindly exposed to an intermittent hypoxic stimulus that oscillated at either a slow or a rapid rate. Ventilatory rate and dyspnea were significantly lower during the rapid cycle. As the degree of hypoxemia was identical during both cycles, the results suggest that dyspnea does not reflect direct cortical perception of chemoreceptor firing.

Rather, dyspnea appears to be linked to the reflex ventilatory response, which is damped during rapid stimulation because less time is available to activate respiratory center neurons. In the second part of this study, hyperventilation was reflexively induced by a hypercapnic stimulus. Subjects were then asked to copy the hyperventilation pattern voluntarily. Dyspnea was significantly lower during the voluntary maneuver despite a similar pattern of muscle use, suggesting that the sensation does not arise from activation of anterior horn cells or lung and chest wall mechanoreceptors. The authors concluded that hypoxemia causes dyspnea via cortical perception of reflex activation of respiratory neurons in the medulla.

The work of other investigators has also supported the hypothesis that hypoxic dyspnea is not a sensation of mechanical ventilatory activity. In a single-blind blind trial involving nine chronic obstructive lung disease patients, Lane et al.[13] demonstrated that supplemental oxygen reduced dyspnea to a proportionately greater degree than ventilation. A randomized, single-blind study by Chronos et al.[14] involving 11 normal volunteers showed that changes in dyspnea induced by hypoxia precede changes in ventilation.

Supplemental oxygen may also alleviate dyspnea through its effects on airway resistance. In an open study involving 12 patients with chronic airflow obstruction, Libby et al.[15] demonstrated that administration of 30% oxygen resulted in increased maximal expiratory flow rates. Comparison of flow rates with and without helium suggested that bronchodilation was occurring at the level of the large airways. Relief of dyspnea may, therefore, reflect reduced work of breathing as well as decreased stimulation of airway mechanoreceptors.

Effects of oxygen on muscle function may also influence dyspnea. In a randomized, single-blind, crossover study, Bye et al.[16] subjected eight patients with chronic obstructive lung disease to air versus 40% oxygen during bicycle exercise. Oxygen use resulted in delayed diaphragmatic fatigue, as measured by abdominal paradox testing and electromyography. This result reflected improved muscle performance rather than decreased ventilation, as demonstrated in a study by Pardy and Bye.[17] Six normal volunteers inspired against a resistance at a fixed ventilatory rate while breathing either air or 100% oxygen in a randomized, single-blind, crossover design. Use of oxygen was associated with a delay in onset of electromyographic evidence of diaphragmatic fatigue, as well as a reduced sensation of respiratory effort.

The significance of the effects of oxygen on muscle metabolism is unclear. Stein et al.[18] randomized nine patients with chronic obstructive lung disease to air versus 30% oxygen during treadmill exercise in a single-blind crossover fashion. While serum lactate levels were lower on oxygen, pH was unchanged due to concomitant carbon dioxide retention so that respiratory drive would not be affected. Also, only two patients were able to exercise to the anaerobic threshold, the remainder being limited in their exercise capacity for reasons unrelated to lactic acidemia.

Theoretically, oxygen may also influence dyspnea via its cardiovascular effects. In an open study of air versus 30% oxygen in 18 patients with chronic obstructive and interstitial lung disease, Olvey et al.[19] demonstrated that oxygen improves the right ventricular exercise ejection fraction. This finding could be explained either by improved myocardial function or reduced pulmonary vascular resistance, the latter having been also demonstrated in other studies.[20] Pressure receptors in the pulmonary vasculature or right atrium, or C fibers in the pulmonary vessels, could potentially mediate dyspnea in this situation.

Clinical Guidelines and Future Research

At present, the only established indication for supplemental oxygen in dyspneic cancer patients is when saturation is less than 90%. However, studies in noncancer populations suggest that nonhypoxemic patients may also benefit from oxygen. Further work in this area is needed. For individual cases, an N of 1 trial may help to determine the usefulness of supplemental oxygen.[21]

The pathophysiology of dyspnea in cancer patients also needs to be better delineated. As airways obstruction and impaired respiratory muscle function are prevalent in this population,[22] the effect of oxygen on these parameters and their relationship to dyspnea merit investigation.

Finally, techniques to induce this often fluctuating symptom reliably in this debilitated population should be developed, as traditional exercise maneuvers are not feasible. Such techniques would enhance the ability to observe treatment effects and help to increase the number of patients eligible for intervention trials.

References

1. Woodcock AA, Gross ER, Geddes DM. Oxygen relieves breathlessness in "pink puffers." *Lancet* 1981;1:907–909.
2. Davidson AC, Leach R, George RJD, et al. Supplemental oxygen and exercise ability in chronic obstructive airways disease. *Thorax* 1988; 43:965–971.
3. Dean NC, Brown JK, Himelman RB, et al. Oxygen may improve dyspnea and endurance in patients with chronic obstructive pulmonary disease and only mild hypoxemia. *Am Rev Respir Dis* 1992; 146:941–945.
4. Liss HP, Grant BJB. The effect of nasal flow on breathlessness in patients with chronic obstructive pulmonary disease. *Am Rev Respir Dis* 1988; 137:1285–1288.
5. Swinburn CR, Mould H, Stone TN, et al. Symptomatic benefit of supplemental oxygen in hypoxemic patients with chronic lung disease. *Am Rev Respir Dis* 1991; 143:913–915.
6. Moore DP, Weston AR, Hughes JMB, et al. Effects of increased inspired oxygen concentrations on exercise performance in chronic heart failure. *Lancet* 1992; 339:850–853.
7. Restrick LJ, Davies SW, Noone L, et al. Ambulatory oxygen in chronic heart failure. *Lancet* 1992; 340:1192–1193.

8. Reuben DB, Mor V. Dyspnea in terminally ill cancer patients. *Chest* 1986; 82(Suppl 2):234–236.
9. Bruera E, de Stoutz N, Velasco-Leiva A, et al. Effects of oxygen on dyspnoea in hypoxaemic terminal-cancer patients. *Lancet* 1993; 342:13–14.
10. Booth S, Kelly MJ, Cox NP, et al. Does oxygen help dyspnea in patients with cancer? *Am J Respir Crit Care Med* 1996; 153:1515–1518.
11. Stulbarg MS, Winn WR. Bilateral carotid body resection for the relief of dyspnea in severe chronic obstructive pulmonary disease. *Chest* 1995; 5:1123–1127.
12. Adams L, Lane R, Shea SA, et al. Breathlessness during different forms of ventilatory stimulation: a study of mechanisms in normal subjects and respiratory patients. *Clin Sci* 1985; 69:663–672.
13. Lane R, Cockcroft A, Adams L, et al. Arterial oxygen saturation and breathlessness in patients with chronic obstructive airways disease. *Clin Sci* 1987; 72:693–698.
14. Chronos N, Adams L, Guz A. Effect of hyperoxia and hypoxia on exercise-induced breathlessness in normal subjects. *Clin Sci* 1988; 74:531–537.
15. Libby DM, Briscoe WA, King TKC. Relief of hypoxia-related bronchoconstriction by breathing 30 per cent oxygen. *Am Rev Respir Dis* 1981; 123:171–175.
16. Bye PTP, Esau SA, Levy RD, et al. Ventilatory muscle function during exercise in air and oxygen in patients with chronic air-flow limitation. *Am Rev Respir Dis* 1985; 132:236–240.
17. Pardy RL, Bye PTP. Diaphragmatic fatigue in normoxia and hyperoxia. *J Appl Physiol* 1985; 58:738–742.
18. Stein DA, Bradley BL, Miller WC. Mechanisms of oxygen effects on exercise in patients with chronic obstructive pulmonary disease. *Chest* 1982; 81:6–10.
19. Olvey SK, Reduto LA, Stevens PM, et al. First pass radionuclide assessment of right and left ventricular ejection fraction in chronic pulmonary disease. *Chest* 1980; 78:4–9.
20. Burrows B. Arterial oxygenation and pulmonary hemodynamics in patients with chronic airway obstruction. *Am Rev Respir Dis* 1972; 110:64–70.
21. Bruera E, Schoeller T, MacEachern T. Symptomatic benefit of supplemental oxygen in hypoxemic patients with terminal cancer: the use of the N of 1 randomized controlled trial. *J Pain Symptom Manage* 1992; 7 (6):365–368.
22. Dudgeon D, Lertzman M. Etiology of dyspnea in advanced cancer patients. *Proceeding of ASCO* 1996; 15:165 (abstract)

15

Treatment of Delirium at the End of Life: Medical and Ethical Issues

ROBIN L. FAINSINGER

Delirium in dying patients is a complicated phenomenon. There is lack of uniformity in descriptors and assessments of what constitutes delirium. It is difficult to define the "end of life" and to determine whether a separate condition called *terminal delirium* or *terminal restlessness* should be delineated. There is also likely to be disagreement over what would be considered a reasonable approach to the assessment, including investigations, and pharmacological management of delirium at the end of life. The frequency with which the treatment of delirium requires sedative pharmacological management is of major importance in understanding this problematic issue. As with many palliative care topics, the medical problems cannot be considered in isolation from the ethical dilemmas that they evoke. In reviewing the literature on these topics, this chapter will attempt to clarify the areas of consensus and controversy.

Medical Issues

Perspectives on delirium in palliative care

Reviews of management perspectives on delirium in dying patients are worth comparing to understand the similarities and differences in the expressed opinions. Our group has noted that it is impossible to work with terminally ill patients and be unaware of the high prevalence of delirium in this population,[1] which has been reported to occur in up to 83% of the patients.[2] The remaining terminally ill patients either experience sudden death or rapid deterioration before the deterioration in their cognition can be detected. The approach to the management of this problem requires a clear understanding and definition of what constitutes delirium in order to minimize the difficulty caused by the bewildering terminology that has often been used in the literature.[3] The Mini-Mental State Examination (MMSE) is recommended as an easily applied tool to assist in the early diagnosis and management of delirium.[4] Emphasis is placed on the need to avoid the "destructive triangle" that can develop as a patient's agitated behavior causes distress for the family, who then exert pressure on both the nursing and medical staffs to relieve their relative's and their own suffering. This may result in premature use of a sedative therapeutic approach. An attempt to determine the cause of the agitation is considered important, as there may be potentially reversible problems. These include medications, metabolic causes, sepsis, hypoxia, and dehydration, all of which can be assessed by a simple examination, review of medications, and basic laboratory investigations. Pharmacological management is not necessary for all patients with delirium, as not all of them exhibit agitated behavior. Haloperidol is recommended as the drug of choice, as it is less sedating than the phenothiazine alternatives such as chlorpromazine or methotrimeprazine. The alternatives to this group of medications, which have some advantages due to their more predictable dose-effect relationship, are the benzodiazepines. Midazolam is recommended as the benzodiazepine of choice due to the rapid onset of its effect short duration of action, and easy titration both to cause rapid sedation and to reverse the sedative effect if any potentially reversible causes for delirium have been addressed. It is emphasized that a few patients do have reversible causes of delirium, which should be excluded and treated, if possible, before the condition is deemed an unavoidable part of the terminal illness.[5]

Caraceni[6] agrees that delirium can be present in 77–83% of dying cancer patients and may be regarded as the hallmark of dying. The diagnosis of delirium relies on clinical criteria as defined by DSM IV.[7] Consistent terminology is extremely importance for both research and clinical reasons. The need to assess carefully for correctable causes is emphasized. A pharmacological approach using haloperidol as the drug of first choice in most situations is recommended. When patients do not respond to haloperidol alone, it may be combined with a benzodiazepine such as lorazepam. Subcutaneous infusion of midazolam is recommended when sedation is necessary.

MacLeod[8] comments that delirium is commonly encountered in palliative care but is often unrecognized, misdiagnosed, and ignored. The specific comment on the difficulty caused in the palliative care literature by referring to delirium as *terminal restlessness* or *terminal anguish* is noted. The cardinal rules for the management of delirium include provision of a safe environment, treatment of the underlying cause, psychological interventions, and pharmacological interventions that may include tranquilization, sedation, or anesthesia. Haloperidol is again described as the drug of choice, its main advantage over phenothiazines being its reduced toxicity. In addition, it is well tolerated when given subcutaneously, and except for its extrapyramidal side effects, adverse reactions are rare. When sedation is required, midazolam is recommended due to its short half-life and its compatibility with other medications. The distress caused by delirium at the end of life requires active management to avoid the unpleasant memories that may endure with the surviving family.

Concern has been expressed that delirium may sometimes lead to the incorrect interpretation that the patient is suffering increasing uncontrolled pain, resulting in escalating doses of opioids that may further exacerbate the delirious behavior.[1,6,9] This problem was well illustrated in a study describing 11 patients who recovered after developing agitated delirium.[10] The pain intensity assessed by the nurse during the delirious phase was significantly higher than the patient's assessment, both before and after the delirium episode. In addition, these patients received a mean of 5 ± 2 extra doses of opioids per day versus 2 ± 1 doses in the three patients who showed no agitation during their delirium. The study concluded that patients who recover from severe agitated delirium have no memory of pain, and that medical and nursing staffs are at risk of overestimating the level of pain of patients with agitated delirium.

Reviews by other authors[11,12] highlight similar issues and management approaches. However, the issue of delirium becomes more complicated by references to "terminal agitation," "terminal anguish," and "terminal restlessness."

Terminal restlessness is an interesting concept in the palliative care literature, and there are a number of publications with this term in the title.[13–16] Back[13] noted that the term is widely used but has never been defined. An accepted definition of terminal restlessness was needed to ensure good communication among health care professionals, as well as adequate consideration of all management options. March[14] defined terminal restlessness "as the thrashing or agitation that may occur in the last days or hours of life." Burke[15] defined it as "agitated delirium in a dying patient, frequently associated with impaired consciousness and multi-focal myoclonus." While it is not clear that all investigators agree that terminal restlessness is a distressing manifestation of delirium in dying patients,[15] a common approach to the management of this problem is generally advocated.[12–16] This includes a consideration of potentially reversible causes identical to those listed in literature reports on the assessment of delirium. In addition, the pharmacological management advocated essentially includes the same antipsychotics and benzodiazepines mentioned in the medical management of delirium, including the possibility of a sedative approach for intractable problems.

Some reports suggest that terminal restlessness may be a manifestation of unresolved psychosocial issues.[14,17] Twycross[12] has described this as *terminal anguish* and claims that it is distinct from either delirium or terminal restlessness. However the pharmacological approach, including the use of heavy sedation, is the same as that described for agitated delirium.

Jones et al.[16] noted the discussion in the palliative care field about the causes of terminal restlessness and whether it is possible to give a defined label to the behavior of patients at the end of life. Noting the need for a clear assessment to improve management, and a reliable and valid measure for attending staff, they attempted to develop an observer-rated instrument to measure terminal restlessness. They concluded that there was significant variation in interpretation of the term *restlessness* among attending staff. In view of the commonly noted disagreement in clinical observation and even interpretation of diagnostic test results, they doubted that bedside observations would ever achieve high levels of consistency. Nevertheless the instrument that they reported did demonstrate moderate reliability.

Whether delirium and terminal restlessness are distinct entities, or merely the same palliative care issue at different times in the natural history of a patient's illness, remains an unresolved issue. Nevertheless, cognitive disorders are commonly associated with a deteriorating illness. A retrospective study reviewed the frequency and clinical course of cognitive failure in patients with advanced cancer admitted to a palliative care unit, as well as the potential value of the MMSE as an indicator and prognosticator of cognitive function.[18] In this study, all 348 patients admitted to the Edmonton General Hospital's palliative care unit over a 26-month period were reviewed. The MMSE was used as a screening tool to assess cognitive function and was administered to all patients at admission and once or twice weekly thereafter. On average, every patient underwent a MMSE every 4.9 ± 3.3 days. As a result, patients whose cognition may have deteriorated during this time prior to death might not have had an abnormal MMSE documented. Nevertheless, of the 231 patients who died on the unit, 157 (68%) had a documented abnormal MMSE prior to death. A further significant finding was that of 87 patients with a documented abnormal MMSE on admission, 25 (29%) were found to have a reversible cause, and their MMSE score rose to normal. Twelve of these 25 patients were discharged from the palliative care unit. It seems reasonable to conclude that cognitive disorders, and delirium in particular, are highly prevalent in palliative care patients. This inevitably causes significant difficulty in symptom assessment and management, and problems with nursing care, as well as significant distress for patients, family members, and staff. As a result, it has been recommended that the cognitive function of palliative care patients be monitored regularly, and that the possibility of a reversible cause be considered as a realistic and worthwhile possibility.

Literature on sedation and delirium

The need to sedate terminally ill patients for uncontrolled symptoms, including delirium, has been frequently reported in palliative care journals.[1,6,8,11,12] Enck[19] commented on the disparity in the medical literature regarding the extent of control of patient symptoms at the end of life, as well as the need for more research and open discussion of this topic to fully define the appropriateness of a sedative approach. Cherny and Portenoy[20] agreed that although outcome data were sparse, clinical experience suggested that good palliative care could effectively manage the symptoms of most cancer patients. However, at the end of life, physical and psychological issues can become more difficult. As a result, some patients can experience symptoms that may be termed *refractory*. The use of sedative drugs can be considered a therapeutic option in the treatment of these refractory symptoms at the end of life. However, the incidence of these refractory symptoms in palliative care patients with advanced cancer is controversial. This problem highlights the need to distinguish between *difficult* and *refractory* symptoms in addressing the needs of palliative care patients.

A clear understanding of the terminology regarding sedation and sedative medications is necessary in comprehending and applying the literature findings on the use of sedatives in palliative medicine.[21,22] *Terminal sedation* has been defined as the intent to deliberately induce and maintain deep sleep, but not to deliberately cause death in specific circumstances.[23] Terminal sedation has also been defined as the prescription of psychotropic agents to control physical and psychological symptoms by making the patient unconscious.[24]

The extent to which sedation is used for the management of agitated delirium or terminal restlessness has been difficult to clarify given the confusing terminology of descriptors and perceived problems. Burke et al.[25] reported that 25% of hospice inpatients required sedation with midazolam for terminal restlessness. Ventafridda et al.[26] stated that 52% of patients required sedation for unendurable symptoms, including dyspnea, pain, delirium, and nausea. McIver et al.[27] reported the use of terminal sedation in about 25% of patients, and they used chlorpromazine for the management of dyspnea and restlessness. Morita et al.[28] required sedation for symptom control in 48% of patients for dyspnea, pain, general malaise, agitation, and nausea. Sanders and Smales[29] noted increased painful tone accompanied by twitches and jerks in 50% of their patients in the last days of life, which required sedating management. Stone et al.[30] reported that 31% of patients in a hospice and 21% of patients in a general hospital required sedation for uncontrolled symptoms, including delirium, mental anguish, pain, and dyspnea. Fainsinger et al.[31] reported that 23 of 76 (30%) patients in a Cape Town hospice required sedating management, 20 patients for delirium, 2 patients for delirium and dyspnea, and 1 patient for dyspnea alone.

The disparity in the literature regarding the symptom complexes requiring sedation is troubling. Some of this might be explained by cultural differences, differing assessments used by palliative care practitioners in defining the uncontrolled symptom, and reports varying from prospective data collections to retrospective chart reviews. Nevertheless, a recurring symptom problem requiring sedation is agitated behavior that is variously described as delirium, terminal restlessness, mental anguish, and agitation. All of these reports suffer from a lack of standardized descriptions of uncontrolled symptoms, which makes comparisons difficult. Midazolam has clearly been the sedating drug of first choice due to its acute onset of action, ease of titration, and rapid reversibility of its effect.[31]

A recent report used a survey of previously identified palliative care practitioners to estimate the frequency of "terminal sedation," as well as the reason for sedating patients, and to identify the prescribed medications and dosages. This resulted in a wide variety of described reasons, including pain (20%), anguish (14%), respiratory distress (12%), agitation/delirium/confusion/hallucinations

(12%), fear/panic/anxiety/terror (10%), emotional/psychological/spiritual distress (10%), restlessness (10%), seizures/twitching (4%), nausea/vomiting/retching (2%), and others (6%). A form of agitated cognitive impairment or delirium appears to be the dominant reason for sedating management. The most common drugs used were midazolam and methotrimeprazine. The limitations of these surveys, as well as those of retrospective chart reviews, have been noted.[23,31] There are limitations in assessing level of consciousness and adequacy of symptom control based on a retrospective review of patient behavior as described by nursing or medical notes. Symptoms such as pain, dyspnea, delirium, and nausea and vomiting requiring medical management may be inadequately described in the notes reviewed. The attending physician's intention to sedate patients cannot always be adequately assessed. The outcome measurement of subsequent patient drowsiness or unresponsiveness, with or without resolution of the initial symptom complex, is also unsatisfactory. It has been suggested that studies could be markedly improved by having the attending physician complete a patient assessment as close as possible to the day of death.[31] This would provide a clearer recollection of the severity of symptoms and the intention to use drugs to achieve sedation. More accurate data collection would enable better characterization of the prevalence of this problem, as well as a better understanding and articulation of the circumstances and problems leading to a decision to use sedation in terminally ill patients. Two multisite studies have attempted to document this problem more clearly.

Four palliative care programs with inpatient units in Israel, South Africa, and Spain participated in a multicenter international study of sedation for uncontrolled symptoms in terminally ill patients.[32] To overcome the difficulty of predicting the last week of life, treating physicians were asked to provide the data at the time of death. The data available for analysis included 387 patients from the four sites. More than 90% of patients required medical management for pain, dyspnea, delirium, and/or nausea in the last week of life. The intent to use sedating management varied from 15% to 36%, with delirium being the most common problem requiring sedation. Of the 387 patients, 97 (25%) required sedation. In 59 of the 97 patients (60%), the reason for this management was recorded as delirium. Midazolam was the most common medication prescribed.

In a second study, our palliative care group in Edmonton attempted to characterize more clearly the prevalence of difficult symptoms at the end of life requiring sedation.[33] Data were collected on the date of death or as close to that date as possible on 50 consecutive patients dying in the tertiary palliative care unit, 50 patients followed by the consulting palliative care program in an acute care hospital, and 50 patients in the three hospice inpatient units in the city. While approximately 80% of the patients in all three settings developed delirium prior to death, the requirement for pharmacological management of this problem varied from 40% in the acute care setting to 80% in the tertiary palliative care unit. This was explained by differences in the characteristics of the patients in the three different settings, highlighting the need to exercise caution when comparing results in different palliative care groups. The percentage of sedated patients ranged from 4% in the hospice setting to 10% in the tertiary palliative care unit. Of the 150 patients, 9 were sedated for delirium and 1 for dyspnea. The prevalence of delirium as well as other symptoms requiring sedation in the Edmonton region was relatively low compared to those in other literature reports. Although it is possible that some of the variability in the use of sedation internationally could be due to patient characteristics, as well as cultural differences, the low prevalence of deliberate use of sedation in Edmonton does suggest the possibility that improved management has resulted in less distressing symptoms at the end of life.

Is delirium reversible?

The relatively short period of time between onset of sedation and death has been consistently reported. Ventafridda et al. reported that, on average, their patients required sedation 2 days before death.[26] Morita et al.[28] reported that, on average, their patients required sedation 3.9 days prior to death. Stone et al.[30] noted that their patients survived for a mean period of 1.3 days after sedation was instituted. The report from the Cape Town Hospice in South Africa noted that, on average, patients were sedated 2.5 days before death (median, 1 day; range, 4 hr to 12 days).[31] The multicenter international study[32] noted that all of the 97 sedated patients were sedated within 1 to 6 days. Our group in Edmonton[33] reported a range for the 10 patients sedated of 1 to 5 days. Comfort has often been taken from the belief that this brief period indicates that the need for sedation is an indicator of impending death rather than a cause of premature death.[30] However, some reports have emphasized that palliative care patients with delirium who may appear extremely ill are not inevitably all dying.[34,35] De Stoutz et al.[36] noted that delirium is a common problem in terminally ill patients and that the poor prognosis for these patients may result in failure to recognize easily treated and reversible conditions. Four patients presenting with delirium were found to have a number of possible reversible causes, including dehydration, hypoxia, sedative drugs, hypercalcemia, renal failure, and infection, resulting in a treatment approach that significantly improved their cognition and quality of life.

Dunlop[37] questioned whether terminal restlessness was sometimes drug-induced in presenting the case of a terminally ill patient on high-dose opioids who proved difficult to control with a number of alternative sedating medications. This patient was receiving diamorphine 2000 mg/day, was anuric, and exhibited agitated delirium and myoclonus. Increasing doses of chlorpromazine and diazepam failed to control the patient's behavior, which eventually responded to high-dose phenobarbital. A similar case was presented by Holdsworth et al.,[38] who described a patient receiving morphine 500 mg/hr, resulting in myoclonus and apparently increasing pain. A continuous infusion of midazolam was started, with the morphine eventually titrated to 1000 mg/hr, and the midazolam was increased to 80 mg/hr.

Coyle et al.[39] reported three patients demonstrating the relationship between delirium and apparently increasing pain. Recognition of this phenomenon, and appropriate management using decreased opioid doses and/or rotation, as well as nonsedating antipsychotics, may have avoided the need to use sedation. De Stoutz et al.[40] described 80/191 palliative care inpatients who underwent opioid rotation for cognitive failure, hallucinations, myoclonus, nausea and vomiting, and uncontrolled pain. The leading symptoms improved in 73% of patients. It was concluded that symptoms of opioid toxicity can often be relieved by a simple switch of opioid.

The report from the hospice in Cape Town, South Africa,[31] compared the mean equivalent daily dose (MEDD) of parenteral morphine in the last week of life for 23 patients who received sedation and the remaining patients who did not need sedative drug management. The MEDD in the last week of life showed a significantly higher mean for the sedated group, and the individual patients in this group were more likely to have had the opioid dose increased. None of the patients in this hospice received parenteral hydration. Two case vignettes in this report describe patients with documented laboratory tests demonstrating renal insufficiency who received ongoing and escalating opioid doses while requiring sedation with midazolam. This resulted in the speculation that the patients with a longer hospice stay, a higher average dose of opioids, and a resulting longer exposure to the accumulation of metabolites were more likely to exhibit agitated behavior resulting in the use of sedatives.

In view of these findings, it seems worthwhile to ask "Can we really feel comfortable that all sedated patients are inevitably dying and do not have any reversible causes for their intractable symptom complex?"[31]

There is general agreement in the literature that some patients need sedative management for a problem commonly described as a form of agitated behavior that arguably fits the criteria for delirium. Nevertheless, the great variation and widespread prevalence of these problems, and the need for sedation as described in the literature, remain a source of concern. Although some of this variation may be due to differing diagnostic criteria for problems such as delirium and dyspnea, as well as cultural variations in coping at the end of life,[41] the self-fulfilling nature of sedative management cannot be ignored. While the majority of sedated patients may well be dying from irreversible causes, some patients may benefit from a careful assessment for reversible conditions, including investigations where necessary.

Ethical Issues

Palliative care and sedation

Increasing literature evidence suggests that problems related to delirium are the most common reasons for the use of sedation in palliative care patients. As a result, it is critical to evaluate the extensive literature on the ethical validity of using sedative management.

Latimer[42] has cautioned that the care of seriously ill and dying patients requires a philosophical and ethical basis to avoid unacceptable patterns of practice. Palliative care should take place within the framework of the four ethical principles of autonomy, beneficence, nonmaleficence, and justice. A focus on the patient's best interests and wishes will help to prevent imposition of the values of others. Inappropriate treatment such as intentional oversedation, or withholding potentially helpful therapies, should not be done in the mistaken belief that palliative care means "do nothing and keep the patient comfortable." Poor care of the dying can be due to a poorly defined philosophy and ethics that deems palliative care patients not sufficiently important to receive thought, attention, and resources. In applying the four ethical principles outlined above, Duff[43] adds the issues of "close-up" or "distant" ethics. Close-up ethics acknowledges the importance of feelings and living conditions, and asserts the freedom to express individual and family conscience. Distant ethics refers mainly to abstract ethical principles and how they are applied. This form of ethics is easier in practice because issues can be resolved simply by rules, with little need for empathy. In applying these principles to terminal sedation in palliative care, a warning to think the issues through carefully can be summed up in the sentence "If it's so damned ethical, why do I feel so bad?"[44]

While there is increasing awareness and acceptance of the use of sedation in the management of refractory symptoms at the end of life,[20,45] the ethical validity of this practice has been criticized. Much of this debate has focused on whether the distinction between assisted suicide or euthanasia and sedation is spurious or valid. Fonderas[24] noted that palliative care has always been dogged by ethical discussions and strong convictions, and that one French association had modified its definition of euthanasia. In 1984 this definition had been: "Euthanasia is understood to mean any action intended to end the life of a person or deprive them of consciousness and lucidity until death." In 1993 this was updated to read: " . . . or to deprive them without *good reason,* until death, of their consciousness and lucidity."

Sedation has been discussed in relation to a number of problematic issues, including poorly controlled pain, psychological distress, withholding of artificial nutrition and hydration, and the use of barbiturates. Cavanaugh[46] addressed the issue of using palliative analgesia to relieve pain while unavoidably hastening or causing the patient's death. Using double-effect reasoning, it was argued that using death-hastening or death-causing palliative analgesia in a terminally ill patient is ethically in the clear and, at times, even obligatory. There are sound ethical arguments based on double-effect reasoning for taking aggressive pallia-tive measures even when these actions may hasten or cause death. In response, Miller[47] argued that patients who request and receive the means of ending their lives because they are suffering without the prospect of satisfactory relief are not harmed but helped, and that intentional acts of physician-assisted death are not necessarily wrong.

Case reports in the literature have also raised the important question of whether sedation is ethically justified in cases of psychological/existential distress.[48,49] Sedation in the management of refractory psychological or existential problems is more difficult to justify, as it may be harder to establish that these conditions are truly refractory.[45]

The use of barbiturates in the terminally ill has been described as potentially problematic from an ethical perspective, as these agents generally hasten the patient's death and have often been used to kill patients intentionally.[50] It was argued that when more traditional approaches to controlling physical suffering are not adequate, barbiturates could be considered as ethically appropriate for the relief of pain and suffering.

Concern has also been raised regarding the use of sedation when artificial nutrition and hydration are withheld. Under these circumstances, death can reasonably be anticipated in a short period of time, due either to the underlying disease, dehydration, the sedative medications, or a combination of these factors.[51]

Much of the debate on this topic can be traced back to the report by Ventafridda et al.[26] outlining the need to sedate more than 50% of their patients in the last days of life due to physical suffering. This resulted in an accompanying editorial by Roy[52] cautioning that resolution of conflicts on matters of fact depends on more comprehensive and methodologically sound research. Further, according to Roy, "those who argue for the ethical and legal justification of euthanasia, would wonder about the clarity or arbitrariness of the distinction between inducing unconsciousness and rapidly terminating life if and when dying persons experience a crescendo of unmanageable suffering in their last days of life."

Double-effect on trial

Numerous articles have argued the value and problems with the double-effect argument as applied to the practice of sedation in palliative care.

Cherny and Portenoy[20] emphasized the need to understand the goals of care of an individual patient; they noted that as prolonging survival and optimizing function become increasingly unachievable, priorities often shift. Under these circumstances, interventions of low or uncertain value may be rejected in favor of more certain approaches even if they further impair cognition or shorten survival. The use of sedation recognizes the right of patients to adequate relief of unendurable symptoms. It was argued that the ethical value of sedation under these circumstances derives from the principle of double-effect. This distinguishes between the compelling primary intent to relieve suffering and the unavoidable consequence of potentially accelerating death.

Dunphy[53] comments that in patients with impaired cognition and agitated behavior, palliative care should strive to improve cognition and reduce agitation without decreasing the level of consciousness. This may involve withdrawing drugs, correcting biochemical abnormalities, treating infections, or initiating other clinical interventions. However, if a point is reached at which no identifiable or reversible cause is found and the patient's confusion and agitation remain problematic, the situation can be described as terminal agitation or delirium. At this point, sedation as an effective clinical intervention should be considered even if it presents ethical problems. The doctrine of double-effect attempts to render actions that have foreseen bad consequences morally permissible within circumscribed criteria. These are[20,53,54]:

1. The action concerned is good or at least morally neutral.
2. The beneficial outcome is intended, and the bad effect, such as the patient's death, may be foreseen but must not be intended.
3. The bad effect must not be a means of bringing out the good effect.
4. There is a sufficiently grave reason for the action in question, and the good effect must outweigh the bad effect.

As this pertains to sedation at the end of life, the adoption of double-effect is considered relevant if the intention is to relieve distress and not kill; the benefit from the distress relieved is proportionate to the potential loss of life; and the result is achieved with minimum effective intervention. It is suggested that as long as the act is not wrong in itself and the benefit obtained is proportionate to the harm, the use of sedation is justified. Dunphy[53] cautions that the suggestion that the double-effect doctrine may be used to justify the possible shortening of life in certain prescribed circumstances should not be used to imply that this embraces euthanasia. Further, in the unusual circumstance where nothing else will be effective, the judicious use of a sedative will relieve the patient's suffering and is covered by the doctrine of double-effect.

Thorns[54] explored the ethical issues surrounding the doctrine of double-effect and noted that this ethical approach appealed to our sense of what is the "right thing to do." This doctrine allowed the health care professional to balance the possible risk of hastening death against the benefits for the patient. One objection to the use of this principle was that it could sometimes intuitively give the wrong answer. In addition, because the intention of the health care professional is central to the justification of this doctrine, we need to recognize that it is impossible to know what is in this individual's mind as he or she carries out a particular course of action. Pressure may be placed on health care professionals to abuse this doctrine, which may be invoked to justify prematurely ending a life rather than consulting a more expert colleague. However, recognizing that end-of-life decisions will always be difficult to make and that there will never be easy answers, the double-effect doctrine does offer some help by providing a framework to guide health care professionals. Finally, abuse of the doctrine would be unlikely if the founding criteria were adhered to.

Hunt[55] examined the morality of palliative treatments that hasten death and highlighted the limitations and weaknesses of the principle of double-effect when used to justify these treatments. The World Health Organization defines palliative care as care that "neither hastens [nor] postpones death." However, there would be no need to invoke the double-effect principle if palliative treatments never hastened death. It was argued that this definition should be revised, and that palliative care clinicians should acknowledge that palliative treatments can affect the duration of the terminal illness, and that they should accept responsibility for discussing this outcome with patients, their families, and their collegues. Further, it was argued that although clinicians' intention may be morally relevant, it is very subjective and should not be the central consideration in judging a treatment to be right or wrong. The application of the double-effect principle, with its narrow focus on clinicians' intention, can lead to "ridiculously divergent results." It was also argued that the basic premise of the double-effect principle—that a hastened death is an unwanted or bad effect—may be false in the setting of intractable terminal suffering. A further problem is that the double-effect principle, which focuses on clinicians' intention regarding the time of death, does not allow for the moral imperative of respect for the patient's autonomy. The ethical framework should involve the patient if competent, or the next of kin or surrogate decision maker if the patient is unable to participate in this discussion. Hunt concluded that the principle of double-effect should not be used to justify the use of death-hastening palliative treatment, which belonged to a paradigm of paternalism that undermined patient autonomy and could lead to patients receiving terminal sedation without their consent. The aim of achieving a consensus on treatment should focus on wishes and interests of the patients rather than the intentions of the clinician.

Quill et al.[56] noted that the double-effect principle is often used to explain why some forms of care at the end of life that result in death are morally permissible and others, such as euthanasia or physician-assisted suicide, are not. This rule is conceptually and psychologically complex in distinguishing between permissible and prohibited actions by relying heavily on the clinicians' intent. It is argued that the double-effect doctrine is of limited assistance in evaluating the practice known as *terminal sedation*. It is argued that terminal sedation inevitably causes death, which in many circumstances may be what the patient desires. Although the goal of terminal sedation may be to relieve uncontrollable suffering, life-prolonging therapies are often withdrawn simultaneously with the intent of hastening death. As a result, terminal sedation would not be permitted under the rule of double-effect, even though it may be considered acceptable according to current legal and medical ethical standards. Finally, Quill et al.[56] concluded that "the rule's absolute prohibitions, unrealistic characterization of physicians' intentions, and failure to account for patients' wishes make it problematic in many circumstances."

This controversy was further highlighted when Billings and Block[57] raised the issue of *slow euthanasia* and criticized the application of the principle of double-effect. Slow euthanasia was defined as the practice of treating a terminal patient in a way that would inevitably lead to a comfortable death, "but not too quickly." It was argued that this form of end-of-life care may be more acceptable to patients, family members, and health professionals than a more rapid approach, although no data were available to document the extent of this practice. In particular, the situation in which terminally ill patients were treated with a continuing and increasing dose of intravenous morphine for poorly documented problems, as well as a case report highlighting the use of sedation for psychological distress,[49] were considered. It was asked why, if we agreed to a request for sedation and acknowledged that in the absence of artificial fluid or nutrition this would inevitably hasten death, this should be done slowly rather than rapidly? Are there other significant differences between treatment options that differ only in whether death occurs instantly or in a few days? Criticizing the intent of the attending staff in using the double-effect doctrine, Billings and Block[57] asked how responsibility can be denied for an act carried out with full awareness of its consequences.

This report resulted in a number of critical responses. Mount[58] pointed out that the definition used for slow euthanasia was in fact a reasonable definition of palliative care. The principle of double-effect was defended as an important ethical distinction between euthanasia and end-of-life sedation. The ethical validity of the principle rests on the two axioms of primary intent as a critical ethical issue in any action, and the ethically significant distinction between foreseeing and primarily intending an unavoidable maleficent outcome. In responding to Billings and Block's question regarding the prolongation of dying as opposed to agreeing to a request for a quick death, Mount commented that first, with sedation, we are accepting the patient's request to die comfortably; second, there are no easy answers to this problem, including the legalization of euthanasia; and third, the most appropriate path is that of making ongoing efforts at symptom control, using sedation if necessary, while we continue to support patients and their families. Dickens,[59] in his response, criticized the lack of respect shown for the distinction between primary and secondary intent and the lack of consideration of the distinction between intent and motive. He concluded that "holding physicians to intend the known effects of the treatment that they administered, and by considering confused, unrealistic, or tiresome the ethical distinctions between a primary purpose of treatment and responsibility for a known but inescapable effect of intended treatment, the authors bypass discussions that have animated ethical discourse for some years."

Portenoy[60] criticized Billings and Block[57] for presenting anecdote as empiricism. In particular, the claim that slow euthanasia was a common practice was criticized due to both lack of data and commonsense observation. Furthermore, terminal sedation as an accepted clinical practice has been openly discussed and was obviously different from euthanasia. The double-effect principle was defended, with the intention of the prescriber noted as the key factor. The practice of palliative care is "truly guided by the principle of double-effect" that was not used to hide the truth, but was an extremely useful ethical principle in guiding bedside practice and decreasing uncomfortable ambiguity in end-of-life care. It was stated that it was a sad reality that the advocates of physician-assisted suicide and euthanasia would misuse the report of Billings and Block.

Conclusion

There is increasing evidence that delirium is a common problem in palliative care and arguably results in the use of sedation in the most problematic clinical situations. This inevitably draws us into complex, divisive, and controversial discussions that will continue to have opposing proponents. Those of us faced with the clinical dilemma of considering the use of sedation in these patients can draw satisfaction from the fact that legal opinions in this area tend to support the doctrine of double-effect as a major ethical foundation for the distinction between palliative care and euthanasia.[61] A Canadian Senate report[61] that included recommendations on palliative care and sedation noted the absence of empirical data and guidelines and called for these to be developed. Although to some extent we now have increasing international knowledge of the use of sedation in palliative care, this does not necessarily assist us in developing universal guidelines or resolving ethical controversies. Clinical practice and opinion internationally will probably continue to be heavily influenced by local social, economic, cultural, and medical circumstances.

Finally, it seems reasonable to consider applying the decision-making approach suggested by Cherny[45] and Rosen.[62] Although their suggestions were in response to the use of sedation for existential distress,[48] the following principles seem valid in sedation for delirium or indeed any other refractory palliative care situation:

1. The designation of a problem as refractory should only follow repeated assessments by skilled clinicians familiar with palliative care, who have established a relationship with the patient and family. All appropriate assessment and management should have been completed and a skilled palliative care physician consulted if appropriate.
2. The suitability of a sedative management approach should be evaluated during a case conference to avoid the influence of individual clinician bias or burnout on the decision.
3. In the hopefully uncommon situation in which sedation is considered appropriate and reasonable, consideration should be given to the temporary use of sedation.
4. A comprehensive clinical evaluation should include a multidisciplinary assessment of the family to ensure that their views are adequately assessed and understood.

References

1. Fainsinger RL, Tapper M, Bruera E. A perspective on the management of delirium in the terminally ill. *J Palliat Care* 1993; 9(3):4–8.
2. Bruera E, Miller L, McCallion J, et al., Cognitive failure in patients with terminal cancer: a prospective study. *J Pain Symptom Manage* 1992; 7(4):192–195.

3. Fainsinger R, Young C. Cognitive failure in a terminally ill patient. *J Pain Symptom Manage* 1991; 6(8):492–494.

4. Folstein MF, Fetting JH, Lobo A, et al. Cognitive assessment of cancer patients. *Cancer* 1984; 53(Suppl 10):2250–2257.

5. Fainsinger RL, Schoeller T, Boiskin M, et al. Cognitive failure (CF) and coma after renal failure in a patient (PT) receiving captopril and hydromorphone. *J Palliat Care* 1993; 9(1):53–55.

6. Caraceni A. Delirium in palliative care. *Eur J Palliat Care* 1995; 2(2):62–67.

7. American Psychiatric Association. *Diagnostic and Statistical Manual of Mental Disorders,* 4th ed. Washington, D.C.: American Psychiatric Association, 1994.

8. MacLeod AD. The management of delirium in hospice practice. *Eur J Palliat Care* 1997; 4(4):116–120.

9. Coyle N, Breitbart W, Weaver S, et al. Delirium as a contributing factor to "crescendo" pain: three case reports. *J Pain Symptom Manage* 1994; 9(1):44–47.

10. Bruera E, Fainsinger RL, Miller MJ, et al. The assessment of pain intensity in patients with cognitive failure: a preliminary report. *J Pain Symptom Manage* 1992; 7(5): 267–270.

11. Bergevin P, Bergevin RM. Recognizing delirium in terminal patients. *Am J Hospice Palliat Care* 1996; 13(2):28–29.

12. Twycross RG. Symptom control: the problem areas. *Palliat Med* 1993; 7(Suppl 1):1–8.

13. Back IN. Terminal restlessness in patients with advanced malignant disease. *Palliat Med* 1992; 6:293–298.

14. March PA. Terminal restlessness. *Am J Hospice Palliat Care* 1998; 15(1):51–53.

15. Burke AL. Palliative care: an update on "terminal restlessness." *Med J Aust* 1997; 166(1):39–42.

16. Jones CL, King MB, Speck P, et al. Development of an instrument to measure terminal restlessness. *Palliat Med* 1998; 12:99–104.

17. Sirois F. Psychosis as a mode of exitus in a cancer patient. *J Palliat Care* 1993; 9(4):16–18.

18. Pereira J, Hanson J, Bruera E. The frequency and clinical course of cognitive impairment of patients with terminal cancer. *Cancer* 1997; 79:835–842.

19. Enck RE. Drug induced terminal sedation for symptom control. *Am J Hospice Palliat Care* 1991; 3:3–5.

20. Cherny NI, Portenoy RK. Sedation and the management of refractory symptoms: guidelines for evaluation and treatment. *J Palliat Care* 1994; 10:31–38.

21. MacLeod AD. Use of sedatives in palliative medicine. *Palliat Med* 1997; 11:493.

22. Stone P. Reply. *Palliat Med* 1997; 11:493–494.

23. Chater S, Viola R, Paterson J, et al. Sedation for intractable distress in the dying — a survey of experts. *Palliat Med* 1998; 12:255–269.

24. Fonderas T. Sedation and ethical contradictions. *Eur J Palliat Care* 1996; 3(1):17–20.

25. Burke AL, Diamond PL, Hulbert J, et al. Terminal restlessness — its management and the role of midazolam. *Med J Aust* 1991; 155:485–487.

26. Ventafridda V, Ripamonti C, deCanno F, et al. Symptom prevalence and control during cancer patients' last days of life. *J Palliat Care* 1990; 6:7–11.

27. McIver B, Walsh D, Nelson K. The use of chlorpromazine for symptom control in dying cancer patients. *J Pain Symptom Manage* 1994; 9:341–345.

28. Morita T, Inoue S, Chihara S. Sedation for symptom control in Japan: the importance

of intermittent use and communication with family members. *J Pain Symptom Manage* 1996; 12:32–38.

29. Sanders H, Smales L. Discomfort and pain associated with paratonia. *Eur J Palliat Care* 1996; 3:54–55.

30. Stone P, Phillips C, Spruit O, et al. A comparison of the use of sedatives in a hospital support team and in hospice. *Palliat Med* 1997; 11:140–144.

31. Fainsinger RL, Landman W, Hoskings, et al. Sedation for uncontrolled symptoms in a South African hospice. *J Pain Symptom Manage* 1998; 16(3):145–152.

32. Fainsinger RL, Waller A, Bercovici M, et al. A multi-centre international study of sedation for uncontrolled symptoms in terminally ill patients. Submitted. *Palliat Med* (in press)

33. Fainsinger RL, deMoissac D, Mancini I, et al. A multi-site study of sedation for delirium and other symptoms in terminally ill patients in Edmonton. Submitted. *J Palliat Care* (in press)

34. Fainsinger RL, Bruera E. Is this opioid analgesic tolerance? *J Pain Symptom Manage* 1995; 10:573–577.

35. Fainsinger RL. Use of sedation by hospital palliative care support team. *J Palliat Care* 1998; 14(1):51–54.

36. de Stoutz ND, Tapper M, Fainsinger RL. Reversible delirium in terminally ill patients. *J Pain Symptom Manage* 1995; 10:249–253.

37. Dunlop RJ. Is terminal restlessness sometimes drug induced? *Palliat Med* 1989; 3:65–66.

38. Holdsworth MT, Adams VR, Chavez CM, et al. Continuous midazolam infusion for the management of morphine-induced myoclonus. *Ann Pharmacother* 1995; 29:25–29.

39. Coyle N, Breitbalt W, Weaver S, et al. Delirium as a contributing factor to "crescendo" pain: three case reports. *J Pain Symptom Manage* 1994; 9:44–47.

40. de Stoutz ND, Bruera E, Suraez-Almazor M. Opioid rotation for toxicity reduction in terminal cancer patients. *J Pain Symptom Manage* 1995; 10:378–384.

41. Centeno-Cortes C, Nunez-Olarte J. Questioning diagnosis disclosure in terminal cancer patients; a prospective study evaluating patient responses. *Palliat Med* 1994; 8:39–44.

42. Latimer E. Caring for seriously ill and dying patients: the philosophy and ethics. *Can Med Soc Assoc J* 1991; 144(7):859–864.

43. Duff RS. "Close-up" versus "distant" ethics: deciding the care of infants with poor prognosis. *Semin Perinatol* 1987; 11(3):344–253.

44. Doka K, Rushton C, Thorstenson TA. Health care ethics forum '94: caregiver distress: if it is so ethical, why does it feel so bad? *AACN* 1994; 5(3):346–352.

45. Cherny NI. Commentary: sedation in response to refractory existential distress: walking the fine line. *J Pain Symptom Manage* 1998; 16(6):404–406.

46. Cavanaugh TA. The ethics of death-hastening or death-causing palliative analgesic administration to the terminally ill. *J Pain Symptom Manage* 1996; 12:248–254.

47. Miller FG. Re: the ethics of death-hastening or death-causing palliative analgesic adminstration. *J Pain Symptom Manage* 1997; 14(1):2.

48. Chaiova L. Case presentation: "terminal sedation" and existential distress. *J Pain Symptom Manage* 1998; 16(6):403–404.

49. Mount BM, Hamilton P. When palliative care fails to control suffering. *J Palliat Care* 1994; 10(2):24–26.

50. Truog RV, Bird CB, Mitchell C, et al. Barbiturates in the care of the terminally ill. *N Engl J Med* 1992; 327(23):1678–1691.
51. Craig G. Is sedation without hydration or nourishment in terminal care lawful? *Med Leg J* 1994; 62:198–201.
52. Roy DJ. Need their sleep before they die? *J Palliat Care* 1990; 6(3):3–4.
53. Dunphy K. Sedation and the smoking gun: double-effect on trial. *Prog Palliat Care* 1998; 6(6):209–212.
54. Thorns A. A review of the doctrine of double-effect. *Eur J Palliat Care* 1998; 5(4): 117–120.
55. Hunt R. A critique of the principle of the double-effect in palliative care. *Prog Palliat Care* 1998; 6(6):213–215.
56. Quill TE, Dresser R, Brock DW. The rule of double-effect — a critique of its role in end of life decision-making. *N Engl J Med* 1997; 337(24):1768–1771.
57. Billings JA, Block SD. Slow-euthanasia. *J Palliat Care* 1996; 12(4):21–30.
58. Mount B. Morphine drops, terminal sedation, and slow-euthanasia: definition and facts, not anecdotes. *J Palliat Care* 1996; 12(4):31–37.
59. Dickens BM. Commentary on "slow-euthanasia." *J Palliat Care* 1996; 12(4):42–43.
60. Portenoy RK. Morphine infusions at the end of life: the pitfalls in reasoning from anecdote. *J Palliat Care* 1996; 12(4):44–46.
61. Ashby M. Palliative care, death causation, public policy and the law. *Prog Palliat Care* 1998; 6(3):69–77.
62. Rosen EG. Commentary: a case of "terminal sedation" in the family. *J Pain Symptom Manage* 1998; 16(6):406–407.

Index

risk factors, 166
systemic interventions, 173, 174*t*
 antifibrinolytic agents, 175–176
 somatostatin analogues, 174–175
 transfusion therapy, 176–177
 vasopressin, 174
 vitamin K, 173–174
Hemostasis
 agents for, 168–170, 169*t*
 dressings for, 168, 169*t*
 packing for, 168
Heparin
 adverse effects, 197
 APTT monitoring, 186, 187, 189*t*
 duration of therapy
  for first DPV episode, 196
  for recurrent DPV episode, 196–197
 efficacy, 186–187
 low-molecular weight. *See* Low-molecular
  weight heparin
 protocol, 187–188, 188*t*
 risks/complications, 188–190
 structure, 186
 therapeutic guidelines, 186
Hip surgery, anticoagulant prophylaxis for, 209
Hodgkin's lymphoma, B symptoms and, 24–25,
 29*t*–30*t*
Hospice
 care, 132
 consultation team. *See* Consultation teams
 historical aspects, 133–134
 patients
  diagnoses, common, 56
  Medicare reimbursement, 56
  survival periods, 4
  symptoms, prognostic significance of, 32,
   34, 41*t*
 referral, timing of, 23
Hospice and Palliative Medicine, Northwestern
 University Medical School, 132–133, 145
 attending physicians, 144–145
 background, 133–134
 clinical program, 134
  consultation service, 134–136
  home program, 137
  inpatient unit, 136–137
 educational outcomes
  fellows, 144
  medical students, 142–143
  residents, 143
 palliative care curriculum, 137–140
 palliative care unit

central role of, 140–142, 141*f*
 patient data, 141–142, 141*f*
 visiting scholars, 145
HRCA-QL (Hebrew Rehabilitation Centre for
 the Aged-Quality of Life), 104*t*, 107
Hydration, withholding, 270
Hydromorphone, epidural, 226
Hypocalcemia, 246
Hypokalemia, 246
Hypomagnesemia, 246
Hypophosphatemia, 246

Immunocompromise, dyspnea and, 246
Inception cohort, 5
Initial Assessment of Suffering, 103, 104*t*
International Normalized Ratio (INR), 194
Intraspinal analgesia, future of, 231–232
Intraspinal procedures, neurolytic, 230
Intrathecal drug delivery, 227–228

Judgment analysis, 109
Juxtapulmonary receptors (J receptors), 239

Karnofsky Performance Status (KPS), 25–26
 criticism of, 26
 functional impairment and, 58–59
 interpretation, 43–44
 interrater reliability, 26–27
 reliability, 10
 results, 9*t*
 survival prediction, 39
 symptom status, quality of life and, 43

Laboratory tests, for dyspnea, 251
Lactate dehydrogenase (LDH), in pleural fluid,
 245
Left ventricular ejection fraction, in heart
 disease, 61
Liver failure, 165
LMWH. *See* Low-molecular weight heparin
Lobectomy, dyspnea and, 247
Local anesthetics, with epidural opioid, 226–227
Low-molecular weight heparin (LMWH)
 clinical trials, 191–193, 192*t*, 193*t*
 commercially available, differences
  between, 190–191
 long-term therapy, 198
 prophylactic, for surgical patients, 208–209
Lung cancer
 non-small cell, 32
 quality-of-life assessments, 38–39
 survival, performance status and, 26